Nutrition and Food Security for All:
A Step Towards the Future

Nutrition and Food Security for All: A Step Towards the Future

Guest Editors

António Raposo
Ariana Saraiva

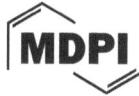 Basel • Beijing • Wuhan • Barcelona • Belgrade • Novi Sad • Cluj • Manchester

Guest Editors

António Raposo
CBIOS (Research Center for Biosciences and Health Technologies)
Universidade Lusófona de Humanidades e Tecnologias
Lisboa
Portugal

Ariana Saraiva
Research in Veterinary Medicine (I-MVET)
Lusófona University
Lisboa
Portugal

Editorial Office
MDPI AG
Grosspeteranlage 5
4052 Basel, Switzerland

This is a reprint of the Special Issue, published open access by the journal *Nutrients* (ISSN 2072-6643), freely accessible at: www.mdpi.com/journal/nutrients/special_issues/843293R79D.

For citation purposes, cite each article independently as indicated on the article page online and using the guide below:

Lastname, A.A.; Lastname, B.B. Article Title. *Journal Name* **Year**, *Volume Number*, Page Range.

ISBN 978-3-7258-3832-5 (Hbk)
ISBN 978-3-7258-3831-8 (PDF)
https://doi.org/10.3390/books978-3-7258-3831-8

© 2025 by the authors. Articles in this book are Open Access and distributed under the Creative Commons Attribution (CC BY) license. The book as a whole is distributed by MDPI under the terms and conditions of the Creative Commons Attribution-NonCommercial-NoDerivs (CC BY-NC-ND) license (https://creativecommons.org/licenses/by-nc-nd/4.0/).

Contents

About the Editors vii

António Raposo and Ariana Saraiva
Nutrition and Food Security for All: A Step Towards the Future
Reprinted from: Nutrients 2025, 17, 1241, https://doi.org/10.3390/nu17071241 1

Sávio Fernandes, Leandro Oliveira, Alda Pereira, Maria do Céu Costa, António Raposo, Ariana Saraiva and Bruno Magalhães
Exploring Vitamin B12 Supplementation in the Vegan Population: A Scoping Review of the Evidence
Reprinted from: Nutrients 2024, 16, 1442, https://doi.org/10.3390/nu16101442 5

Ewa Duda
Understanding Health-Related Motivations for Urban Food Self-Production in the Light of Semantic Fields Analysis
Reprinted from: Nutrients 2024, 16, 1533, https://doi.org/10.3390/nu16101533 25

Jayna M. Dave, Tzuan A. Chen, Alexandra N. Castro, Mamie A. White, Elizabeth A. Onugha, Sloane Zimmerman and Debbe Thompson
Urban–Rural Disparities in Food Insecurity and Weight Status among Children in the United States
Reprinted from: Nutrients 2024, 16, 2132, https://doi.org/10.3390/nu16132132 41

Farooq Ahmed, Najma Iqbal Malik, Shamshad Bashir, Nazia Noureen, Jam Bilal Ahmad and Kun Tang
Political Economy of Maternal Child Malnutrition: Experiences about Water, Food, and Nutrition Policies in Pakistan
Reprinted from: Nutrients 2024, 16, 2642, https://doi.org/10.3390/nu16162642 51

Teeranut Harnirattisai, Sararud Vuthiarpa, Lisa Renee Pawloski, Kevin Michael Curtin, Eden Blackwell, Jenny Nguyen and Sophia Madeleine Bourgeois
Nutritional Health Risk (Food Security) in Thai Older Adults and Related Factors
Reprinted from: Nutrients 2024, 16, 2703, https://doi.org/10.3390/nu16162703 71

Martín del Valle M, Kirsteen Shields and Sofía Boza
Using Household Dietary Diversity Score and Spatial Analysis to Inform Food Governance in Chile
Reprinted from: Nutrients 2024, 16, 2937, https://doi.org/10.3390/nu16172937 83

Priscila Claudino De Almeida, Eduardo Yoshio Nakano, Ivana Aragão Lira Vasconcelos, Renata Puppin Zandonadi, António Raposo, Ariana Saraiva, et al.
Food Neophobia in Children: A Case Study in Federal District/Brazil
Reprinted from: Nutrients 2024, 16, 2962, https://doi.org/10.3390/nu16172962 106

Shuxian Hua, Vicky Vong, Audrey E. Thomas, Yeeli Mui and Lisa Poirier
Barriers and Enablers for Equitable Healthy Food Access in Baltimore Carryout Restaurants: A Qualitative Study in Healthy Food Priority Areas
Reprinted from: Nutrients 2024, 16, 3028, https://doi.org/10.3390/nu16173028 118

Mateusz Rozmiarek
The Role of Nutrition in Maintaining the Health and Physical Condition of Sports Volunteers
Reprinted from: Nutrients 2024, 16, 3336, https://doi.org/10.3390/nu16193336 134

Yasemin Ertaş Öztürk, Sevtap Kabalı, Yasemin Açar, Duygu Ağagündüz and Ferenc Budán
Adaptation of the Food Literacy (FOODLIT) Tool for Turkish Adults: A Validity and Reliability Study
Reprinted from: *Nutrients* 2024, 16, 3416, https://doi.org/10.3390/nu16193416 144

Diana Melo Ferreira, Susana Machado, Liliana Espírito Santo, Maria Antónia Nunes, Anabela S. G. Costa, Manuel Álvarez-Ortí, et al.
Defatted Flaxseed Flour as a New Ingredient for Foodstuffs: Comparative Analysis with Whole Flaxseeds and Updated Composition of Cold-Pressed Oil
Reprinted from: *Nutrients* 2024, 16, 3482, https://doi.org/10.3390/nu16203482 154

Mateusz Rozmiarek
Nutritional Education Needs and Preferences of Sports Volunteers: Access, Expectations, and Forms of Support
Reprinted from: *Nutrients* 2024, 16, 3568, https://doi.org/10.3390/nu16203568 171

Leandro Oliveira, Ariana Saraiva, Maria João Lima, Edite Teixeira-Lemos, Jwaher Haji Alhaji, Conrado Carrascosa and António Raposo
Mediterranean Food Pattern Adherence in a Female-Dominated Sample of Health and Social Sciences University Students: Analysis from a Perspective of Sustainability
Reprinted from: *Nutrients* 2024, 16, 3886, https://doi.org/10.3390/nu16223886 182

Angélica Hernández-Moreno, Olga Vásquez-Palma, Leonardo Castillo-Cárdenas, Juan Erices-Reyes, Alexsa Guzmán-Jiménez, Carlos Domínguez-Scheid, et al.
Food Security in the Rural Mapuche Elderly: Analysis and Proposals
Reprinted from: *Nutrients* 2024, 16, 4042, https://doi.org/10.3390/nu16234042 197

Katarzyna Czarnek, Małgorzata Tatarczak-Michalewska, Grzegorz Wójcik, Agnieszka Szopa, Dariusz Majerek, Karolina Fila, et al.
Nutritional Risks of Heavy Metals in the Human Diet—Multi-Elemental Analysis of Energy Drinks
Reprinted from: *Nutrients* 2024, 16, 4306, https://doi.org/10.3390/nu16244306 214

Odysseas Androutsos, George Saltaouras, Michail Kipouros, Maria Koutsaki, Athanasios Migdanis, Christos Georgiou, et al.
Comparative Analysis of Dietary Behavior in Children and Parents During COVID-19 Lockdowns in Greece: Insights from a Non-Representative Sample
Reprinted from: *Nutrients* 2025, 17, 112, https://doi.org/10.3390/nu17010112 235

Brittany M. Repella and Greta Jakobsdottir
Dietary Intakes Among University Students in Iceland: Insights from the FINESCOP Project
Reprinted from: *Nutrients* 2025, 17, 432, https://doi.org/10.3390/nu17030432 245

About the Editors

António Raposo

António Raposo is an Assistant Professor at Universidade Lusófona de Humanidades e Tecnologias, and he is an Integrated Member of CBIOS (Research Center for Biosciences and Health Technologies). He graduated in Nutritional Sciences from the Instituto Superior de Ciências da Saude Egas Moniz, Portugal, in 2009 and obtained his Ph.D. with a European Mention in Animal Health and Food Safety from the University Institute of Animal Health and Food Safety, University of Las Palmas de Gran Canaria, Spain, in 2013. His main research interests are studies on the utilization of Catostylus tagi jellyfish in health sciences, particularly as a food ingredient, food habits, food safety evaluation, food innovation, natural food products, food security, and sustainability. He is a member of the editorial boards and an invited reviewer of relevant international peer-reviewed journals in his research field. He has published more than 180 papers in indexed JCR journals, as well as scientific book chapters and a patent model, and co-authored a book in English with a special focus on nutrition, food security, and food safety sciences. He has been a Guest Editor of several Special Issues published in high-impact JCR journals such as *Foods*, *Sustainability*, and the *International Journal of Environmental Research and Public Health*. He has collaborated as a Visiting Professor at Portuguese, Spanish, Chilean, and Vietnamese universities.

Ariana Saraiva

Ariana Saraiva is an Assistant Professor at Research in Veterinary Medicine (I-MVET), Faculty of Veterinary Medicine, Lusófona University, and she is an Integrated Member of CECAV. She graduated in Nutritional Sciences from the Egas Moniz Higher Institute of Health Science, Portugal, and obtained her Ph.D. in Animal Health and Food Safety from the University of Las Palmas de Gran Canaria, Spain. Her main research interests are food safety evaluation, food innovation, sensory analysis, and natural food products. She has published more than 40 papers in indexed JCR journals and co-authored a book with Professor Antonio Raposo in English. She has been acting as Guest Editor of Special Issues published in the *International Journal of Environmental Research and Public Health* and *Nutrients*.

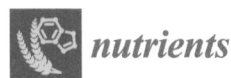

Editorial

Nutrition and Food Security for All: A Step Towards the Future

António Raposo [1,*] and Ariana Saraiva [2,3]

1. CBIOS (Research Center for Biosciences and Health Technologies), Universidade Lusófona de Humanidades e Tecnologias, Campo Grande 376, 1749-024 Lisboa, Portugal
2. Research in Veterinary Medicine (I-MVET), Faculty of Veterinary Medicine, Lisbon University Centre, Lusófona University, Campo Grande 376, 1749-024 Lisboa, Portugal; ariana.saraiva@ulusofona.pt
3. Veterinary and Animal Research Centre (CECAV), Faculty of Veterinary Medicine, Lisbon University Centre, Lusófona University, Campo Grande 376, 1749-024 Lisboa, Portugal
* Correspondence: antonio.raposo@ulusofona.pt

Ensuring food and nutritional security has been a top concern on the global development agenda. Even so, about 600 million people are projected to suffer from chronic undernourishment by 2030 [1]. Because the associated difficulties and growth goals have evolved over time, the necessary action has not been carried out in this field. A more comprehensive agreement that safeguards food security and lowers hunger and malnourishment in all its forms has been approved, in order to support strong economies, healthy populations, and sustainable growth [2–7]. Promoting a positive outlook on food, nutrition, and health is essential to eradicate food insecurity in many nations [8]. This may be accomplished by educating individuals about healthy eating choices at a young age through the media, schools, and family. Understanding the importance of a diverse, balanced, and nutrient-rich diet is essential to achieve the second Sustainable Development Goal (SDG) of the global agenda [9]. Furthermore, when creating policies to achieve the SDG 2's objectives, factors pertaining to security, culture, society, economy, and environment must be taken into account.

When producing food, it is crucial to take into account both the waste generated in the food chain as a result of environmental degradation, and the food waste that could be otherwise consumed by members of society. Finding strategies to boost local and regional food production and consumption is also crucial for promoting sustainable availability, food security, and healthy diets [10]. Other objectives include lowering animal illness rates and producing enough high-quality food in adequate amounts with little waste.

Taking into account these ideas, this Special Issue presents 17 papers published by researchers from 16 different countries all over the world, including Brazil, Chile, China, Greece, Hungary, Iceland, Pakistan, Poland, Portugal, Saudi Arabia, Spain, Thailand, Turkey, the UK, Uruguay, and the USA.

Regarding the review articles included in this Special Issue, it is possible to find one work (scoping review) that addresses the following theme: vitamin B12 supplementation in the vegan population [11]. Because vegans consume less animal products, the researchers came to the conclusion that vitamin B12 insufficiency is prevalent among vegans.

In terms of research articles, we mention 16 relevant works that focus on different areas common to the objectives of this Special Issue: the research conducted by Duda [12] to understand the health-related motivations for urban food self-production in light of semantic field analysis, where the results showed that the inadequate availability of healthy vegetables to residents makes their health concerns a major determinant of their willingness to take part in urban food self-production initiatives; the investigations on urban–rural disparities in food insecurity and weight status among children in the USA, which emphasize

Received: 27 January 2025
Revised: 18 February 2025
Accepted: 1 April 2025
Published: 2 April 2025

Citation: Raposo, A.; Saraiva, A. Nutrition and Food Security for All: A Step Towards the Future. *Nutrients* 2025, 17, 1241. https://doi.org/10.3390/nu17071241

Copyright: © 2025 by the authors. Licensee MDPI, Basel, Switzerland. This article is an open access article distributed under the terms and conditions of the Creative Commons Attribution (CC BY) license (https://creativecommons.org/licenses/by/4.0/).

the significance of integrating food security interventions into future obesity prevention programs, given the association between food insecurity and increased obesity rates, especially among urban children [13]; and Ahmed et al. [14] published a study on the political economy of maternal child malnutrition: experiences about water, food, and nutrition policies in Pakistan. Nutrition programs encounter challenges including underfunding, weak monitoring, the exclusion of those with low social and cultural capital, corruption in the health system, and the influence of formula milk businesses that are affiliated with the medical community and bureaucracy. In order to increase nutrition security in Pakistan, this study suggests that tackling the macropolitical and economic factors that contribute to undernutrition should be given top priority. Harnirattisai et al. [15] investigated nutritional health risks (food security) in older Thai adults and the related factors, and found that, in Thailand, elderly persons seem to be at a greater risk of malnutrition, especially those with underlying medical conditions and poor incomes. Moreover, using Household Dietary Diversity Scores and spatial analysis to inform food governance in Chile was the topic of the work conducted by del Valle, M. et al. [16]. They stressed how crucial it is to use data insights such as the Household Dietary Diversity Score and spatial visualization to improve food security and guide food governance strategies. Furthermore, a case study in the Federal District of Brazil about food neophobia in children revealed that children from the Federal District exhibit higher levels of neophobia than Brazilian children overall, underscoring the need for more research on the factors that contribute to food phobia in this demographic and nutritional education initiatives to lessen food phobias in the children from this region [17], whilst a qualitative study on healthy food priority areas, barriers, and enablers for equitable healthy food access in Baltimore restaurants was carried out [18]. This study highlights that policies and interventions should demonstrate cultural awareness, give financial support, and provide more precise instructions to assist these companies in overcoming obstacles and gaining access to the resources required for a fair, wholesome food environment. In the works developed by Rozmiarek on the role of nutrition in maintaining the health and physical condition of sports volunteers [19], where it emerged that a large number of volunteers in sports are unaware of how their diet affects their health and fitness, the author pointed out that nutritional education is required to help this population better understand the value of a balanced diet in the context of increasing physical activity. Better nutritional conditions for sporting events should also be provided, and professional sources of knowledge on healthy eating should be encouraged, as well as on the nutritional education needs and preferences of sports volunteers, including access, expectations, and forms of support [20]. Although the volunteers indicated a desire for better nutritional education, more research is required to verify the connection between this knowledge and possible improvements in their health and performance. In another work on the adaptation of the food literacy (FOODLIT) tool for Turkish adults: a validity and reliability study [21], the findings demonstrated the validity and reliability of this adaption. The authors believe that this will be a good tool to measure the level of food literacy among people living in Turkey, and to find out how food literacy affects culinary skills, food production and quality, planning and selection, environmental safety, and food origin. Moreover, the investigation carried out by Ferreira et al. [22] on defatted flaxseed flour as a new ingredient for foodstuffs is a comparative analysis with whole flaxseeds and an updated composition of cold-pressed oil. In line with consumer preferences for natural, low-fat meals, the flour's importance in promoting food security, the circular economy, and sustainability goals was highlighted by explorations into its role as a minimally processed food ingredient. An analysis from the perspective of sustainability on Mediterranean food pattern adherence in a female-dominated sample of health and social sciences university students [23] highlighted the need for focused initiatives meant to encourage university students to follow Mediterranean food patterns, since this might lead to better health outcomes and more environmental sustainability. Another key piece of research was that conducted by Hernández-Moreno et al. [24] on food security in the rural Mapuche elderly; their analysis and proposals concluded that although rural Mapuche elders continue to follow important practices for their food security, there are major obstacles due to weak policies, migration, and environmental deterioration, while a multi-elemental analysis of energy drinks regarding the nutritional risks of heavy metals in the human diet demonstrated that there may be carcinogenic risks connected to the hazardous element content of energy drinks, in addition to health effects based on their caffeine level. Significant variations in trace element levels between different energy drink products, which may have significant effects on the health and well-being of consumers [25], are also highlighted in this study. Another important study was the comparative analysis of dietary behaviors in children and parents during COVID-19 lockdowns in Greece: insights from a non-representative sample [26]. According to the COVEAT study's findings, the dietary habits of children and adolescents, as well as those of their parents, were affected differently by each lockdown period. Less positive changes were seen in the second COVID-19 lockdown, which raises the possibility that the introduction of more lockdowns may have had a detrimental effect on people's lifestyles. Finally, insights from the FINESCOP project on dietary intakes among university students in Iceland were of crucial significance [27]. In this study, Icelandic university students' food intakes and the relationships between dietary components were investigated. To further comprehend the eating practices of Icelandic university students and investigate the possibility of drawing causal conclusions, more research is required.

Due to the added value provided by all these works, the editors believe that this Special Issue can contribute to deepening the knowledge on nutrition and food security from a global perspective, both for the scientific community and for populations all over the world, and that great steps can be made towards a better future in this context.

Author Contributions: This Special Issue was edited jointly by A.R. and A.S. This editorial was written jointly by the editors. All authors have read and agreed to the published version of the manuscript.

Acknowledgments: The authors would like to extend a very special thanks for the commitment and dedication of all researchers who published their works in this Special Issue. Only in this way was it possible to carry out this successful project.

Conflicts of Interest: The authors declare no conflicts of interest.

References

1. Food and Agriculture Organization of the United Nations. The State of Food Security and Nutrition in the World 2023: Urbanization, Agrifood Systems Transformation and Healthy Diets Across the Rural–Urban Continuum. Available online: https://www.fao.org/documents/card/en/c/cc3017en (accessed on 27 January 2025).
2. Barrett, C.B. Overcoming global food security challenges through science and solidarity. *Am. J. Agric. Econ.* **2021**, *103*, 422–447. [CrossRef]
3. Hariram, N.P.; Mekha, K.B.; Suganthan, V.; Sudhakar, K. Sustainalism: An Integrated Socio-Economic-Environmental Model to Address Sustainable Development and Sustainability. *Sustainability* **2023**, *15*, 10682. [CrossRef]
4. Raposo, A.; Ramos, F.; Raheem, D.; Saraiva, A.; Carrascosa, C. Food Safety, Security, Sustainability and Nutrition as Priority Objectives of the Food Sector. *Int. J. Environ. Res. Public Health* **2021**, *18*, 8073. [CrossRef]
5. Raposo, A.; Han, H. The Multifaceted Nature of Food and Nutrition Insecurity around the World and Foodservice Business. *Sustainability* **2022**, *14*, 7905. [CrossRef]
6. Raposo, A.; Zandonadi, R.P.; Botelho, R.B.A. Challenging the Status Quo to Shape Food Systems Transformation from a Nutritional and Food Security Perspective. *Foods* **2022**, *11*, 604. [CrossRef] [PubMed]
7. Raposo, A.; Zandonadi, R.P.; Botelho, R.B.A. Challenging the Status Quo to Shape Food Systems Transformation from a Nutritional and Food Security Perspective: Second Edition. *Foods* **2023**, *12*, 1825. [CrossRef] [PubMed]

8. Onyeaka, H.; Ejiohuo, O.; Taiwo, O.R.; Nnaji, N.D.; Odeyemi, O.A.; Duan, K.; Nwaiwu, O.; Odeyemi, O. The Intersection of Food Security and Mental Health in the Pursuit of Sustainable Development Goals. *Nutrients* **2024**, *16*, 2036. [CrossRef]
9. Oluwole, O.; Ibidapo, O.; Arowosola, T.; Raji, F.; Zandonadi, R.P.; Alasqah, I.; Lho, L.H.; Han, H.; Raposo, A. Sustainable transformation agenda for enhanced global food and nutrition security: A narrative review. *Front. Nutr.* **2023**, *10*, 1226538. [CrossRef]
10. Lins, M.; Puppin Zandonadi, R.; Raposo, A.; Ginani, V.C. Food Waste on Foodservice: An Overview through the Perspective of Sustainable Dimensions. *Foods* **2021**, *10*, 1175. [CrossRef]
11. Fernandes, S.; Oliveira, L.; Pereira, A.; Costa, M.d.C.; Raposo, A.; Saraiva, A.; Magalhães, B. Exploring Vitamin B12 Supplementation in the Vegan Population: A Scoping Review of the Evidence. *Nutrients* **2024**, *16*, 1442. [CrossRef]
12. Duda, E. Understanding Health-Related Motivations for Urban Food Self-Production in the Light of Semantic Fields Analysis. *Nutrients* **2024**, *16*, 1533. [CrossRef] [PubMed]
13. Dave, J.M.; Chen, T.A.; Castro, A.N.; White, M.A.; Onugha, E.A.; Zimmerman, S.; Thompson, D. Urban–Rural Disparities in Food Insecurity and Weight Status among Children in the United States. *Nutrients* **2024**, *16*, 2132. [CrossRef] [PubMed]
14. Ahmed, F.; Malik, N.I.; Bashir, S.; Noureen, N.; Ahmad, J.B.; Tang, K. Political Economy of Maternal Child Malnutrition: Experiences about Water, Food, and Nutrition Policies in Pakistan. *Nutrients* **2024**, *16*, 2642. [CrossRef]
15. Harnirattisai, T.; Vuthiarpa, S.; Pawloski, L.R.; Curtin, K.M.; Blackwell, E.; Nguyen, J.; Bourgeois, S.M. Nutritional Health Risk (Food Security) in Thai Older Adults and Related Factors. *Nutrients* **2024**, *16*, 2703. [CrossRef] [PubMed]
16. del Valle, M.M.; Shields, K.; Boza, S. Using Household Dietary Diversity Score and Spatial Analysis to Inform Food Governance in Chile. *Nutrients* **2024**, *16*, 2937. [CrossRef]
17. De Almeida, P.C.; Nakano, E.Y.; Vasconcelos, I.A.L.; Zandonadi, R.P.; Raposo, A.; Saraiva, A.; Alturki, H.A.; Botelho, R.B.A. Food Neophobia in Children: A Case Study in Federal District/Brazil. *Nutrients* **2024**, *16*, 2962. [CrossRef]
18. Hua, S.; Vong, V.; Thomas, A.E.; Mui, Y.; Poirier, L. Barriers and Enablers for Equitable Healthy Food Access in Baltimore Carryout Restaurants: A Qualitative Study in Healthy Food Priority Areas. *Nutrients* **2024**, *16*, 3028. [CrossRef]
19. Rozmiarek, M. The Role of Nutrition in Maintaining the Health and Physical Condition of Sports Volunteers. *Nutrients* **2024**, *16*, 3336. [CrossRef]
20. Rozmiarek, M. Nutritional Education Needs and Preferences of Sports Volunteers: Access, Expectations, and Forms of Support. *Nutrients* **2024**, *16*, 3568. [CrossRef]
21. Ertaş Öztürk, Y.; Kabalı, S.; Açar, Y.; Ağagündüz, D.; Budán, F. Adaptation of the Food Literacy (FOODLIT) Tool for Turkish Adults: A Validity and Reliability Study. *Nutrients* **2024**, *16*, 3416. [CrossRef]
22. Ferreira, D.M.; Machado, S.; Espírito Santo, L.; Nunes, M.A.; Costa, A.S.G.; Álvarez-Ortí, M.; Pardo, J.E.; Alves, R.C.; Oliveira, M.B.P.P. Defatted Flaxseed Flour as a New Ingredient for Foodstuffs: Comparative Analysis with Whole Flaxseeds and Updated Composition of Cold-Pressed Oil. *Nutrients* **2024**, *16*, 3482. [CrossRef]
23. Oliveira, L.; Saraiva, A.; Lima, M.J.; Teixeira-Lemos, E.; Alhaji, J.H.; Carrascosa, C.; Raposo, A. Mediterranean Food Pattern Adherence in a Female-Dominated Sample of Health and Social Sciences University Students: Analysis from a Perspective of Sustainability. *Nutrients* **2024**, *16*, 3886. [CrossRef] [PubMed]
24. Hernández-Moreno, A.; Vásquez-Palma, O.; Castillo-Cárdenas, L.; Erices-Reyes, J.; Guzmán-Jiménez, A.; Domínguez-Scheid, C.; Girona-Gamarra, M.; Cáceres-Senn, M.; Hochstetter-Diez, J. Food Security in the Rural Mapuche Elderly: Analysis and Proposals. *Nutrients* **2024**, *16*, 4042. [CrossRef] [PubMed]
25. Czarnek, K.; Tatarczak-Michalewska, M.; Wójcik, G.; Szopa, A.; Majerek, D.; Fila, K.; Hamitoglu, M.; Gogacz, M.; Blicharska, E. Nutritional Risks of Heavy Metals in the Human Diet—Multi-Elemental Analysis of Energy Drinks. *Nutrients* **2024**, *16*, 4306. [CrossRef] [PubMed]
26. Androutsos, O.; Saltaouras, G.; Kipouros, M.; Koutsaki, M.; Migdanis, A.; Georgiou, C.; Perperidi, M.; Papadopoulou, S.K.; Kosti, R.I.; Giaginis, C.; et al. Comparative Analysis of Dietary Behavior in Children and Parents During COVID-19 Lockdowns in Greece: Insights from a Non-Representative Sample. *Nutrients* **2025**, *17*, 112. [CrossRef]
27. Repella, B.M.; Jakobsdottir, G. Dietary Intakes Among University Students in Iceland: Insights from the FINESCOP Project. *Nutrients* **2025**, *17*, 432. [CrossRef]

Disclaimer/Publisher's Note: The statements, opinions and data contained in all publications are solely those of the individual author(s) and contributor(s) and not of MDPI and/or the editor(s). MDPI and/or the editor(s) disclaim responsibility for any injury to people or property resulting from any ideas, methods, instructions or products referred to in the content.

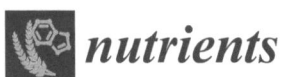

Review

Exploring Vitamin B12 Supplementation in the Vegan Population: A Scoping Review of the Evidence

Sávio Fernandes [1], Leandro Oliveira [1,2], Alda Pereira [3,4], Maria do Céu Costa [1,5,*], António Raposo [1,*], Ariana Saraiva [6] and Bruno Magalhães [7,8,9]

1. CBIOS (Research Center for Biosciences and Health Technologies), Universidade Lusófona de Humanidades e Tecnologias, Campo Grande 376, 1749-024 Lisboa, Portugal; saviof.nt@gmail.com (S.F.); leandroliveira.nut@gmail.com (L.O.)
2. Coimbra Health School, Polytechnic Institute of Coimbra, Rua 5 de Outubro—S. Martinho do Bispo, Apartado 7006, 3046-854 Coimbra, Portugal
3. Institute for Preventive Medicine and Public Health, Faculty of Medicine, University of Lisbon, 1649-028 Lisboa, Portugal; aldapsilva@medicina.ulisboa.pt
4. University Clinic of General and Family Medicine, Ecogenetics and Human Health Unity, Institute for Environmental Health, Instituto de Saúde Ambiental (ISAMB), 1649-028 Lisboa, Portugal
5. Núcleo de Investigação em Ciências e Tecnologias da Saúde (NICiTeS), Polytechnic Institute of Lusophony, ERISA—Escola Superior de Saúde Ribeiro Sanches, 1900-693 Lisboa, Portugal
6. Department of Animal Pathology and Production, Bromatology and Food Technology, Faculty of Veterinary, Universidad de Las Palmas de Gran Canaria, Trasmontaña s/n, 35413 Arucas, Spain; ariana_23@outlook.pt
7. School of Health, University of Trás-os-Montes and Alto Douro (UTAD), 5000-801 Vila Real, Portugal; brunomm@utad.pt
8. RISE—Health Research Network, Faculty of Medicine, University of Porto, 4099-002 Porto, Portugal
9. Clinical Academic Centre of Trás-os-Montes and Alto Douro (CACTMAD), 5000-801 Vila Real, Portugal
* Correspondence: maria.costa@ulusofona.pt (M.d.C.C.); antonio.raposo@ulusofona.pt (A.R.)

Abstract: With a significant portion of the population adopting veganism and conflicting views among nutrition professionals regarding the necessity of vitamin B12 supplementation, this review aims to explore existing studies evaluating interventions through food supplementation. It focuses on the impact of vitamin B12 deficiency across different demographics. The present study seeks to understand how research has addressed the relationship between the rise in veganism and vitamin B12 deficiency over the past decade. A scoping review was conducted following the PRISMA flow diagram. Studies from 2010 to 2023 were identified using Boolean operators and key terms in electronic databases such as PubMed/MEDLINE, Web of Science, and EBSCO (Library, Information Science & Technology Abstracts, and Academic Search Complete). Out of 217 articles identified, 70 studies were included. The topical analysis categorized the studies into three groups: those associating vitamin B12 deficiency with diseases ($n = 14$), those analyzing the dietary habits of vegetarian individuals (vegan or not) without a specific focus on vitamin B12 ($n = 49$), and those addressing food guides and nutrition institution positions ($n = 7$). The authors concluded that vitamin B12 deficiency is prevalent among vegans due to limited consumption of animal products. For vegetarians, supplementation is an efficient means of treating and preventing deficiency; a daily dose of 50 to 100 micrograms is advised. There are still significant gaps in the research, nevertheless, such as the absence of randomized controlled trials evaluating various forms or dosages of vitamin B12 among vegetarians and the requirement for more information and awareness of the vitamin's significance in vegan diets.

Keywords: cobalamin; food supplements; plant-based diet; vegan diet; vegetarianism; vitamin B12

Citation: Fernandes, S.; Oliveira, L.; Pereira, A.; Costa, M.d.C.; Raposo, A.; Saraiva, A.; Magalhães, B. Exploring Vitamin B12 Supplementation in the Vegan Population: A Scoping Review of the Evidence. *Nutrients* **2024**, *16*, 1442. https://doi.org/10.3390/nu16101442

Academic Editor: Anna Maria Marconi

Received: 1 April 2024
Revised: 7 May 2024
Accepted: 9 May 2024
Published: 10 May 2024

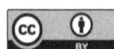

Copyright: © 2024 by the authors. Licensee MDPI, Basel, Switzerland. This article is an open access article distributed under the terms and conditions of the Creative Commons Attribution (CC BY) license (https://creativecommons.org/licenses/by/4.0/).

1. Introduction

Considering rapid population growth and inevitable pressures on the global food supply, such as the projected 44% increase in demand for animal products by 2050 to meet current global consumption levels, plant-based diets present a potentially healthier and more sustainable alternative [1].

"Vegetarian" is a term that defines a person who abstains from eating meat, fish, shellfish, and products made from these foods, optionally including other animal derivatives such as dairy, eggs, and honey in their diet [2,3]. Vegans, on the other hand, exclude any type of food or derivative of animal origin from their diet [2,3]. Choosing vegetarianism goes beyond food selection and reflects a philosophy aimed at reducing animal exploitation and cruelty, especially in food production. Additionally, this practice may be motivated by potential benefits for both health and the environment, making it an appealing option for many people [4,5]. Vegetarian diets are associated with a reduced risk of cardiovascular diseases by lowering modifiable risk factors like abdominal obesity, blood pressure, serum lipid profile, and blood glucose levels [6]. Additionally, these diets reduce inflammation markers, decrease oxidative stress, and protect against atherosclerotic plaque development, resulting in a lower risk of ischemic heart disease development and mortality [3,6].

Vegetarian diets are deemed beneficial for health, as they encourage diversity and stability of intestinal microbiota. This microbial diversity is significantly associated with body mass index (BMI), obesity, and cardiovascular protection [7]. Scientifically robust evidence suggests that vegan or vegetarian diets are linked to reductions in weight and BMI, and in certain instances, alterations in fat mass distribution [8].

In fact, well-designed vegetarian diets, including vegan diets, are considered healthy and nutritionally adequate, and may offer health advantages in preventing and managing specific disease risks. However, plant-based foods naturally lack a reliable source of vitamin B12, requiring individuals following a vegan diet to incorporate fortified foods or take vitamin B12 supplements to meet their dietary needs [9]. Inadequate vegetarian diets may lead to deficiencies in iron, calcium, zinc, vitamin D, and B12, as well as some amino acids. In some cases, this can result in hyperhomocysteinemia, protein deficiency, anemia, and decreased muscle creatinine [6,10].

The European Food Safety Authority (EFSA) proposes utilizing biomarkers such as serum cobalamin, holotranscobalamin, methylmalonic acid, and plasma total homocysteine, to establish Dietary Reference Values for cobalamin [11]. Despite uncertainties in defining cutoff values for vitamin B12 insufficiency and limited data, consistent evidence indicates that a daily intake of vitamin B12 at 4 µg/day or higher in adults is associated with adequate vitamin B12 status. Consequently, EFSA recommends an adequate intake (AI) of 4 µg/day for vitamin B12 in the European population, taking into account various biomarkers and observed intakes ranging from 4.2 to 8.6 µg/day in several EU countries [11].

Vitamin B12 deficiency varies depending on both the severity and the cause, being classified as mild, moderate, or severe, depending on measurable pathophysiological factors. The deficiency classified as mild generally arises as a result of inadequate intake, mainly among the differentiated population of vegans, vegetarians, individuals with low cobalamin consumption, and breastfeeding mothers with vitamin B12 deficiency. The body absorbs 1–5 mg of vitamin B12 daily and stores it substantially in the liver. However, noticeable clinical symptoms of deficiency arise only when vitamin levels fall significantly below the required limit. Determining serum vitamin B12 concentration is the main test to assess vitamin B12 status and risk of deficiency [12].

Some studies point to a deficient concentration of vitamin B12 (<156 pmol/L) as having a prevalence of 52% in vegan individuals and only 1% in omnivorous individuals [13]. Subnormal vitamin B12 status is prevalent (50–70%) in vegetarians or vegans in Austria, Germany, Italy, Australia, India, and China [14].

In this context, this scoping review aims to identify current studies concerning interventions through dietary supplementation of vitamin B12. It seeks to examine how this topic has evolved in recent years to address the genuine necessity for individual supplementation. Additionally, the present study aims to explore potential interventions tailored to specific vulnerable populations.

2. Methods

2.1. Study Design

To achieve the objectives, a scoping review of the scientific literature on vitamin B12 supplementation in vegan individuals was designed and the PRISMA model (Preferred Reporting Items for Systematic Reviews and Meta-Analyses) [15] was used to organize the information.

The formulation of the research question was based on the acronym PCC (population, context, and concept): What is known, from the existing literature, about vitamin B12 supplementation in vegan individuals?

The inclusion criteria for the articles are summarized in Table 1 and were defined based on the population, contexts and concepts, type of study, language, and date of publication.

Table 1. Definition of inclusion criteria.

	Inclusion Criteria
Population (P)	Studies in adults aged 18 years and older on a vegan diet
Context (C)	Studies in which participants receive oral vitamin B12 supplementation
Concept (C)	Studies that address the effects of vitamin B12
Types of Studies	All primary or secondary, qualitative or quantitative studies
Language	Studies published in English, Spanish, or Portuguese
Publication date	Studies published between January 2010 and December 2023

The first methodological approach to identifying publications consisted of an exploratory search in electronic databases using previously defined keywords. In the next stage, the most relevant articles were consulted, the main phrases and search keywords were identified, and the terms of the Boolean phrases were defined to systematically carry out the final search. The respective descriptors in English were identified using the MeSH terms identified in the PubMed/MEDLINE, Web of Science, and EBSCO databases (Library, Information Science & Technology Abstracts, and Academic Search Complete).

Combinations of descriptors/medical subject headings (MeSH), subject headings, and subject terms were then applied to each of the databases, implementing the Boolean method operators "OR" and "AND" and the "*" tool, which leveraged research by creating new variations of the same word (Table S1).

2.2. Eligibility, Exclusion Criteria, and Selection Process

For original studies on the need for vitamin B12 supplementation, the following eligibility criteria were adopted for the included studies:

- Observation studies of individuals with a vegan diet;
- Studies that contain in their results an explicit, positive or negative, recommendation or indication of vitamin B12 supplementation.

All studies in which participants were involved in other studies without the participation of a population with a restricted vegan diet were excluded, as well as all studies in which there was supplementation by means other than oral administration, studies focused only on the development of new supplements on the market, studies on animals and, finally, studies that had been published in languages other than Portuguese, English, or Spanish.

For the selection process, two independent reviewers took on this task, reading in full the content available on the rayyan.ai® platform (https://www.rayyan.ai/, accessed on 10 January 2024), and after analysis, they determined the study to be adequate or not (included or excluded). If the two reviewers simultaneously opted for the inclusion of an article, it was selected; in the same way, if one of the reviewers excluded the study while the other chose to include it, it was automatically classified as "perhaps," with a third reviewer appointed as responsible for arbitrating the final decision on inclusion or non-inclusion.

None of the studies needed to be classified in this way, and it was not necessary to appoint a third reviewer.

2.3. Data Collection/Extraction Process

As the selected studies repeatedly presented results or developments that were only partially conclusive on the topic, the data considered necessary for the soundness of the discussion and conclusion of this review were taken from the original texts based on the expertise of the reviewers. Data were extracted regarding the direct association of the vegan diet with possible vitamin B12 deficiency and their respective recommendations for supplementation or not. This process was carried out by three reviewers, the first being responsible for collecting information from study groups 2 (G2) and 3 (G3), and the second reviewer responsible for group 1 (G1). The third reviewer oversaw the revision of the final text, including all groups.

The data researched and considered relevant to the study came from the question "Is vitamin B12 supplementation necessary in vegan individuals?" To elucidate the question, the parameters described in this section were established. The articles and studies should then have been clear in terms of whether they recommend vitamin supplementation at any age, for any gender, and without violating the ethical principles of exclusion.

2.4. Synthesis Method

The process used to determine the eligible studies was carried out jointly by two reviewers, analyzing the complete studies in general but especially the results obtained and the discussion about the recommendation of vitamin B12 supplementation. Studies were selected if they deliberately mentioned a positive or negative recommendation for supplementation. All selected studies have full text. After the eligibility selection, relevant data were removed from each study, such as the authors' names, country where it was carried out, year of publication, objective, abstract, and scope of the study.

This scoping review did not collect data for meta-analysis, as it was deemed unnecessary for the authors and the reviewers.

3. Results

Considering the described procedures, the research results were refined, according to the previously established criteria and processes, until the final number of articles included in this review was reached. Figure 1 describes each one of the steps to reach the final number of articles included within the flowchart for the identification and selection of studies.

Using the outlined search strategy, a total of 218 articles were initially identified across various databases. Among these, 70 were found to be duplicates and thus were excluded.

The remaining bibliographic sample consisted of 156 articles. However, upon closer examination, 15 articles were in languages other than the primary language of the review, 42 were deemed irrelevant due to incorrect population or background, and 5 articles focused on animal studies, which were deemed ethically discordant with the scope of this review. Additionally, 11 articles were related to specific commercial drugs, and 8 were rejected after a thorough reading of the full text. These findings were organized and summarized in Table 2, with the summaries prepared by the reviewers following a comprehensive analysis of the relevant information extracted from the full texts.

From the thematic analysis of all selected articles, three distinct groups of studies were defined as a posteriori by the researchers.

The first group consists of studies that focus on associating vitamin B12 deficiency with a disease ($n = 14$). A second group was formed by studies that analyzed the dietary intake of vegetarian individuals (vegan or not) without specifically focusing on vitamin B12 ($n = 49$). A third group was formed by studies on the composition of food guides and positions of nutrition institutions ($n = 7$).

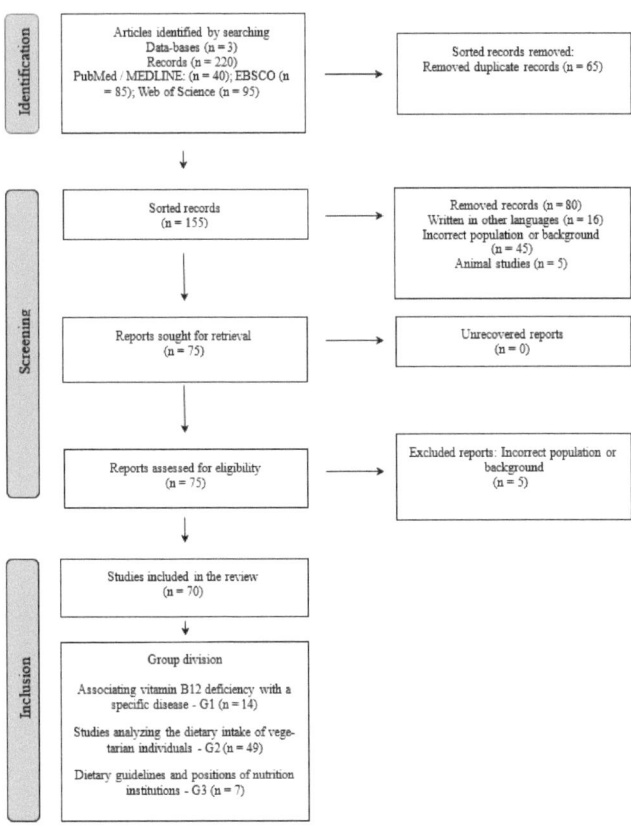

Figure 1. Process of identification and inclusion of articles—PRISMA diagram flowchart.

Table 2. Studies selected for the literature review.

Study	Objectives	Type of Study
E1 [16]	Associating atherosclerosis and the occurrence of vitamin B12 inadequacy	Randomized controlled trial
E2 [17]	Comparing the amounts of vitamin B12 and homocysteine in vegetarians and omnivores	Systematic review and meta-analysis
E3 [18]	Investigating the food intake of groups of 30–90-year-old carnivores, fish eaters, vegetarians, and vegans using semiquantitative diet frequency questionnaires	Analytical cross-sectional study
E4 [19]	Comparing standards of dietary intake and nutritional status of Finnish long-term vegans and non-vegetarians	Analytical cross-sectional study
E5 [20]	Examining prevalence values of cobalamin deficiency among vegetarian individuals assessed for serum vitamin B12	Systematic review
E6 [21]	Discussing vitamin B12 status of vegetarians with a focus both on the detection of cobalamin deficiency and appropriate sources for sufficient intake	Narrative review
E7 [22]	Guiding as to recommended nutrient (folate, vitamin B12, and vitamin B6) intake during pregnancy	Narrative review
E8 [23]	Using vitamin B12 and MMA markers to show the cobalamin status of Spanish vegetarians, along with the results of a plant-based diet and vitamin B12 supplementation	Analytical cross-sectional study
E9 [24]	Determining the impact of maternal diets on the levels of vitamin B12, ferritin, hemoglobin, and folic acid in mother's blood and umbilical cord blood	Analytical cross-sectional study

Table 2. *Cont.*

Study	Objectives	Type of Study
E10 [25]	Analyzing breast milk vitamin B12 concentration and vitamin B12 supplement use patterns among women who adhered to vegan, vegetarian, and nonvegetarian different dietary patterns	Analytical cross-sectional study
E11 [26]	Establishing practical parameters of micronutrient consumption for children involved with vegan diets	Practice guidelines
E12 [27]	Analyzing serum status of folate and vitamin B12 in vegan and ovo-lacto vegetarians	Analytical cross-sectional study
E13 [28]	Investigating any association between the plasma concentration of vitamin B12 and the use of animal-based meals, fortified foods, and supplements by non-vegetarians and vegetarians	Analytical cross-sectional study
E14 [29]	Reviewing literature to provide recommendations for how to construct a vegan diet for athletes and exercisers	Narrative review
E15 [30]	Outlining the metabolism of vitamin B12 and assessing the causes and effects of subclinical B12 insufficiency	Narrative review
E16 [31]	Discussing the nutrients potentially related to major concerns in a vegetarian diet along with the health benefits of following a vegetarian diet	Narrative review
E17 [32]	Obtaining insights on the benefits and risks of vegetarianism, with emphasis on vegetarian child nutrition profiles	Narrative review
E18 [33]	Potential nutritional deficiencies can be avoided by carefully choosing meals, fortifying foods, or using supplements to assist in maintaining good bone condition and lower the risk of fracture in those who follow vegetarian diets	Narrative review
E19 [34]	Determining any extent to which the reason for following a vegan diet has been associated with healthy behaviors	Analytical cross-sectional study
E20 [9]	Position of the Academy of Nutrition and Dietetics about several aspects of vegetarian diets	Institution position
E21 [35]	Clarifying the myths and facts of vegetarian and gluten-free diets, according to the existing evidence	Narrative review
E22 [14]	Evaluating the overall intake and the status on selected vitamins and minerals among vegetarians and vegan adults living in Switzerland	Analytical cross-sectional study
E23 [13]	Position of the Working Group of the Italian Society of Human Nutrition about several aspects of vegetarian diets	Institution position
E24 [36]	Reporting on vitamin B-12 (B12) as part of the Biomarkers of Nutrition for Development (BOND) Project, providing advice and state of the art on the selection, use, and interpretation of biomarkers for nutrient exposure, function, and status, and also including a section on vegetarian diets	Narrative review
E25 [37]	Analyzing the nutritional sustainability of the vegetarian diet of professional dancers	Narrative review
E26 [38]	Position of the Working Group of the Nutrition Committee, German Society for Pediatric and Adolescent Medicine (DGKJ) about vegetarian diets in childhood and adolescence	Institution position
E27 [39]	Developing vegan meal plans that focus on nutrients commonly lacking in the diet for children	Analytical cross-sectional study
E28 [40]	Tracing the profile of consumed micronutrients and related biomarkers for vegetarian and vegan athletes	Cohort study
E29 [41]	Exploring the vitamin B12 status of toddlers living in high-poverty areas of China and observing the effects of different complementary foods on the cognitive level of these toddlers and vitamin B12 status	Analytical cross-sectional study
E30 [42]	Creating theoretical plant-based, whole-food meal plans that are vegan and based on popular nutrition and cookery sources that were found through a thorough web questionnaire	Analytical cross-sectional study

Table 2. *Cont.*

Study	Objectives	Type of Study
E31 [43]	Comparing the nutritional consumption of recreational runners who are omnivores, lacto-ovo vegetarians, and vegans with the intake guidelines recommended for the general public by the Austrian, German, and Swiss Nutrition Societies	Cohort study
E32 [44]	Comparing macro- and micronutrient availability among vegetarian and traditional healthy diets	Narrative review
E33 [45]	Summarizing existing knowledge on the variability of defined nutrients in the breastmilk of mothers who reported to adhere to a plant-based diet	Systematic review
E34 [12]	Determining the status of cobalamin between Australian vegetarians and vegans	Narrative review
E35 [46]	Presenting advantages and disadvantages of vitamin supplementation and the indications for it in diverse life situations	Narrative review
E36 [47]	Examining the primary visual representations of food-based vegetarian diet recommendations from many nations in order to develop a new guide tailored to this particular Spanish demographic	Narrative review
E37 [48]	Position of the Committee on Nutrition and Breastfeeding in The Spanish Paediatric Association on vegetarian diets in infants and children	Institution position
E38 [49]	Systematic review of the evidence of associations between seasonal affective disorder and diet, eating behavior, and nutrition intervention	Systematic review
E39 [50]	Evaluation of vitamin B12 status of apparently healthy Indian children 6–23 months of age	Analytical cross-sectional study
E40 [51]	Studying the impact in vegetarians of vitamin B12 supplementation on arterial function	Randomized study
E41 [52]	Identifying the prevalence of vitamin B12 deficiency in vegetarian Indians	Epidemiological study
E42 [53]	Identifying the prevalence of vitamin B12 deficiency in vegans who do not use supplements in the Czech Republic	Epidemiological study
E43 [54]	Determining whether a vegetarian diet is healthy for children	Narrative review
E44 [55]	Reviewing literature to provide recommendations for how to construct a vegan diet for special populations of athletes and exercisers	Narrative review
E45 [56]	Presenting data on the influence of maternal vitamin B12 deficiency in infant psychomotor retardation	Case study
E46 [57]	Reporting a case of a 10-month-old infant with developmental regression secondary to vitamin B12 deficiency	Case study
E47 [58]	Describing the vitamin B12 status of South Asian women residing in Auckland who are primarily overweight or obese and linking the relationship between insulin resistance and blood vitamin B12 and vegetarian status	Epidemiological study
E48 [59]	Concentrating information necessary for the successful planning of vegetarian food introduction in children	Narrative review
E49 [60]	Estimating dietary B12 intake in the population of women originating from South Asia	Epidemiological study
E50 [61]	Verifying if the vegan diet exempt from food of animal origin still supplies the nutritional recommendations of supporters	Narrative review
E51 [62]	Reporting on a patient whose etiological and diagnostic work-up revealed delirium caused by a vitamin B12 deficiency	Case study
E52 [63]	Reviewing literature to indicate the influence of mineral and vitamin supplements on pregnancy outcome	Narrative review
E53 [64]	Examining the effect of vitamin B deficiency on the adult nervous system and other clinical manifestations of vitamin B deficiency	Narrative review
E54 [65]	Examining and contrasting the health and demographic traits of Australian women of reproductive age who follow a vegan diet with those of the general population, finding sources and amounts of vitamin B12 and comparing them to current guidelines, and looking for correlations between participant attributes and sufficient vitamin B12 intake	Epidemiological study

Table 2. Cont.

Study	Objectives	Type of Study
E55 [66]	Analyzing the existing literature on the growth and health impact of selected nutrients in the vegan child population	Narrative review
E56 [67]	Reviewing the literature dealing with potential associations between religious food rules and potential nutritional outcomes	Narrative review
E57 [68]	Reviewing the literature on the association between pregnancy in vegan and vegetarian populations and vitamin B12 deficiency	Narrative review
E58 [69]	Examining the prevalence and typical forms of vitamin B12-deficient presentations among non-vegetarian patients aged 20 to 80 who visited a tertiary care hospital in the state of Eastern India	Analytical cross-sectional study
E59 [70]	Analyzing a population of women during early pregnancy in Nepal for cobalamin and folate status	Randomized controlled trial
E60 [71]	Analyzing the impact of two forms of vitamin B12 supplements (methylcobalamin and cyanocobalamin) on the amount of active blood vitamin (holotranscobalamin) in a group of Romanians who ate a plant-based, vegan diet	Analytical cross-sectional study
E61 [72]	Identifying if vitamin B12 insufficiency in newborns is caused by dietary issues or an inherited defect in absorption and metabolism	Case study
E62 [73]	Describing the role of vitamin B12 deficiency in cardiovascular disease development among vegetarians	Systematic review and meta analysis
E63 [74]	Reviewing the literature on issues of pregnancy in vegans	Narrative review
E64 [75]	Investigating the vegan diet as a cause of severe megaloblastic anemia and psychosis	Case study
E65 [76]	Estimating the impact of a vegan diet over time on blood B12 concentrations in healthy omnivorous individuals by contrasting the effects of eating natural products with those enriched with B12	Prospective analytical cross-sectional study
E66 [77]	Assessing the adequacy of vitamin B12 supplementation in Australian vegan study participants by comparing intake to RDI, outlining the range of supplementation habits, and commenting on appropriate supplementation regimens	Analytical cross-sectional study
E67 [78]	Finding out how common cobalamin insufficiency is and how often vegetarian and vegan children in the Czech Republic use vitamin B12 supplements	Analytical cross-sectional study
E68 [79]	Evaluating the nutritional status of healthy, young, and physically active individuals who followed different types of diets (omnivores, vegetarians, and vegans) in terms of various nutrients, including vitamin B12	Analytical cross-sectional study
E69 [80]	Identifying the prevalence of regular and irregular vitamin B12 supplementation in Slovak and Czech vegans	Analytical cross-sectional study
E70 [81]	Investigating health and supplementation behavior on vitamin B12 supplementation, and demographically characterizing the community of Austrian adult vegans. Additional aim: to evaluate adherence to check-ups and vitamin B12 supplementation among Austrian vegans, and the prevalence of healthy behaviors	Analytical cross-sectional study

3.1. Group 1—Association of Vitamin B12 Deficiency with Any Disease

3.1.1. Illnesses in Infants

A vitamin B12 deficit in children is related to megaloblastic anemia from the mother or from a vegan and vegetarian diet without adequate supplementation [56,57]. The low level of this vitamin is only possible to transmit to the child when the mother exclusively breastfeeds until 6 months of age. In two studies, inappropriate levels of cobalamin were reported due to the type of diet of the vegan mother. One of the studies was about a 10-month-old child, and the other study related to a 6-month-old child. Both were female [56,57]. The children had identical symptoms: They could not stabilize their necks when sitting or grasping objects, and there was a regression in neurodevelopment and psychomotor activity [56,57].

Vitamin B12 deficiency in the first stage of life is rare, but it can be cured [57]. The treatment involves a scheme of cobalamin medicinal injections, the first stage of which consists of weekly injections for 4 weeks, then once a month for 3 months, and finally, once every 3 months for 6 months [57].

It is concluded that breastfeeding mothers who are vegetarian/vegan must pay special attention to their levels of vitamin B12 and take supplementation, if necessary, to avoid deficits of the same vitamin in infants.

3.1.2. Childhood Illnesses

A recent study [54] had two objectives: (1) to find out the consequences of vegetarianism and veganism in children from conception to the end of the growth period and (2) to study the interaction potential of certain foods with physical and cognitive development. Through a controlled study design, where the target population was children who were vegetarian due to poverty, they studied whether milk, soy, and eggs would be equivalently good substitutes for meat. They divided the children into four groups: meat, milk, energy, and control. The first three groups were offered a dish based on products of vegetable origin with a supplementation of 60 g of meat, 200 mL of milk, or an extra 3 g of oil. In contrast, children who were part of the control group did not receive extra meals. Among the four study groups, the group in which there was an extra meat meal presented the best results, with improved physical activity during recess, an improvement in leadership activities, and a sense of initiative [54].

The relationship with acne was also investigated, for which diet is the crucial factor for its appearance. Acne is induced by hyperinsulinemia, and together with low insulin response and high protein doses, it has been deduced that these factors increase acne symptoms in child and adolescent patients [54].

Overall, this study concludes that a diet without food of animal origin or proper supplementation and care is neither beneficial nor safe for children's health since it is associated with various risks to children's growth, such as the risk of having a vitamin B12 deficiency, which can lead to delayed physical and cognitive development [54].

3.1.3. Osteoporosis

Osteoporosis is recognized as a chronic disease that is associated with a progressive loss of bone mineral density, leading to a higher risk of fractures. To help combat or delay the development of this disease, calcium in the daily diet is foreseen as important, especially from foods such as milk and cheese. Vegetarian diets are poor in this mineral and in other vitamins such as cobalamin, since it is excluded from the diet. Nevertheless, it is determined that these diets are rich in other nutrients with a protective character, allowing vegetarians to have a low risk of bone fracture [33].

Osteoporosis risk increases with elevated serum methylmalonic acid levels, serving as a reliable indicator of insufficient vitamin B12 levels. Conversely, low vitamin B12 levels are linked to decreased mineral density, contributing to osteoporosis development [33].

Several studies have been carried out on vitamin B12 in association with low bone mineral density and consequently with osteoporosis. Studies in the target vegetarian population showed that a low concentration of cobalamin was associated with better bone remodeling and could lead to the acceleration of bone loss. In addition to this conclusion it was also discovered that a European study in which ovolactovegetarians, vegans, and omnivores were compared found that the prevalence of vitamin B12 deficiency was 77%, 92%, and 11%, respectively [33].

A vegetarian or vegan diet provides not only benefits for health but also risks, which can lead to malnutrition, that is, a deficit of certain nutrients such as vitamin B12, which can lead to neural or physical diseases such as osteoporosis and a higher risk of fractures [33]. However, if the individual is properly supplemented and followed by a professional, the health risk is lower and a healthy life may be achieved.

3.1.4. Cardiovascular Diseases

The main reason a vegan diet is followed is the belief that it is better for health, as this type of diet has been reported as being potentially cardiac protective. The literature proves that there is a lower prevalence of hypercholesterolemia, hypertension, diabetes mellitus, and mortality due to heart attack among vegetarians [16]. As a rule, it is believed that vegetarian diets are protective of cardiovascular pathologies, although numerous studies prove the opposite [51]. The population following a vegetarian diet has a high prevalence of cobalamin deficiency, excessive salt consumption, and increased serum concentration of triglycerides, which may lead to certain pathologies such as arteriosclerosis [51]. To assess the impact of vitamin B12 supplementation, 50 vegetarian communities were studied, with an average of 14 years; non-smokers; no known kidney, vascular, or liver diseases; and no medication or supplementation taken [51]. A food frequency questionnaire was applied to estimate food intake over one week [51]. After applying this questionnaire, individuals were randomly assessed and received 500 μg of vitamin B12 orally per day for 12 weeks [51].

Research has shown that supplementing vitamin B12 in deficient vegetarians enhances arterial endothelial function compared to those receiving a placebo. Vegetarian diets, rich in plant-based compounds, are often linked with cardiovascular health benefits, including lower serum cholesterol levels and potentially reduced blood pressure [51]. However, cohort studies indicate that vegetarian diets may not significantly lower mortality rates from cardiovascular disease, particularly among strict vegetarians [51]. Notably, vitamin B12 deficiency is prevalent among two demographic groups: the elderly and vegetarians, often without noticeable symptoms. Nonetheless, a more advanced stage of cardiovascular disease can be prevented through vitamin B12 supplementation and adequate consumption of dairy products, eggs, and fortified cereals [51].

It is reasonable to assert that vegetarian diets offer protection for cardiovascular health. Moreover, vegan diets, when compared to lacto-ovo-vegetarian diets, demonstrate protective effects against high body mass index (BMI) and the prevalence of diabetes mellitus, hypertension, and hyperlipidemia [16]. It is also believed that vitamin B12 supplementation in vitamin B12-impaired but asymptomatic vegetarians may lead to a significant improvement in arterial endothelial function and carotid intimal thickness with possible potential to improve cardiovascular health [51]. Thus, one may conclude that the consumption of dairy products and eggs combined with the consumption of vegetables, fruits, cereals, and vitamin C can alleviate the adverse metabolic and vascular effects, resulting in a beneficial outcome for cardiac health [16].

3.1.5. Delirium (Clinical Case)

Cobalamin deficiency affects about 20% of the elderly population and is considered a public health problem, and its symptoms can manifest at a neuropsychiatric, gastrointestinal, and hematological level, or in this case, symptoms such as depression, dementia, and delirium [62].

Cobalamin deficiency occurs due to poor absorption and pernicious anemia, making food play a fundamental role in preventing the problem. Therefore, it is necessary to pay attention to vegetarians as a risk group for contracting this type of condition [62]. Neuropsychiatric problems derive from the involvement of vitamin B12 with folate and homocysteine [62]. In this article, a case of a patient who contracted a psychological pathology due to cobalamin deficiency was studied [62].

The clinical case refers to a 62-year-old woman of Argentine origin who was admitted to the emergency room of a hospital. She was found lost on the street and showed signs of confusion. The patient complained that she suffered from insomnia, fatigue, and lack of concentration. After some tests, it was concluded that she had a psychomotor delay, anxiety, and depression [62].

This patient had a history of vitamin B12 deficiency but no reported neuropsychiatric symptoms potentially causing deficiency. The cause was found to be the vegetarian diet that the patient followed, which led to cases of delirium [62]. Weekly injections of 1000 μg of cyanocobalamin were applied to treat the patient. The levels of vitamin B12 normalized after a week and after 2 weeks. After psychiatric examination, the cognitive impairment had decreased as well as a part of the remission of the symptoms of depression [62]. Four weeks after the incident, tests showed that the patient was mentally stable and in complete remission of her depression symptoms [62].

3.2. Group 2—Studies Analyzing the Food Consumption of Vegetarian Individuals (Vegan or Not) without a Specific Focus on Vitamin B12

It has been demonstrated that vegans are deficient in vitamin B12, and it is generally agreed upon that this vitamin has to be supplemented [44]. Indicators of vitamin B12 deficiency (homocysteine, plasma methylmalonic acid, and holotranscobalamin II) show that vegans have lower levels of vitamin B12, but relatively few report clinical symptoms [34]. Compared with non-vegetarians, vegetarians have lower mortality from ischemic heart disease and lower BMI, serum glucose, serum cholesterol, and blood pressure [21]. Although long-term intake of a vegan diet is associated with these benefits, concentrations of essential nutrients are compared with baseline values [19]. Studies using plant-based foods to increase cobalamin intake are promising, but more data are needed [21]. The frequency of vitamin B12 deficiency is higher in people who do not take supplements or consume foods fortified with B12 than those who follow other vegetarian diets [20,27].

The vitamin B12 status of predominantly overweight or obese people is low, especially when they are vegetarians, as has been seen [58]. However, a well-planned vegetarian diet is healthy if nutritionally adequate and may help prevent and treat certain chronic diseases [31]. Since a vegan diet provides adequate nutritional recommendations for all nutrients except vitamins B12 and D, as well as calcium, in these cases, the use of fortified foods or food supplements becomes essential to ensure adequate nutritional support [61,76]. Dietary/food supplements containing vitamin B12 contribute significantly to plasma vitamin B12 levels, especially in vegans and ovolactovegetarians, followed by vitamin-fortified milk replacers in non-supplemented users. Milk replacer significantly impacts plasma vitamin B12 concentrations among individuals who are not receiving any type of supplementation [28]. This situation would be of particular importance for women of reproductive age to prevent the risks associated with maternal–fetal vitamin B12 deficiency [52].

Public health services, nutritionists, complementary and alternative therapists, and medical professionals must consider the needs of vegans, especially concerning monitoring cobalamin status to prevent cobalamin deficiency [53]. In Schüpbach et al. [14], it is noted that despite the relatively low consumption of vitamin B12 among vegans in Switzerland, deficiency rates remain low due to the prevalent use of dietary supplements. Likewise, Chandra-Hioe et al. [12] conducted a study in Australians seeking to understand the consumption of foods that provide adequate vitamin B12 for individuals on an omnivore diet, such as dairy products and meat. However, there seems to be a lack of knowledge about the consumption of foods such as vitamin B12-enriched foods and beverages by the general population, where vegan diets, even occasionally, are becoming more common. Data available from the Australian Health Survey on the consumption of fortified foods (such as soy milk) are limited to consumption by different age groups of the population and provide the only distinction between the sexes. This information can serve as a valuable resource in designing nutritionally balanced diets for both vegetarians and non-vegetarians. Additionally, it can inform the design of future clinical trials aimed at investigating the efficacy of various dietary sources of vitamin B12 in preventing deficiency among individuals who are not aware of the use of vitamin B12 supplements [28].

Regarding a more specific audience referring to puerperal women, infants, and children in early childhood, it was noted that vitamin B12 deficiency is a preventable cause of maternal and childhood diseases. As evidenced by Cruchet et al. [35], who sought to elucidate the myths and facts of vegetarian and gluten-free diets concerning infant feeding, vegetarianism does not represent any nutritional threat, as it normally includes egg and milk. Under expert supervision and with the appropriate vitamin B12 dosage, children get all the nutrients they need. However, vegan diets are not advised for everyone at any age, especially in vulnerable periods of life. If followed under the guidance of a professional, a vegetarian diet might be an effective alternative. Bandyopadhyay et al. [69] state that the UK NSC (National Safety Council) should consider including vitamin B12 deficiency in prenatal and neonatal screening in high-risk groups [69].

Mearns et al. [60] developed a semi-quantitative food frequency questionnaire (vitamin B12 FFQ) that is a non-invasive, easy-to-administer tool with moderate predictive ability to screen inadequate dietary vitamin B12 intake in South Asian women. Identifying women of childbearing age at low risk of vitamin B12 deficiency due to inadequate dietary intake offers the opportunity to offer dietary advice to prevent vitamin B12 deficiency or, where appropriate, to intervene with low-dose oral vitamin B12 supplements to treat early depletion or vitamin B12 deficiency. This is a significant public health announcement that can help lower the dangers to the health of mothers and their unborn children that come with a mother's lack of vitamin B12 during pregnancy and lactation. It is especially relevant to communities in South Asia.

Chouraqui et al. [67] investigated possible associations of religious dietary rules, including strict vegetarian diets, with potential nutritional consequences. The conclusion was that, when implemented according to prescribed rules, most religious dietary precepts may be classified as not harmful to health, as evidenced by their historical adherence over millennia. However, some practices can lead to nutritional inadequacies, leading to vitamin B12 deficiencies. Patients with low socioeconomic status, the child population, and women of reproductive age are at particular risk of such deficiencies.

Another important point observed was the different forms of presentation of vitamin B12 in the food supplement market. The most common forms are cyanocobalamin (cyanCbl) and methylcobalamin (methylCbl). Manufacturers advise using methylCbl, as it is a ready-to-use form of the vitamin, whereas cyanCbl needs to be activated before being used in metabolism. The lowest amounts of holotranscobalamin were seen in vegans who attempted to supplement with other foods (seaweed, kombucha, and other fermented items), consistently falling short of the necessary intake. Hence, it is recommended that vegan individuals should be instructed about vitamin B12 supplementation, the pharmaceutical forms available on the market and their actions, and choosing the ideal plan to avoid the appearance of vitamin B12 deficiency [71].

Finally, Costantino et al. [47] investigated dietary guides from different countries to establish an opinion pattern to compose a Spanish guide for the vegetarian population. This led to the conclusion that vegetarians differ in their dietary group composition and position. Every image featured stressed the need to consume grains, vegetables, fruits, legumes, soy products, and nuts daily. Even after reviewing 11 guides, it was concluded that there is no consensus regarding the needs regarding amounts and portions of vita-min B12 supplementation. Karlsen et al. [42] investigated the nutritional content of meals based on common dietary guidelines, such as the MyPlate program from the US Department of Agriculture, using the Nutrition Data System for Research (NDSR). They aimed to assess the food and nutrient levels of whole-food plant-based (WFPB) and vegan diets over a 30-day period, sourced from popular cookbooks and recipe websites. Their study also compared these findings to US dietary recommendations like dietary reference intakes (DRIs) and MyPlate meal guidelines. Using NDSR analyses, they found that WFPB diets differed significantly from MyPlate recommendations, providing a more nutrient-rich diet with lower amounts of refined grains and added sugars compared to typical American diets. However, they recommended supplementation with vitamins B12 and D [42].

3.3. Group 3—Studies on the Composition of Food Guides and Positions of Nutrition Institutions

The third category comprises publications from nutrition institutions, which encompass additional studies supplementing food guides and established stances regarding the necessity of vitamin B12 supplementation for vegetarians or vegans. These publications, including references [13,18,26,35,36,38,48], may delve into topics such as vitamin B12 deficiency among vegetarians and vegans, its causes and repercussions, factors influencing vitamin B12 absorption, and various methods of vitamin B12 supplementation. In addition, these studies could also discuss the available evidence on the use of vitamin B12 supplements in vegetarians and vegans and formulate alternatives to help nutrition and health professionals provide more accurate and scientifically supported information about the nutritional needs of vegetarians and vegans.

The EPIC-Oxford [18], the Oxford component of the European Prospective Investigation into Cancer and Nutrition (EPIC), verified the difference between omnivores, pescatarians, ovolactovegetarians, and restricted vegans, and it was observed that the last group has the lowest levels of vitamin B12, of which only 20.8% make use of vitamin B12 supplements, either on its own (exclusive supplements with the vitamin) or as a multivitamin, which do not contain sufficient amounts for adequate vitamin supplementation.

The Biomarkers of Nutrition for Development (BOND) Project study by Allen et al. [36] investigated the vitamin B12 state of the art. It was found that enough of the vitamin can be obtained through fortified foods such as breakfast cereals. Therefore, the Vegan Society in the UK recommends the consumption of various fortified foods in different meals of the day. Nutritional yeasts should not be considered fortified because they do not present sufficient amounts for supplementation [9]. In addition, infants of vegan mothers are at greater risk of developing vitamin deficiency, and only 50% of them take supplementation. With these facts, the Institute of Medicine (IOM) of the United States concluded that babies of vegan mothers should be supplemented with adequate intake (AI) of vitamin B12 starting at birth because their reserves will be low, as will the concentrations of vitamin B12 in breast milk. Within this context, another study by Rudloff et al. [38] carried out specifically in vegan children and adolescents indicated that this type of diet, when prolonged, can lead to vitamin deficiency. The type of vitamins added to fortified products should also be characterized, since the most recommended form is cyanocobalamin, which is more stable in this type of food [9].

In conclusion, vitamin B12 plays a crucial role in maintaining the normal functioning of the brain and nervous system, as well as in the formation of blood cells. The authors observed that insufficient intake of these nutrients among vegans can result in health issues such as fatigue, anemia, depression, and cognitive impairment. In addition, it is important to regularly monitor the serum amounts of vitamin B12 in the vegan population, and responsible professionals should always recommend supplementation when vitamin amounts are not reached with fortified foods alone [13,48].

4. Discussion

The data presented allow us to conclude that there are no long-term prospective studies evaluating the effect of a vegan diet on vitamin B12 status. To explore the evidence regarding the rise in veganism and its association with vitamin B12 deficiency across different demographics, we identified 70 studies. These included narrative reviews (24, 34.3%), cross-sectional analytical studies (25, 35.7%), institutional positions on vegetarian diets (4, 5.7%), systematic reviews (3, 4.3%), systematic reviews and meta-analyses (2, 2.9%), randomized controlled trials (2, 2.9%), cohort studies (2, 2.9%), case studies (5, 7.1%), practice guidelines (1, 1.4%), a randomized trial (1, 1.4%), and a randomized clinical trial (1, 1.4%).

These studies assessed interventions involving food supplementation, with consistently positive outcomes. Primarily, due to vitamin B12 being sourced from animal products, its deficiency is prevalent among vegans who do not consume animal products or who consume insufficient amounts of fortified foods containing the vitamin. For the general population, vitamin B12 is well recognized as an essential nutrient that plays a crucial role in DNA formation, the production of red blood cells, and the proper functioning of the nervous system. The EFSA Panel on Dietetic Products and Allergies [11] has established a cause-and-effect relationship between dietary vitamin B12 intake and several health benefits. These include the regulation of homocysteine metabolism, the promotion of normal neurological and psychological functions, and a reduction in fatigue and tiredness. Also recognized is the claim that it "supports folic acid metabolism, in succession: DNA synthesis" for the general population in terms of cell division. The consolidated list of health claims according to Article 13 of Regulation (EC) No. 1924/2006 [82] submitted by Member States contains other additional entry claims with corresponding conditions of use as follows:

- Vitamin B12 contributes to normal energy-yielding metabolism;
- Vitamin B12 contributes to the normal functioning of the nervous system;
- Vitamin B12 contributes to normal homocysteine metabolism;
- Vitamin B12 contributes to normal psychological function;
- Vitamin B12 contributes to normal red blood cell formation;
- Vitamin B12 contributes to the normal function of the immune system;
- Vitamin B12 contributes to a reduction in tiredness and fatigue;
- Vitamin B12 has a role in the process of cell division.

The Institute of Medicine (IoM) [83] and the EFSA Panel on Dietetic Products and Allergies [11] offer recommendations for vitamin B12 intake in healthy adults. The IoM suggests a daily intake of 2.4 micrograms of vitamin B12 for adults, while the EFSA recommends a daily intake of 4 micrograms for the same demographic. Regarding children, the IoM provides varying daily intake recommendations: 0.9 micrograms for ages 1 to 3 years, 1.2 micrograms for ages 4 to 8 years, and 1.8 micrograms for ages 9 to 13 years. Meanwhile, the EFSA advises daily intake ranges of 0.5 to 1.5 micrograms for ages 1 to 3 years, 1.0 to 2.0 micrograms for ages 4 to 8 years, and 2.0 to 4.0 micrograms for ages 9 to 13 years. Regarding pregnancy and lactation, the IoM recommends 2.6 micrograms of vitamin B12 daily for pregnant women and 2.8 micrograms for lactating women. In contrast, the EFSA suggests a higher daily intake of 4.5 micrograms for pregnant and breastfeeding women. It is relevant that daily intake recommendations may vary according to gender, age, physiological status, and other factors associated with individual health conditions. It is always recommended to consult a healthcare professional before starting any vitamin B12 supplementation or making dietary changes.

Regularly monitoring blood levels is a crucial preventive step that everyone should undertake. This allows healthcare providers to assess whether supplementation or dosage adjustments are necessary. Common recommendations for preventive vitamin B12 supplementation in adults include taking a daily single dose of 50–100 µg [13,21], three daily doses of 2 µg [13], or a weekly dose of 2000 µg, either as a single intake or divided into two doses of 1000 µg each, taken twice a week [21].

A clinical study compared the effectiveness of taking a daily dose of 50 µg versus taking a single weekly dose of 2000 µg in improving vitamin B12 levels in vegetarians and vegans with mild deficiency. Surprisingly, no differences were observed between the groups, indicating that, despite higher doses potentially being associated with lower absorption, supplementation appears to be equally effective when the dose and frequency are appropriate, whether as a daily dose of 50 µg or a weekly dose of 2000 µg [84]. There is no recommended upper limit for vitamin B12 intake because it is a water-soluble vitamin, meaning that part of it is excreted in urine. Therefore, to date, no adverse effects associated with excessive supplement intake have been reported in healthy individuals [11].

Data on the cobalamin dose required to maintain normal hematological status and serum cobalamin levels in vegetarians have shown that daily losses of ca. 0.2% of body stores are possible irrespective of the size of the body pool. Those with pernicious anemia in remission are expected to have depleted stores and thus lower absolute daily losses than healthy individuals. Thus, an intake of 1.5–2 µg/day may be considered to represent a minimum requirement for the maintenance of normal hematological status, linked with low body stores of 1 to 2 mg. Higher body stores (2–3 mg) are currently observed in healthy individuals, whose maintenance would require higher concentrations of intake [11].

Also important is that there are inherited causes of deficiency (Imerslund–Gräsbeck syndrome) or acquired defects such as pernicious anemia because of problems of malabsorption or due to the impairment of transport of vitamin B12 within the body. Insufficient dietary intake is rare in adults living in developed countries but is more often reported in vegans [73]. Within this context, Bärebring et al. highlighted that no conclusions can be drawn on whether habitual B12 intake or an intake in line with guidelines is enough to prevent a deficiency status in vegetarians and vegans because of an absence of published prospective cohort studies relating to B12 intake to status among vegetarians and vegans [85].

Key concepts/definitions are well clarified in the literature: There are two known reactions in humans that need vitamin B12 as a coenzyme. One is the conversion of succinyl-CoA from methylmalonyl-coenzyme A (CoA) by methylmalonyl CoA mutase in mitochondria during propionate metabolism. The other is homocysteine cytosolic trans-methylation by 5-methyl-tetrahydrofolate (5-methyl-THF) to methionine synthase-produced methionine [86,87]. Vitamin B12 and folate interact in the latter reaction. Insufficient levels of both vitamins hinder the synthesis of methionine and its derivative S-adenosyl-methionine (SAM), leading to significant disruptions in normal cellular function. Methionine, an essential amino acid, relies heavily on recycling through the remethylation pathway for its various metabolic functions. SAM is the universal methyl donor in over 100 transmethylation reactions involving neurotransmitter nucleotide, amino acid, and phospholipid metabolism, as well as detoxification reactions. Tetrahydrofolate (THF), the fully reduced form of folate, is another product of the methionine synthase reaction [88]. Case studies on infants from mothers with undetected pernicious anemia or adhering to strict veganism indicate that clinical symptoms of deficiency may appear in infants at around four to seven months of age [89].

When examining how research has been conducted on this topic, we recall the EFSA's recommendations [11] for researchers to pursue studies on vitamin B12 biomarkers as a function of habitual intake in adults, children, and infants, including during pregnancy and lactation, comparing vegans with other populations. Also, outcomes are still scarce for vegan populations, and further investigation is needed into the relationships between vitamin B12 intake, biomarkers, and health. Data should be gathered systematically through national programs on the bioavailability of vitamin B12 from various foods and dietary intake patterns about age and physiological states (e.g., pregnancy, lactation), namely, for vegetarians.

We have focused the aim of this review on looking for key characteristics or factors related to existing studies that evaluated interventions through food supplementation, whether the result was favorable or not, in the different target audiences, with a focus on vitamin B12 and the consequent effects of the deficiency of this essential nutrient. In this respect, the present review has identified considerable knowledge gaps.

This scoping review demonstrates several strengths. We rigorously adhered to best practices, such as prospectively registering the protocol, and followed the PRISMA statement for reporting systematic reviews and meta-analyses. Additionally, the review benefited from systematic execution by three independent reviewers and the inclusion of a diverse range of article types, facilitating comprehensive data synthesis. While robust in many aspects, this scoping review also presents several limitations. Firstly, there is a possibility of publication bias, wherein unpublished studies or those not available in the languages covered by the review might have been missed, potentially skewing the results. Secondly, despite our systematic approach, there is always a risk of selection bias, where certain studies might have been inadvertently overlooked or chosen with bias. Thirdly, the included studies exhibit heterogeneity in terms of design, methodology, and population, which could impact the synthesis of findings and the general applicability of the results. Additionally, the quality of the included studies varies, potentially influencing the reliability of our conclusions. Furthermore, some studies may lack sufficient data, limiting the depth of analysis and the certainty of the conclusions drawn. Lastly, there is a limitation regarding the time frame, as the review might not capture the most recent evidence due to constraints on literature search cutoff dates.

Future research endeavors should aim to fill these knowledge gaps, thereby offering improved guidance. The management of vitamin B12 deficiency in vegans is imperative, necessitating educational efforts, a general heightened awareness, and regular monitoring. Additionally, careful consideration of potential risks linked to excessive vitamin B12 supplementation is crucial in further studies. Furthermore, there is a pressing need for enhanced public education regarding the significance of vitamin B12 in vegan diets. This could entail the implementation of campaigns and outreach initiatives aimed at advocating for a balanced vegan diet that fulfills all nutritional needs.

5. Conclusions

This scoping review sheds light on the relationship between veganism and vitamin B12 deficiency. It aimed to find out how dietary supplementation affects different groups regarding vitamin B12 deficiency. The findings reveal that vitamin B12 deficiency is common among vegans due to their limited intake of animal products. The review identified 70 relevant studies, including various types such as reviews, trials, and guidelines. There are commercially available sources of vitamin B12 for vegans, such as fortified cereals, plant-based drinks, and nutritional yeast. Supplementation has been shown to effectively prevent and treat vitamin B12 deficiency in vegetarians, with daily doses ranging from 50 to 100 micrograms being sufficient. It is noteworthy that data on the dose of cobalamin required to maintain normal hematological status and serum cobalamin concentrations in vegetarian populations or individuals with low cobalamin intake have also been considered by some specialized bodies, but systematic data collection is lacking regarding cobalamin, with few references concerning the criteria (endpoints) on which dietary reference values are based, namely, indicators of the need for cobalamin to maintain a balanced hematological status. Healthcare professionals must educate vegan patients on monitoring and supplementing their vitamin B12 levels to prevent developmental delays. However, there are gaps in the research, such as the lack of randomized trials on vitamin B12 doses and the long-term effects of vegetarianism on health.

Supplementary Materials: The following supporting information can be downloaded at: https://www.mdpi.com/article/10.3390/nu16101442/s1, Table S1: Indexers used to select publications. Used Boolean phrases.

Author Contributions: Conceptualization, S.F., A.P., M.d.C.C. and B.M.; methodology, S.F., A.P., M.d.C.C. and B.M.; validation, M.d.C.C. and A.R.; formal analysis, S.F., A.P., M.d.C.C. and B.M.; investigation, S.F., A.P., M.d.C.C. and B.M.; data curation, S.F., A.P., M.d.C.C. and B.M.; writing—original draft preparation, S.F.; writing—review and editing, S.F., A.P., M.d.C.C., L.O., A.R., A.S. and B.M.; visualization, M.d.C.C. and A.R.; project administration, M.d.C.C. and A.R.; funding acquisition, A.R. and A.S. All authors have read and agreed to the published version of the manuscript.

Funding: This research was funded by national funds through the FCT—Foundation for Science and Technology, I.P. (Portugal), under the projects DOI 10.54499/UIDB/04567/2020 and DOI 10.54499/UIDP/04567/2020.

Conflicts of Interest: The authors declare no conflict of interest.

References

1. Smart Protein Project. Plant-Based Foods in Europe: How Big Is the Market? 2020. Available online: https://www.novozymes.com/en/plant-based-foods?utm_source=google&utm_medium=cpc&utm_campaign=pl_gl_plantbasedfoods&utm_content=ge_defensivesem&gad_source=1&gclid=Cj0KCQjwk6SwBhDPARIsAJ59GwdubsQZMl_axfKEh3p61O-PWsSZBrdIR_L-XymlZEADmJxfAy2mw44aApcXEALw_wcB (accessed on 31 March 2024).
2. Chen, C.; Chaudhary, A.; Mathys, A. Dietary Change Scenarios and Implications for Environmental, Nutrition, Human Health and Economic Dimensions of Food Sustainability. *Nutrients* **2019**, *11*, 856. [CrossRef]
3. Bali, A.; Naik, R. The Impact of a Vegan Diet on Many Aspects of Health: The Overlooked Side of Veganism. *Cureus* **2023**, *15*, e35148. [CrossRef] [PubMed]

4. Alnasser, A.; Alomran, N. The motivations and practices of vegetarian and vegan Saudis. *Sci. Rep.* **2023**, *13*, 9742. [CrossRef] [PubMed]
5. Miki, A.J.; Livingston, K.A.; Karlsen, M.C.; Folta, S.C.; McKeown, N.M. Using Evidence Mapping to Examine Motivations for Following Plant-Based Diets. *Curr. Dev. Nutr.* **2020**, *4*, nzaa013. [CrossRef] [PubMed]
6. Łuszczki, E.; Boakye, F.; Zielińska, M.; Dereń, K.; Bartosiewicz, A.; Oleksy, Ł.; Stolarczyk, A. Vegan diet: Nutritional components, implementation, and effects on adults' health. *Front. Nutr.* **2023**, *10*, 1294497. [CrossRef] [PubMed]
7. Tomova, A.; Bukovsky, I.; Rembert, E.; Yonas, W.; Alwarith, J.; Barnard, N.D.; Kahleova, H. The Effects of Vegetarian and Vegan Diets on Gut Microbiota. *Front. Nutr.* **2019**, *6*, 47. [CrossRef]
8. Fontes, T.; Rodrigues, L.M.; Ferreira-Pêgo, C. Comparison between Different Groups of Vegetarianism and Its Associations with Body Composition: A Literature Review from 2015 to 2021. *Nutrients* **2022**, *14*, 1853. [CrossRef] [PubMed]
9. Melina, V.; Craig, W.; Levin, S. Position of the Academy of Nutrition and Dietetics: Vegetarian Diets. *J. Acad. Nutr. Diet.* **2016**, *116*, 1970–1980. [CrossRef]
10. Pilis, W.; Stec, K.; Zych, M.; Pilis, A. Health benefits and risk associated with adopting a vegetarian diet. *Rocz. Panstw. Zakl. Hig.* **2014**, *65*, 9–14.
11. EFSA Panel on Dietetic Products, Nutrition, and Allergies (NDA). Scientific Opinion on Dietary Reference Values for cobalamin (vitamin B12). *EFSA J.* **2015**, *13*, 4150.
12. Chandra-Hioe, M.V.; Lee, C.; Arcot, J. What is the cobalamin status among vegetarians and vegans in Australia? *Int. J. Food Sci. Nutr.* **2019**, *70*, 875–886. [CrossRef] [PubMed]
13. Agnoli, C.; Baroni, L.; Bertini, I.; Ciappellano, S.; Fabbri, A.; Papa, M.; Pellegrini, N.; Sbarbati, R.; Scarino, M.; Siani, V.; et al. Position paper on vegetarian diets from the working group of the Italian Society of Human Nutrition. *Nutr. Metab. Cardiovasc. Dis.* **2017**, *27*, 1037–1052. [CrossRef] [PubMed]
14. Schüpbach, R.; Wegmüller, R.; Berguerand, C.; Bui, M.; Herter-Aeberli, I. Micronutrient status and intake in omnivores, vegetarians and vegans in Switzerland. *Eur. J. Nutr.* **2017**, *56*, 283–293. [CrossRef] [PubMed]
15. Page, M.J.; McKenzie, J.E.; Bossuyt, P.M.; Boutron, I.; Hoffmann, T.C.; Mulrow, C.D.; Shamseer, L.; Tetzlaff, J.M.; Akl, E.A.; Brennan, S.E.; et al. The PRISMA 2020 statement: An updated guideline for reporting systematic reviews. *Syst. Rev.* **2021**, *10*, 89. [CrossRef] [PubMed]
16. Woo, K.S.; Kwok, T.C.Y.; Celermajer, D.S. Vegan diet, subnormal vitamin B-12 status and cardiovascular health. *Nutrients* **2014**, *6*, 3259–3273. [CrossRef] [PubMed]
17. Obersby, D.; Chappell, D.C.; Dunnett, A.; Tsiami, A.A. Plasma total homocysteine status of vegetarians compared with omnivores: A systematic review and meta-analysis. *Br. J. Nutr.* **2013**, *109*, 785–794. [CrossRef] [PubMed]
18. Sobiecki, J.G.; Appleby, P.N.; Bradbury, K.E.; Key, T.J. High compliance with dietary recommendations in a cohort of meat eaters, fish eaters, vegetarians, and vegans: Results from the European Prospective Investigation into Cancer and Nutrition-Oxford study. *Nutr. Res.* **2016**, *36*, 464–477. [CrossRef] [PubMed]
19. Elorinne, A.-L.; Alfthan, G.; Erlund, I.; Kivimäki, H.; Paju, A.; Salminen, I.; Turpeinen, U.; Voutilainen, S.; Laakso, J. Food and nutrient intake and nutritional status of Finnish vegans and non-vegetarians. *PLoS ONE* **2016**, *11*, e0148235. [CrossRef] [PubMed]
20. Pawlak, R.; Lester, S.E.; Babatunde, T. The prevalence of cobalamin deficiency among vegetarians assessed by serum vitamin B12, a review of literature. *Eur. J. Clin. Nutr.* **2014**, *68*, 541–548. [CrossRef]
21. Rizzo, G.; Laganà, A.S.; Rapisarda, A.M.C.; La Ferrera, G.M.G.; Buscema, M.; Rossetti, P.; Nigro, A.; Muscia, V.; Valenti, G.; Sapia, F.; et al. Vitamin B12 among vegetarians: Status, assessment and supplementation. *Nutrients* **2016**, *8*, 767. [CrossRef]
22. Simpson, J.L.; Bailey, L.B.; Pietrzik, K.; Shane, B.; Holzgreve, W. Micronutrients and women of reproductive potential: Required dietary intake and consequences of dietary deficiency or excess. Part I–Folate, Vitamin B12, Vitamin B6. *J. Matern. Fetal Neonatal Med.* **2010**, *23*, 1323–1343. [CrossRef] [PubMed]
23. Gallego-Narbón, A.; Zapatera, B.; Álvarez, I.; Vaquero, M.P. Methylmalonic acid levels and their relation with cobalamin supplementation in Spanish vegetarians. *Plant Foods Hum. Nutr.* **2018**, *73*, 166–171. [CrossRef] [PubMed]
24. Avnon, T.; Anbar, R.; Lavie, I.; Ben-Mayor Bashi, T.; Paz Dubinsky, E.; Shaham, S.; Yogev, Y. Does vegan diet influence umbilical cord vitamin B12, folate, and ferritin levels? *Arch. Gynecol. Obstet.* **2020**, *301*, 1417–1422. [CrossRef] [PubMed]
25. Pawlak, R.; Vos, P.; Shahab-Ferdows, S.; Hampel, D.; Allen, L.H.; Perrin, M.T. Vitamin B-12 content in breast milk of vegan, vegetarian, and nonvegetarian lactating women in the United States. *Am. J. Clin. Nutr.* **2018**, *108*, 525–531. [CrossRef] [PubMed]
26. Lemale, J.; Mas, E.; Jung, C.; Bellaiche, M.; Tounian, P. Vegan diet in children and adolescents. Recommendations from the French-speaking Pediatric Hepatology, Gastroenterology and Nutrition Group (GFHGNP). *Arch. Pediatr.* **2019**, *26*, 442–450. [CrossRef] [PubMed]
27. Gallego-Narbón, A.; Zapatera, B.; Barrios, L.; Vaquero, M.P. Vitamin B12 and folate status in Spanish lacto-ovo vegetarians and vegans. *J. Nutr. Sci.* **2019**, *8*, e7. [CrossRef]
28. Damayanti, D.; Jaceldo-Siegl, K.; Beeson, W.L.; Fraser, G.; Oda, K.; Haddad, E.H. Foods and supplements associated with vitamin B12 biomarkers among vegetarian and non-vegetarian participants of the Adventist Health Study-2 (AHS-2) calibration study. *Nutrients* **2018**, *10*, 722. [CrossRef] [PubMed]
29. Rogerson, D. Vegan diets: Practical advice for athletes and exercisers. *J. Int. Soc. Sports Nutr.* **2017**, *14*, 36. [CrossRef] [PubMed]
30. O'Leary, F.; Samman, S. Vitamin B_{12} in health and disease. *Nutrients* **2010**, *2*, 299–316. [CrossRef]
31. Craig, W.J. Nutrition concerns and health effects of vegetarian diets. *Nutr. Clin. Pract.* **2010**, *25*, 613–620. [CrossRef]

32. Van Winckel, M.; Vande Velde, S.; De Bruyne, R.; Van Biervliet, S. Clinical practice: Vegetarian infant and child nutrition. *Eur. J. Pediatr.* **2011**, *170*, 1489–1494. [CrossRef] [PubMed]
33. Tucker, K.L. Vegetarian diets and bone status. *Am. J. Clin. Nutr.* **2014**, *100*, 329S–335S. [CrossRef] [PubMed]
34. Radnitz, C.; Beezhold, B.; DiMatteo, J. Investigation of lifestyle choices of individuals following a vegan diet for health and ethical reasons. *Appetite* **2015**, *90*, 31–36. [CrossRef] [PubMed]
35. Cruchet, S.; Lucero, Y.; Cornejo, V. Truths, Myths and Needs of Special Diets: Attention-Deficit/Hyperactivity Disorder, Autism, Non-Celiac Gluten Sensitivity, and Vegetarianism. *Ann. Nutr. Metab.* **2016**, *68*, 42–50. [CrossRef] [PubMed]
36. Allen, L.H.; Miller, J.W.; De Groot, L.; Rosenberg, I.H.; Smith, A.D.; Refsum, H.; Raiten, D.J. Biomarkers of Nutrition for Development (BOND): Vitamin B-12 Review. *J. Nutr.* **2018**, *148*, 1995S–2027S. [CrossRef] [PubMed]
37. Brown, D.D. Nutritional Considerations for the Vegetarian and Vegan Dancer. *J. Danc. Med. Sci.* **2018**, *22*, 44–53. [CrossRef] [PubMed]
38. Rudloff, S.; Bührer, C.; Jochum, F.; Kauth, T.; Kersting, M.; Körner, A.; Koletzko, B.; Mihatsch, W.; Prell, C.; Reinehr, T.; et al. Vegetarian diets in childhood and adolescence: Statement of the Nutrition Committee of the German Society for Pediatric and Adolescent Medicine (DGKJ). *Monatsschrift Kinderheilkd.* **2018**, *166*, 999–1005. [CrossRef]
39. Menal-Puey, S.; Martínez-Biarge, M.; Marques-Lopes, I. Developing a food exchange system for meal planning in vegan children and adolescents. *Nutrients* **2019**, *11*, 43. [CrossRef]
40. Nebl, J.; Schuchardt, J.P.; Ströhle, A.; Wasserfurth, P.; Haufe, S.; Eigendorf, J.; Tegtbur, U.; Hahn, A. Micronutrient status of recreational runners with vegetarian or non-vegetarian dietary patterns. *Nutrients* **2019**, *11*, 1146. [CrossRef]
41. Sheng, X.; Wang, J.; Li, F.; Ouyang, F.; Ma, J. Effects of dietary intervention on vitamin B12 status and cognitive level of 18-monthold toddlers in high-poverty areas: A cluster-randomized controlled trial. *BMC Pediatr.* **2019**, *19*, 334. [CrossRef]
42. Karlsen, M.C.; Rogers, G.; Miki, A.; Lichtenstein, A.H.; Folta, S.C.; Economos, C.D.; Jacques, P.F.; Livingston, K.A.; McKeown, N.M. Theoretical food and nutrient composition of whole-food plant-based and vegan diets compared to current dietary recommendations. *Nutrients* **2019**, *11*, 625. [CrossRef] [PubMed]
43. Nebl, J.; Schuchardt, J.P.; Wasserfurth, P.; Haufe, S.; Eigendorf, J.; Tegtbur, U.; Hahn, A. Characterization, dietary habits and nutritional intake of omnivorous, lacto-ovo vegetarian and vegan runners—A pilot study. *BMC Nutr.* **2019**, *5*, 51. [CrossRef] [PubMed]
44. García-Maldonado, E.; Gallego-Narbón, A.; Vaquero, M.P. Are vegetarian diets nutritionally adequate? A revision of the scientific evidence. *Nutr. Hosp.* **2019**, *36*, 950–961. [PubMed]
45. Karcz, K.; Królak-Olejnik, B. Vegan or vegetarian diet and breast milk composition—A systematic review. *Crit. Rev. Food Sci. Nutr.* **2021**, *61*, 1081–1098. [CrossRef] [PubMed]
46. Jungert, A.; Lötscher, K.Q.; Rohrmann, S. Vitamin substitution beyond childhood: Requirements and risks. *Dtsch. Arztebl. Int.* **2020**, *117*, 14–22. [PubMed]
47. Costantino, C.; Morante, L. Vegetarian dietary guidelines: A comparative dietetic and communicational analysis of eleven international pictorial representations. *Rev. Española Nutr. Humana Dietética* **2020**, *24*, 120–132. [CrossRef]
48. Redecilla Ferreiro, S.; Moráis López, A.; Moreno Villares, J.M.; en Representación del Comité de Nutrición y Lactancia Materna de la AEP. Position paper on vegetarian diets in infants and children. Committee on Nutrition and Breastfeeding of the Spanish Paediatric Association. *An. Pediatr.* **2020**, *92*, 306.e1–306.e6. [CrossRef]
49. Yang, Y.; Zhang, S.; Zhang, X.; Xu, Y.; Cheng, J.; Yang, X. The Role of Diet, Eating Behavior, and Nutrition Intervention in Seasonal Affective Disorder: A Systematic Review. *Front. Psychol.* **2020**, *11*, 1451. [CrossRef] [PubMed]
50. Kalyan, G.B.; Mittal, M.; Jain, R. Compromised Vitamin B12 Status of Indian Infants and Toddlers. *Food Nutr. Bull.* **2020**, *41*, 430–437. [CrossRef]
51. Kwok, T.; Chook, P.; Qiao, M.; Tam, L.; Poon, Y.K.P.; Ahuja, A.T.; Woo, J.; Celermajer, D.S.; Woo, K.S. Vitamin B-12 supplementation improves arterial function in vegetarians with subnormal vitamin B-12 status. *J. Nutr. Health Aging* **2012**, *16*, 569–573. [CrossRef]
52. Naik, S.; Mahalle, N.; Bhide, V. Identification of Vitamin B 12 deficiency in vegetarian Indians. *Br. J. Nutr.* **2018**, *119*, 629–635. [CrossRef] [PubMed]
53. Selinger, E.; Kühn, T.; Procházková, M.; Anděl, M.; Gojda, J. Vitamin B12 deficiency is prevalent among Czech vegans who do not use vitamin B12 supplements. *Nutrients* **2019**, *11*, 3019. [CrossRef] [PubMed]
54. Cofnas, N. Is vegetarianism healthy for children? *Crit. Rev. Food Sci. Nutr.* **2019**, *59*, 2052–2060. [CrossRef] [PubMed]
55. Constantin, E.-T.; Cretu, A.; Apostu, M.; El Bsat, R.; Predescu, C. Vegetarian diet in aerobic sports. Particularities, necessities and recommendations. *Discobolul Phys. Educ. Sport Kinetotherapy J.* **2019**, *57*, 63–70.
56. Dubaj, C.; Czyż, K.; Furmaga-Jabłońska, W. Vitamin B12 deficiency as a cause of severe neurological symptoms in breast fed infant—A case report. *Ital. J. Pediatr.* **2020**, *46*, 1–6. [CrossRef] [PubMed]
57. Subramani, P.; Saranya, C.G.; Chand, G.M.; Narayani, R.S.; James, S.; Vinoth, P.N. Neuroregression in an infant: A rare cause. *S. Afr. J. Child Health* **2015**, *9*, 59–60.
58. Gammon, C.S.; von Hurst, P.R.; Coad, J.; Kruger, R.; Stonehouse, W. Vegetarianism, vitamin B12 status, and insulin resistance in a group of predominantly overweight/obese South Asian women. *Nutrition* **2012**, *28*, 20–24. [CrossRef] [PubMed]
59. Ali, A.B.; Pessoa, B.; Oliveira, M.; Kashiwbara, T. Introdução alimentar em crianças vegetarianas—Revisão de literatura. *Food Release Veg. Child.* **2014**, *20*, 82–87.

60. Mearns, G.J.; Rush, E.C. Screening for inadequate dietary vitamin B-12 intake in South Asian women using a nutrient-specific, semi-quantitative food frequency questionnaire. *Asia Pac. J. Clin. Nutr.* **2017**, *26*, 1119–1124.
61. Siqueira, É.P.; Martins, J.A.; Silva, M.A.; Marques, P.F.; Rodrigues, D. Avaliação da oferta nutricional de dietas vegetarianas do tipo vegana. *Nutr. Eval. Offer. Veg. Diets Type Vegan* **2016**, *33*, 44–64.
62. Mavrommati, K.; Sentissi, O. Delirium as a result of vitamin B12 deficiency in a vegetarian female patient. *Eur. J. Clin. Nutr.* **2013**, *67*, 996–997. [CrossRef]
63. Hovdenak, N.; Haram, K. Influence of mineral and vitamin supplements on pregnancy outcome. *Eur. J. Obstet. Gynecol. Reprod. Biol.* **2012**, *164*, 127–132. [CrossRef]
64. Sechi, G.; Sechi, E.; Fois, C.; Kumar, N. Advances in clinical determinants and neurological manifestations of B vitamin deficiency in adults. *Nutr. Rev.* **2016**, *74*, 281–300. [CrossRef]
65. Benham, A.J.; Gallegos, D.; Hanna, K.L.; Hannan-Jones, M.T. Intake of vitamin B-12 and other characteristics of women of reproductive age on a vegan diet in Australia. *Public Health Nutr.* **2021**, *24*, 4397–4407. [CrossRef]
66. Sutter, D.O.; Bender, N. Nutrient status and growth in vegan children. *Nutr. Res.* **2021**, *91*, 13–25. [CrossRef]
67. Chouraqui, J.-P.; Turck, D.; Briend, A.; Darmaun, D.; Bocquet, A.; Feillet, F.; Frelut, M.-L.; Girardet, J.-P.; Guimber, D.; Hankard, R.; et al. Religious dietary rules and their potential nutritional and health consequences. *Int. J. Epidemiol.* **2021**, *50*, 12–26. [CrossRef]
68. Rashid, S.; Meier, V.; Patrick, H. Review of Vitamin B12 deficiency in pregnancy: A diagnosis not to miss as veganism and vegetarianism become more prevalent. *Eur. J. Haematol.* **2021**, *106*, 450–455. [CrossRef]
69. Bandyopadhyay, D.; Choudhury, J.; Mukherjee, K. Vitamin B12 Deficiency in Eastern India: A Hospital Based Cross-sectional Study. *J. Clin. Diagn. Res.* **2021**, *15*, 1–4. [CrossRef]
70. Schwinger, C.; Sharma, S.; Chandyo, R.K.; Hysing, M.; Kvestad, I.; Ulak, M.; Ranjitkar, S.; Shrestha, M.; Shrestha, L.P.; McCann, A.; et al. Cobalamin and folate status in women during early pregnancy in Bhaktapur, Nepal. *J. Nutr. Sci.* **2021**, *10*, 1–9. [CrossRef]
71. Zugravu, C.-A.; Macri, A.; Belc, N.; Bohiltea, R. Efficacy of supplementation with methylcobalamin and cyancobalamin in maintaining the level of serum holotranscobalamin in a group of plant-based diet (vegan) adults. *Exp. Ther. Med.* **2021**, *22*, 993. [CrossRef]
72. Guez, S.; Chiarelli, G.; Menni, F.; Salera, S.; Principi, N.; Esposito, S. Severe vitamin B12 deficiency in an exclusively breastfed 5-month-old Italian infant born to a mother receiving multivitamin supplementation during pregnancy. *BMC Pediatr.* **2012**, *12*, 85. [CrossRef]
73. Pawlak, R. Is vitamin B12 deficiency a risk factor for cardiovascular disease in vegetarians? *Am. J. Prev. Med.* **2015**, *48*, e11–e26. [CrossRef]
74. Pawlak, R. To vegan or not to vegan when pregnant, lactating or feeding young children. *Eur. J. Clin. Nutr.* **2017**, *71*, 1259–1262. [CrossRef]
75. Bachmeyer, C.; Bourguiba, R.; Gkalea, V.; Papageorgiou, L. Vegan diet as a neglected cause of severe megaloblastic anemia and psychosis. *Am. J. Med.* **2019**, *132*, e850–e851. [CrossRef]
76. Mądry, E.; Lisowska, A.; Grebowiec, P.; Walkowiak, J. The impact of vegan diet on B-12 status in healthy omnivores: Five-year prospective study. *Acta Sci. Pol. Technol. Aliment.* **2012**, *11*, 209–212.
77. Benham, A.J.; Gallegos, D.; Hanna, K.L.; Hannan-Jones, M.T. Vitamin B12 supplementation adequacy in Australian Vegan Study participants. *Nutrients* **2022**, *14*, 4781. [CrossRef]
78. Světnička, M.; Sigal, A.; Selinger, E.; Heniková, M.; El-Lababidi, E.; Gojda, J. Cross-sectional study of the prevalence of cobalamin deficiency and vitamin B12 supplementation habits among vegetarian and vegan children in the Czech Republic. *Nutrients* **2022**, *14*, 535. [CrossRef]
79. Storz, M.A.; Müller, A.; Niederreiter, L.; Zimmermann-Klemd, A.M.; Suarez-Alvarez, M.; Kowarschik, S.; Strittmatter, M.; Schlachter, E.; Pasluosta, C.; Huber, R.; et al. A cross-sectional study of nutritional status in healthy, young, physically-active German omnivores, vegetarians and vegans reveals adequate vitamin B12 status in supplemented vegans. *Ann. Med.* **2023**, *55*, 2269969. [CrossRef]
80. Latal, R.; Habanova, M.; Selinger, E.; Bihari, M.; Hamulka, J. Cross sectional study of vitamin B12 supplementation in Slovak and Czech vegans. *Rocz. Panstw. Zakl. Hig.* **2023**, *74*, 195–205. [PubMed]
81. Fuschlberger, M.; Putz, P. Vitamin B12 supplementation and health behavior of Austrian vegans: A cross-sectional online survey. *Sci. Rep.* **2023**, *13*, 3983. [CrossRef] [PubMed]
82. European Commission. Commission Regulation (EU) No 432/2012 of 16 May 2012 establishing a list of permitted health claims made on foods, other than those referring to the reduction of disease risk and to children's development and health. *Off. J. Eur. Union* **2012**, L 136/1. Available online: https://eur-lex.europa.eu/LexUriServ/LexUriServ.do?uri=OJ:L:2012:136:0001:0040:en:PDF (accessed on 1 April 2024).
83. Institute of Medicine FaNB. *Dietary Reference Intakes for Thiamin, Riboflavin, Niacin, Vitamin B(6), Folate, Vitamin B(12), Pantothenic Acid, Biotin, and Choline*; National Academies Press: Washington, DC, USA, 1998.
84. Del Bo', C.; Riso, P.; Gardana, C.; Brusamolino, A.; Battezzati, A.; Ciappellano, S. Effect of two different sublingual dosages of vitamin B12 on cobalamin nutritional status in vegans and vegetarians with a marginal deficiency: A randomized controlled trial. *Clin. Nutr.* **2019**, *38*, 575–583. [CrossRef]

85. Bärebring, L.; Lamberg-Allardt, C.; Thorisdottir, B.; Ramel, A.; Söderlund, F.; Arnesen, E.K.; Nwaru, B.I.; Dierkes, J.; Åkesson, A. Intake of vitamin B12 in relation to vitamin B12 status in groups susceptible to deficiency: A systematic review. *Food Nutr. Res.* **2023**, *67*, 1–15. [CrossRef]
86. Ludwig, M.L.; Matthews, R.G. Structure-based perspectives on B12-dependent enzymes. *Annu. Rev. Biochem.* **1997**, *66*, 269–313. [CrossRef]
87. Matthews, R.G.; Sheppard, C.; Goulding, C. Methylenetetrahydrofolate reductase and methionine synthase: Biochemistry and molecular biology. *Eur. J. Pediatr.* **1998**, *157*, S54–S59. [CrossRef]
88. Scott, J.M. Folate and vitamin B12. *Proc. Nutr. Soc.* **1999**, *58*, 441–448. [CrossRef]
89. Dror, D.K.; Allen, L.H. Effect of vitamin B12 deficiency on neurodevelopment in infants: Current knowledge and possible mechanisms. *Nutr. Rev.* **2008**, *66*, 250–255. [CrossRef]

Disclaimer/Publisher's Note: The statements, opinions and data contained in all publications are solely those of the individual author(s) and contributor(s) and not of MDPI and/or the editor(s). MDPI and/or the editor(s) disclaim responsibility for any injury to people or property resulting from any ideas, methods, instructions or products referred to in the content.

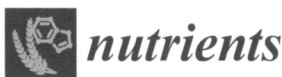

Article

Understanding Health-Related Motivations for Urban Food Self-Production in the Light of Semantic Fields Analysis

Ewa Duda

Institute of Education, Maria Grzegorzewska University, 02-353 Warsaw, Poland; eduda@aps.edu.pl

Abstract: One of the contemporary challenges facing urban areas is the necessity to identify novel approaches to resident involvement in solution creation, with a particular focus on ensuring the best possible nutrition. By investigating the process of co-participation of city dwellers in a unique education project, this paper aims to gain a deeper understanding of the health-related motivations that underpin the decision of early adopters of the implemented technological innovations to join the social experiment. The qualitative study employed purposive sampling and in-depth interviews conducted in two waves, the first between October and November 2022 and the second between September 2023 and January 2024. The study comprised 42 participants drawn from two communities of residents in Łódź and Warsaw, Poland. Transcriptions of the interviews were carried out using semantic field analysis, employing a quantitative approach that counts the frequency of keyword occurrences. Three categories of semantic fields were identified: associations, oppositions, and actions toward the subject, including positive, neutral, and negative temperatures. The findings demonstrate that the health concerns of residents are a pivotal factor in their decision to participate in urban food self-production initiatives, given their limited access to nutritious and healthy vegetables. This is related to several factors, including restrictions related to urbanization and the displacement of local suppliers, lifestyle, and the fast pace of urban life. The dissemination of innovative solutions for growing food in urban environments could, therefore, facilitate awareness-raising and motivation to alter the dietary habits of inhabitants.

Keywords: environmental literacy; food-growing intention; green transformation; health education; healthy foods; public health and nutrition; pro-environmental behaviors; technology-enhanced education; urban gardening; Urban Living Lab

Citation: Duda, E. Understanding Health-Related Motivations for Urban Food Self-Production in the Light of Semantic Fields Analysis. *Nutrients* **2024**, *16*, 1533. https://doi.org/10.3390/nu16101533

Academic Editors: Ariana Saraiva and António Raposo

Received: 21 April 2024
Revised: 13 May 2024
Accepted: 14 May 2024
Published: 20 May 2024

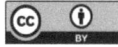

Copyright: © 2024 by the author. Licensee MDPI, Basel, Switzerland. This article is an open access article distributed under the terms and conditions of the Creative Commons Attribution (CC BY) license (https://creativecommons.org/licenses/by/4.0/).

1. Introduction

The topic of urban development has recently gained renewed attention, particularly in the context of creating green, competitive, and inclusive living spaces, as well as providing quality food [1]. That is particularly relevant given the increasing prevalence of actions that contradict the concept, such as the removal of green spaces to facilitate the construction of additional buildings or the creation of areas that, due to the predominance of concrete, appear to be more easily maintained. The increasingly common elimination of greenery from urban spaces, including fruit orchards and vegetable gardens, not only results in limited access to nature but also has wider implications for the environment. There is a lack of such green spaces that could effectively promote a positive attitude towards gardening and serve as venues for organizing educational interventions promoting food security, diverse and balanced nutrition, and health, while simultaneously maximizing the health benefits associated with plant cultivation in urban spaces [2].

This study forms part of a larger project that is investigating novel approaches to engaging urban residents in the development of solutions that optimize their access to nutritious foods while addressing the challenges posed by climate change. The intention of the paper is to contribute to the ongoing academic discussion on fostering green urban development by elucidating the health-related motivations that underpin the decision of early adopters of the implemented technological innovations to join the social experiment. The qualitative research conducted among the participants of the presented project aimed to ascertain how they determine health issues, their nutrient supply needs, and their motivations, attitudes, intentions and expectations towards the educational intervention tools created. The findings of the study can inform the design and development of innovative educational tools that promote pro-environmental behavior and foster the development of environmental literacy [3]. This can bring multiple benefits to society and contribute to the creation of more sustainable future cities.

This article comprehensively analyzes the statements of participants in a unique educational experiment, drawing insights from interdisciplinary research, the results of which are presented in subsequent sections of the article. The "Current Study" section introduces theoretical aspects related to the article's topic, introducing the reader to the subject of urban gardening, its connections to health issues, food security, and the introduction of innovative educational tools for the development of urban gardening. The "Materials and Methods" section defines the overarching goals and theoretical frameworks underlying this study, outlining its assumptions and course. The "Results" section delves into a meticulous analysis of the participants' statements, emphasizing health issues that emerged during responses to questions about participants' previous gardening experiences and their expectations for upcoming activities. The following section elaborates on the research findings in relation to the achievements of other authors and presents practical implications and recommendations for the project implementation team, as well as other researchers and practitioners interested in the research topic. The final section briefly summarizes the study, delineates its main contribution to the development of the discipline, presents the study's limitations, and outlines plans for further research.

2. Current Study

Urban gardening, often associated with aesthetics and relaxation [4,5], has become a significant aspect of public health with rapid urbanization and population growth [6]. The development of urban gardening can significantly contribute to improving the quality of life for residents, supporting efforts to enhance societal well-being, including health [7]. Improving air quality, promoting physical activity, and ensuring access to healthy food are key aspects that can be incorporated into the development of urban green spaces.

Urban gardening promotes physical activity and a healthy lifestyle [8]. Cultivating vegetables, fruits, and herbs in urban allotment gardens or on balconies encourages greater activity, including outdoor activities. Regular gardening can improve physical fitness and stamina, and reduce stress, contributing to overall physical and mental health improvement [9]. Community urban gardens, squares, or parks with edible gardens provide residents with access to fresh and healthy agricultural products [10]. Consuming fresh fruits and vegetables from one's cultivation can contribute to maintaining a balanced diet rich in vitamins, minerals, and antioxidants, thereby improving overall health and immunity [11].

However, despite these benefits, there are also health challenges associated with urban gardening. One of the main issues is soil contamination. Cities often have chemical pollutants, such as heavy metals and pesticides, which can accumulate in the soil and be transferred to cultivated plants. Consuming such products can pose a health risk to people [12]. Another challenge is the presence of pests and plant diseases. In urban conditions, where gardens are usually densely packed, there is a greater risk of problems related to pests and plant diseases. The use of pesticides to control these pests can have negative effects on human health and the environment [13]. There is also a risk associated with the quality of water used for watering plants. In some urban areas, water quality may be low due to chemical and biological pollutants. Using such water for watering plants can lead to the contamination of agricultural products and pose a health risk [14].

In response to these challenges, efforts are being made to introduce innovative solutions that would mitigate the negative impact of urban gardening on human health. One of them is hydroponic food cultivation [15]. One of the major advantages of hydroponics is its efficiency in resource utilization. This may be a significant factor in encouraging urban dwellers to utilize hydroponic techniques for the cultivation of food. In traditional agriculture, a large amount of water is lost through evaporation and absorption by the soil, whereas in hydroponics, water is directly supplied to the plant roots. This process allows for water conservation, which is essential not only in the context of human health but also in the context of climate change and global water resource shortages [16].

Secondly, the pursuit of food self-sufficiency can serve as a motivating factor for the utilization of hydroponic cultivation [17]. In urban areas where access to fresh produce may be limited, the ability to cultivate vegetables or herbs in one's own home or on a balcony can be a highly appealing proposition. The implementation of hydroponics allows for the efficient management of space and resources, which is of particular importance in urban environments where land availability is limited. Future users may be encouraged by the fact that plants in hydroponics can be grown in a variety of locations, including indoors, on rooftops, in vacant lots, or even in desert areas where soil conditions are unfavorable. This gives the opportunity to produce food locally, reducing the need for long-distance transportation and the associated greenhouse gas emissions.

An additional rationale for utilizing alternative methods of cultivating food in urban environments is the ability to exert control over the environmental conditions that influence plant growth. Technological advances, including the development of advanced hydroponic systems, also influence the motivation to use this form of cultivation. The advent of modern technology has enabled the automation of the agricultural growing process, rendering it more accessible and easier to manage even for individuals lacking prior farming experience. In hydroponics, pH level, nutrient solution composition, temperature, and humidity can be precisely controlled, allowing for optimal growth conditions for different plant species. This, in turn, leads to faster growth and better crop quality. The products in question are typically greener, free of harmful chemicals and pesticides, and therefore safer for human health, more palatable, and nutritionally superior [18].

However, hydroponics is not without drawbacks, negatively influencing the decision to use it. One of the main issues with this system is the initial investment cost. Building and maintaining a hydroponic system can be more expensive than traditional soil cultivation, especially initially. The hydroponic installation constituted a research contribution, funded by a grant, which enabled the realization of this unique project. Consequently, an analysis of the cost-effectiveness of hydroponic solutions in the city was not carried out as part of the project. However, it is worth noting that these issues are important when implementing innovative solutions requiring a significant financial contribution. Another challenge is maintaining balance in the nutrient solution. The regular monitoring and adjustment of pH level and nutrient solution composition are necessary to provide plants with adequate nutrition. Improper balancing can lead to nutrient deficiencies or excesses, which in turn can negatively affect plant growth [19].

Despite the aforementioned limitations, the implementation of urban farming through hydroponic installations can provide a response to the challenges faced by contemporary cities in ensuring healthy and sustainable food for increasingly diverse and growing urban populations. Urban hydroponic farming represents an innovative strategy that not only promotes local food production but also alters the way residents make decisions regarding their diet and healthy lifestyle. It is therefore important to consider whether residents are inclined to adopt this strategy.

One of the key motivational factors could be the growing health awareness among urban residents. There is a growing recognition that a healthy diet based on fresh, local products can contribute to overall health improvements, reduce chronic disease risks such as obesity, diabetes and heart diseases, or support preventive actions. Previous studies on traditional farming have demonstrated that urban food cultivation in community gardens, school gardens, and backyard gardens provides residents with direct access to fresh vegetables, fruits, and herbs, which can encourage them to make healthier dietary choices [20].

The pursuit of food self-sufficiency can be a significant motivating factor for engaging in traditional urban food cultivation. The capacity to cultivate one's own vegetables or fruits engenders a sense of autonomy and gratification. Individuals value the ability to control the quality of their food and to avoid the use of artificial pesticides or herbicides, which are often employed in commercial agriculture. Fresh, locally grown products are richer in nutrients and vitamins than those available in supermarkets, which are often subjected to lengthy storage and transportation processes. Consuming fresh fruits and vegetables from one's own garden is beneficial to one's health, which in turn affects the overall physical and mental well-being of residents [21].

In the case of traditional gardens, urban food cultivation can become a means of spending active time outdoors for a significant proportion of the population. The act of working in a garden provides a multitude of benefits, including physical exercise, relaxation, and a means of disconnecting from the urban environment. The combination of physical activity and food production serves as a motivating factor for individuals to engage in regular care of their garden or plot, as well as their health [22].

Building a local community is also identified as a motivation that attracts individuals to engage in food production within urban areas. The health benefits associated with the consumption of collectively cultivated products contribute to the overall improvement of residents' health and facilitate the modification of their dietary habits. Urban food cultivation is therefore not only a means of attaining a healthier lifestyle but also fosters the development of a health-oriented local community. Those who engage in this activity frequently establish connections with their neighbors and other enthusiasts of a healthy lifestyle. Community gatherings in community gardens or local farmers' markets facilitate social integration and the exchange of experiences [23].

The main goal of the presented study is therefore to gain a deeper understanding of the health-related motivations that influenced the decision of early adopters of technological innovations oriented towards self-food production. The research will aim to examine how they perceive health issues and their nutritional needs, and through them motivations, attitudes, intentions, and expectations related to the educational intervention tools being created. The intention of the study is therefore to deepen the understanding of whether the health-related motivations underpinning the unique project are analogous to those of conventional urban food gardens, or whether motivations and attitudes diverge when urban food growing is linked to innovative technology. These objectives are expressed through the following research questions:

RQ1—How do positive-emotional networks of semantic fields reveal the perception of health-related motivations by city residents planning to engage in innovative food self-production?

RQ2—How do neutral-emotional networks of semantic fields reveal the perception of health-related motivations by city residents planning to engage in innovative food self-production?

RQ3—How do negative-emotional networks of semantic fields reveal the perception of health-related motivations by city residents planning to engage in innovative food self-production?

3. Materials and Methods

3.1. Theoretical Framework of the Study

The study was conducted based on Rogers' Diffusion of Innovations Theory [24]. This approach focuses on the experiences of early adopters, who are crucial in the diffusion of innovations. It is through their openness that new, innovative ideas are tested and then transferred between different peer groups. Early adopters are a social group that engages in the acceptance of new ideas or technologies, often preceding the majority of society. They stand out for their readiness to test and their openness to innovations. They frequently act as opinion leaders within their communities and derive satisfaction from experimenting with new solutions. An important factor determining the behavior of early adopters is their ability to assess the value of innovations. Perceived value, or the subjective belief in the utility of innovations, plays a crucial role in the adoption process. Early adopters are capable of quickly evaluating the benefits of a new technology or idea and making swift decisions regarding its adoption. Their willingness to try something new often stems from a belief in the potential benefits of a given solution [24].

Furthermore, social networks play a significant role in shaping the behaviors of early adopters. These individuals often connect with others sharing common goals, facilitating information exchange, and encouraging decisions to adopt new innovations. Early adopters can also be inspired by other members of their social group who are more open to novelties and serve as role models. However, early adopters bear greater risks than those who wait for later stages of innovation diffusion. New technologies or ideas may still be underdeveloped or unreliable, carrying a risk of failure. Additionally, the early adoption of innovations can be time-consuming and may require additional effort in learning and adapting to new practices. Overcoming these initial challenges, the engagement of early adopters can accelerate societal acceptance of innovation, creating a snowball effect where positive experiences attract subsequent groups to adopt the innovation. Simultaneously, their actions can provide valuable feedback to innovation creators, enabling the improvement and customization of products to meet user needs [24].

3.2. Procedure, Participants

Addressing the challenges of contemporary cities, this study is part of a project aimed at implementing innovative tools based on sustainable food consumption and production patterns, promoting healthy dietary habits, social inclusion, and reducing food waste. The project is likely the first such experiment conducted in Poland. As part of a controlled social experiment carried out in a selected residential block, residents participate in hydroponic food cultivation located in the corridors of their block [25]. Due to the high installation costs, the project involves 20 residents responsible for individual hydroponic cabins.

The study involved two groups of respondents. The first group of residents selected for the project originated from Łódź, but due to legal constraints pertaining to the guarantee of an inhabited building, the experimental phase in this location was not feasible. Consequently, the first research group did not participate in the experiment, and a second residential community had to be selected. The second group of residents came from the city of Warsaw. Both cities are among the largest cities in Poland and are located in central Poland. The experimental phase of the project took place in a selected residential block in Warsaw, in the Mokotów district.

The study participants are owners or tenants of residential premises who expressed a willingness to participate in an innovative social experiment. Due to the need to understand their needs and expectations regarding project activities, the research sample was purposively selected. Here, 37 individual in-depth interviews lasting from 1.5 to 2 h were conducted with them. The interviews were conducted by a team of four professionals, all members of the research team. Two of the team members hold doctoral degrees, while the remaining two are PhD candidates. Prior to their participation in the interviews, the participants were informed of the nature of the study and gave informed consent to participate in the interviews. Participants were compensated with a monthly amount of approximately EUR 22 for participating in project activities. The first set of interviews was conducted from October to November 2022, while the second set was conducted from September 2023 to January 2024. The time gap between interviews was due to the need to select a second project site that met certain technical requirements.

The interviews were conducted prior to the commencement of the experimental phase of the project. At this stage, the participants had limited knowledge of the implementation of the project. They were aware of the purpose of the experiment and the benefits they would receive from participating in it. The project required the insertion of 20 hydroponic cabins in the corridors of the block, the installation of a photovoltaic system on the roof of the building to power the cabins and the installation of a water supply system for the cabins with the possibility of using rainwater. At the finished stage of the project, the residents' community was presented with a choice: to keep the hydroponic cabins or to uninstall them. In contrast, the photovoltaic installation was to be permanently installed in the block. The planned interviews were intended to facilitate an early understanding of the project applicants, regarding their expectations, intentions, and needs, prior to the commencement of the experimental activities.

The interviews covered the following thematic areas: (1) introductory information, (2) neighborly relations, (3) issues related to participation in the project, (4) food waste. A total of 42 respondents participated in the interviews (Mage = 43.7, SD = 14.6, range 27–78), including 26 women (Mage = 46.1, SD = 16.1, range 27–78) and 16 men (Mage = 40.1, SD = 11.8, range 28–77). Eighteen participants were childless, eighteen had one child, including twelve minors, four participants had two children, including three minors, and one participant had three minors. Four participants had completed secondary education, 37 participants had obtained university degrees, and one participant did not specify their level of education. Four participants had received education in agriculture, while six participants had received education in healthcare. The remaining participants represented a range of other professions. Of the 19 individuals who participated in the initial interview phase and were subsequently deemed eligible for inclusion in the project, 19 ultimately did not take part in the project. The remaining 23 participants from the second wave of interviews proceeded with the project. The participants constituted the full experimental group.

3.3. Data Analysis

Participants' statements were analyzed and interpreted according to the semantic field analysis method [26]. This method involves selecting the object of study represented by a keyword (in this study, the keyword is "health"), and then analyzing statements containing this word (the so-called semantic field) based on their belonging to the selected network of meanings. This method allows for a more in-depth analysis of respondents' perceptions of the issues relevant to the study. While this method is not commonly employed in non-linguistic disciplines, a number of valuable analyses conducted using it can be found in the literature [27]. The presented study represents a novel research approach, employing methods originally developed for other disciplines in new areas.

Robin [26] identifies six distinct networks of meanings. Three of them were selected for analysis in the context of this study: (1) network of associations with the analyzed keyword "health"; (2) network of opposites to the keyword "health"; (3) network of actions towards the subject, i.e., a set of words or phrases that describe actions or consequences of actions taken by others towards the analyzed keyword "health".

The advantage of employing this methodology is that it not only provides insight into the specific health-related motivations that prompted the participants to engage with the project, but also allows for the observation of the contexts in which these motivations are discussed. The capacity to observe the context in which a given motive is discussed allows for the interpretation of the attitudes and intentions held by the participants. Statements belonging to the "associations" category, namely, what a keyword is associated with and what it accompanies, are interpreted differently. This is also true of statements belonging to the "oppositions" category, namely, what the respondents perceive as the opposite of health, and what health is opposed to. Conversely, statements belonging to the category of "actions towards the subject" permit the interpretation of the actions taken by respondents towards the subject, namely, their attitudes towards health.

The analysis also utilized the method of assigning one of the three emotional temperatures [23] to each semantic field of the analyzed keyword "health": (1) positively charged field; (2) negatively charged field; or (3) neutrally charged field. The classification of positively valued fields was based on the terms in the semantic field that indicated such a character of the utterance, for example, "I like to eat" and "it is nice to eat lettuce". Conversely, negatively valued fields were classified based on terms such as "I can't convince myself to eat these things". Finally, statements that could not be considered positive or negative were classified as neutral.

In addition to the qualitative approach, the study employed quantitative methods of data analysis. The number of individual semantic fields categorized was counted and presented in descending order of frequency of occurrence. The analysis was conducted using MAXQDA 2022 Analytics Pro software. The research material used for analysis, in the form of interview transcripts, was prepared in Polish, in the language of the interviews.

4. Results

4.1. Characteristics of Positive-Emotional Networks

4.1.1. Actions towards the Subject

Among the most frequently mentioned positive opinions regarding health-related issues were those belonging to the category of "Actions toward the subject". They constituted 39.6% of all statements (Figure 1). Among them, those concerning dietary habits predominated (19 statements, Figure 2). Participants stated that their decision to modify their diet was usually influenced by aspects related to healthcare through proper nutrition. Access to their own vegetables results in a feeling that the food consumed is clean and healthy. Participants pointed out the need to consume balanced and healthy meals as direct regulators of the overall state of the body or hormone levels. Some participants declared that they take care of the quality of the food they consume, for example, by eating "a healthier variety of pasta" (TG25:249) or maintaining a healthy diet by avoiding supermarkets and shopping at local vendors.

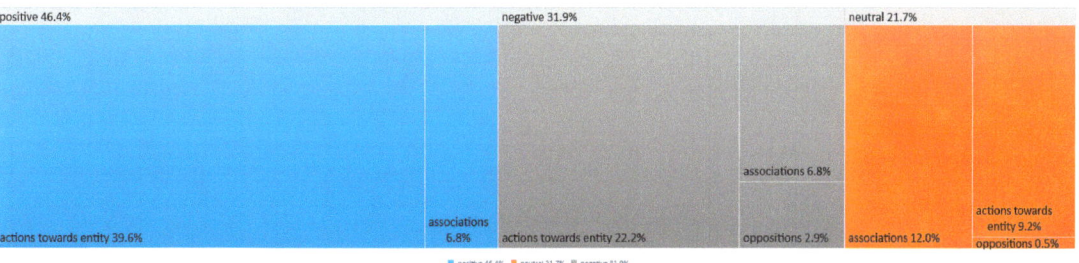

Figure 1. Statements with positive/neutral/negative emotional temperature.

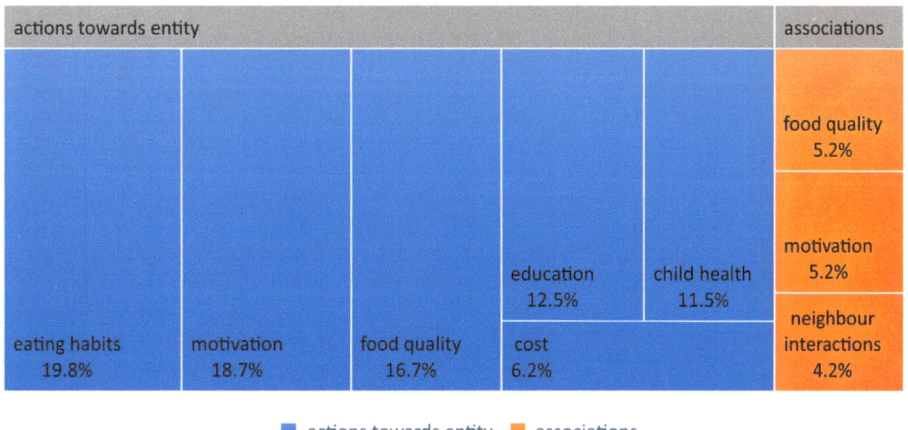

Figure 2. Statements with positive emotional temperature.

Participants in the interviews also emphasized the impact of their diet on health-related issues associated with appearance. An example could be a statement regarding the practice of drinking celery juice for six months as a "brilliant treatment" (TG30:41) for the skin or the need to "regain part of the wardrobe" (TG37:120). Equally important for this group of participants was the preparation of meals themselves, which is perceived as control over what goes into the proverbial pot, equivalent to perceiving the food consumed as healthy (TG40:193).

Another dominant set of statements concerned motivation to participate in the project (18 statements). Experiment participants indicated that easy access to vegetables would be a reason to change their dietary habits and eat more healthily. Interviewees believed that having access to homegrown vegetables would lead to actual consumption of those vegetables, as there would be no need to buy them, and their freshness and self-grown nature would make them more desirable to eat. Participants also expressed the belief that if such organizational solutions were more popular, more people would be persuaded to adopt healthier eating habits by consuming more vegetables daily.

Another aspect related to motivation to participate in the project that participants declared was the desire to take part in an interesting project. Due to increasing media interest in the topic of growing vegetables and edible plants in urban settings, such as on balconies or terraces, the opportunity to participate in a hydroponic cultivation project served as an incentive to engage in activities related to growing plants, which were perceived as healthy in this respect, "I will just produce healthy food myself" (TG27:161). The attractiveness of the project, in the opinion of the block residents participating in the experiment, lies in recognizing the potential health benefits associated with their "small oasis of nature" (TG37:270).

Due to their frequency, another important health-related aspect was actions related to ensuring good quality food products, mentioned 16 times. Participants were convinced that the vegetables they grow themselves, observing how they grow, are definitely healthy (TG3:149). In the participants' opinion, these vegetables represent a "cumulation of all mineral nutrients and vitamins" (TG39:186). Another cited method of verifying the quality of the product was using a mobile application supporting healthy shopping choices (TG15:147).

According to the values and beliefs passed down from generation to generation, they defined healthy food as unprocessed (TG4:35). Fruits and vegetables from local suppliers also enjoy high trust. Interview participants talked about practices where they collectively order organic products from such suppliers. Based on the cooperative established by the residents, vegetables and fruits were regularly delivered to them directly from farmers (TG11:315). Examples of actions aimed at obtaining healthy products also included buying flour directly from the producer (TG15:143) or purchasing healthy food at local markets (TG26:459).

Among the participants' statements, aspects related to learning were also important. This constituted every eighth positive statement. One participant even specified that they are excessively interested in what is inside their food. They regularly read or listen to broadcasts about various nutrients, where they come from, why they are important, what products should be combined, and when they are recommended. They try to incorporate appropriate fats into their diet, avoid excessive carbohydrates, and maintain a balanced diet (TG28:72). Another participant declared that they try to dedicate time to reading about products, especially about health novelties. They have a habit of searching for such products under the influence of suggestions from the Internet or Instagram, for example, while observing dedicated dietary profiles, and then searching for and buying those products in local stores (TG29:55).

One of the participants noticed that the trend of growing edible plants on balconies or terraces is increasing because residents do not want to consume chemically sprayed vegetables. They want access to clean and healthy food. In their opinion, although these people do not have the necessary knowledge about self-cultivation, "they don't even do it wrong" (TG6:25). For many people, participation in the project is an opportunity not only to acquire knowledge about growing edible plants and gardening skills, but also knowledge about the cultivated plants and how they affect human health (TG30:119).

Educational issues were important regarding participation in the project. Participation in the project may lead participants to read more about healthy food and try various other ways to gain interesting knowledge, not only about growing edible plants but also about the nutrients they contain (TG24:34). Another important action for children's health undertaken by the interview participants was activities related to caring for children. Among the positive statements, aspects related to children's health appeared 11 times. These statements emphasize a change in priorities regarding healthy eating habits when a child is born (TG22:358), especially when the child has health problems, for example, allergies (TG15:42). Showing concern for the quality of children's nutrition is their health, represented by resistance to potential diseases (TG22:358). But also, the health of the child is seen as a response to their food preferences. Parents see good health in children as a result of meeting their expectations by buying the kind of food the child likes and enjoys eating, such as ham without skin and soft bread (TG37:120).

Another significant action for children's health is their education. Taking care of their health means teaching them how to eat. From the perspective of participating in the project, it is an opportunity to teach children about the growth cycle of plants, and how to take care of plants. As a result, children can learn practically how to produce food without the use of chemicals (TG23:101).

Another positive aspect of perceiving health issues was through the prism of saving money in the household budget (these statements numbered six). In their opinion, consuming healthier food will result in not having to spend money on vegetables (TG27:199). Furthermore, as the participants note, many stores currently have sections with food from organic farming, but they are much more expensive, so growing vegetables themselves will positively affect household expenses (TG30:57). An example cited by one of the participants is the price of watercress, which is considered the healthiest plant. However, it is only available in some stores and at a high price. Participation in the project will thus enable greater access to this particularly appreciated source of nutrients (TG39:233).

4.1.2. Associations

Among the most frequently mentioned opinions regarding health issues, which can be classified as having a positive emotional temperature, were those belonging to the category of "Associations". They accounted for 14.6% of all positive statements. Among them, those related to statements about factors motivating participation in the experiment predominated (five statements). Among these statements, connections were seen amongst participants' desire to grow their own edible plants, which equals healthier eating (TG8:205), and the desire of residents to obtain their own vegetables, which will have a positive impact on their health or nutrition (TG22:346), including more diverse vegetables (TG13:279).

Further associations regarding health issues can be made with participants' statements regarding the quality of food products (five statements). Here, among other things, participants pointed out that it is important for them to have contact with healthy food, i.e., unprocessed food that can be observed growing (TG14:81). It is important for vegetables to be chemical-free and as organic as possible, simply to be as healthy as possible (TG23:101). Also important were aesthetic issues, so that dishes prepared with homegrown vegetables would be well presented (TG37:188). The quality of products was also evaluated based on the association with the form of sale; self-grown will surely be better than packaged (TG40:570).

Health issues also appeared in four statements from residents regarding their neighborly interactions. Topics related to health, healthy eating, and nutrients are often discussed during short encounters in the hallway or in front of the block (TG31:179), or during newly established acquaintanceships (TG15:147). Participation in the experiment is also seen as an opportunity to talk to neighbors about topics such as a healthier lifestyle, reducing chemicals in products, consuming vegetables, and herbs (TG37:138).

Among the statements with a positive emotional temperature, there were none that could be assigned to the category of "Oppositions".

4.2. Characteristics of Neutral-Emotional Networks

4.2.1. Associations

Among the most frequently mentioned opinions regarding health issues, which can be classified as having a neutral emotional temperature, were those belonging to the category of "Associations". It contained 45 such statements (Figure 3). Interestingly, most issues related to healthy food appeared in the context of responses to the question of what sustainable food consumption is. Participants responded that it is consumption where people eat healthily and consciously, without buying excessive amounts of food that they then throw away (TG14:100). Sustainable food consumption is such that if it is healthy and green, it does not harm (TG40:488). But there were also associations with sustainable consumption, such as healthy eating consisting of "providing the body with what it needs and in the quantities that are needed" (TG38:257).

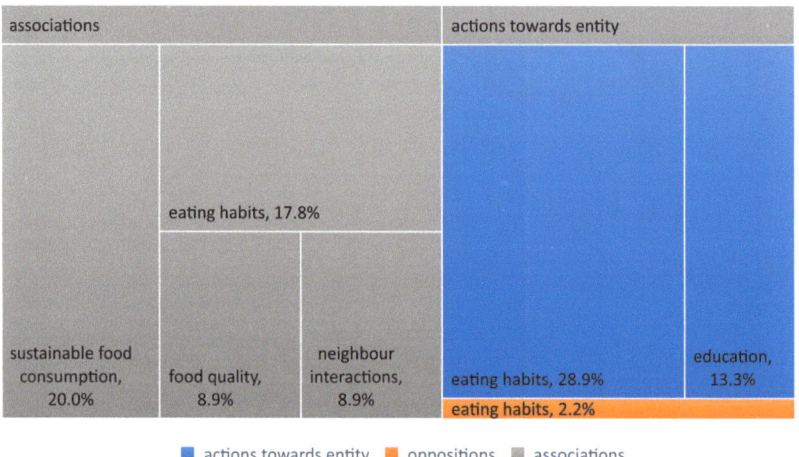

Figure 3. Statements with neutral emotional temperature.

Next, a significant group (nine statements) consisted of opinions that could be classified into the category of "Eating Habits". In the participants' statements, there were fragments indicating that healthy eating is associated with consuming less sugar (TG19:215), more vegetables (TG16:188), longevity (TG22:358), and traditional Polish dishes, as one of the participants believed that good, Polish, healthy cuisine is the best and healthiest (TG37:180).

The next group of statements with a neutral emotional temperature concerned "Neighborly Interactions". Just like in the case of clearly positive statements, they mainly revolved around health topics discussed during conversations between neighbors during chance encounters. Health issues also arose in relation to the "quality of products". Here, statements appeared regarding vegetables grown as part of the project, as healthy plants, i.e., those that contain vitamins, are not sprayed with chemicals, so they can be eaten without harm (TG6:94).

4.2.2. Actions towards the Subject

The next most frequently mentioned opinions regarding health issues with a neutral connotation belonged to the category of "Actions toward the subject". This category contained 19 statements. Among them, the largest group (13 statements) consisted of opinions that could be classified into the "Eating Habits" group. They included participants' experiences regarding the influence of other people or factors on their eating habits. For some, these included a doctor's recommendation (TG6:90) or a partner's suggestion (TG40:512), while for others, they were concern for the state of our planet (TG14:187), general concern for their own health (TG22:358), a specific disease like diabetes, requiring a specific diet (TG40:209), proximity to good health food stores (TG28:148), but also the decision to participate in the project as a stimulus for change (TG16:186).

Another group of statements related to educational activities (six statements). They were mostly concerned with motivation to participate in the project. Within it, participants declared that they mainly want to find out what the proportion of meat, vegetables, and fruits is in their daily diet, what proportion vegetables should occupy in it, and whether they eat healthily as a result. Participants would like to verify their existing knowledge and confirm whether what they think is healthy is indeed healthy (TG5:163). The necessity of caring for plants, and responsibility for them, will motivate them to acquire knowledge about them (TG19:189).

4.2.3. Oppositions

Among the least frequently mentioned opinions regarding health issues, which can be classified as having a neutral emotional temperature, were those belonging to the category of "Oppositions". There was one statement regarding eating habits. One of the interviewees described times when he ate improperly, and did not follow any diet, as unhealthy times. However, he still retains habits related to eating spicy products such as hot peppers, radishes, horseradish, and garlic. This participant hopes that during the project, his daughter will see him eating such vegetables from his own cultivation and will also want to try them, thus learning about different tastes (TG37:120).

4.3. Characteristics of Negative-Emotional Networks

4.3.1. Actions towards the Subject

Among the most frequently mentioned opinions regarding health issues, which can be classified as having a negative emotional temperature, were those belonging to the category of "Actions towards the subject". It contained 46 such statements (Figure 4). Among them, the largest group (20 statements) consisted of opinions that could be classified into the "Eating Habits" group. Predominant among them were statements about the lifestyle and eating habits of the interview participants. They declare that even though they try to maintain a healthy diet, from time to time they consume meals that are not healthy (TG16:188), meaning heavy, mainly fried meals, with large amounts of meat, and especially sweets (TG25:248), or their diet is not rich in vegetables (TG18:116). Some respondents expressed the opinion that although they like to eat healthily, they do not like to prepare meals or do not have time for it. They buy unhealthy products to save time (TG22:354), or consume unhealthy meals that are easy and quick to prepare (TG33:151). Participants also question the quality of purchased products. Although they try to read labels, they either do not fully trust the content of the product to match the description on the label, or buy a particular product despite the ingredients not meeting their expectations (TG21:107), often not bringing good food from home and buying something quickly during a break at work (TG36:158).

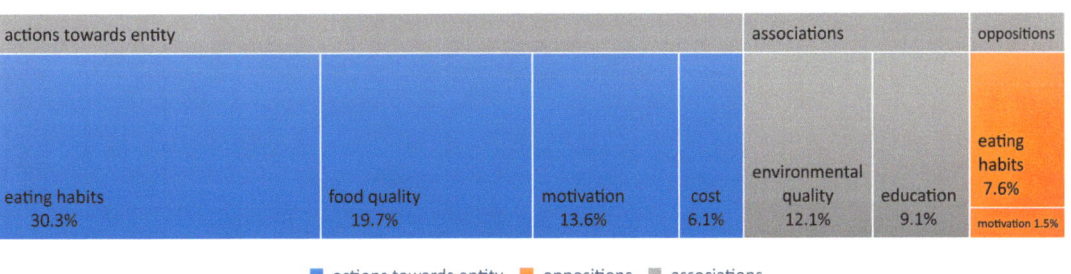

Figure 4. Statements with negative emotional temperature.

Among these are statements regarding the difficulties in selecting diets for individuals with health issues. Just as devising a diet for a healthy person usually does not involve significant obstacles, it is challenging for those who are ill to find specialists who specialize in tailoring diets for specific medical conditions (TG9:149). According to participants, taking medications can pose a challenge, as some of them may interact. For example, one participant presented the possibility of adverse reactions when taking blood pressure medication and consuming large amounts of chokeberry juice (TG30:55). Another participant pointed out the difficulty in selecting a diet for hormonal issues (TG32:105).

Another group of statements referencing health issues pertained to the quality of products (13 statements). Participants were critical of the offerings in stores. For instance, participants observed that contemporary jams contain a significant amount of enhancers, while sugar is replaced with substances that are carcinogenic (TG6:105). Deli meats and meats are unhealthy because they contain substantial amounts of chemicals and antibiotics, and are fatty, which adversely affects cholesterol levels, leading participants to abstain from these products (TG11:119). According to participants, vegetables are currently sprayed with chemicals, so buying, for example, tasty tomatoes, is almost impossible (TG37:266). Another example cited a television program whereby a reporter was employed at a bakery and witnessed improper food practices, such as adding chemical agents to baked goods (TG40:207).

Nine statements with a negative emotional temperature appeared regarding the motivation to grow edible plants as part of participating in the experiment. One participant expressed uncertainty about the project's nature, particularly regarding healthy eating, so they could not determine if the project could change anything in their daily lives. They doubted that merely growing edible green plants as residents would alter their eating habits. According to them, everyone has such strong habits that they are rather difficult to change (TG3:274). Another participant expressed concern about her husband. She assessed that her participation in the project would probably not encourage her husband to join gardening activities because he prefers urban life and would rather spend his free time cycling (TG15:153).

Some statements regarding health appeared in responses regarding motivation to grow plants in general. Participants indicated impatience with plants, and even if they wanted access to healthy food, the plants they grew wilted very quickly, so they preferred to buy them ready-made at the store, such as basil (TG30:49).

Another group of statements with a negative emotional temperature concerned the cost of products. Participants pointed out the very high cost of organic products. Even if they are healthier, they indicated that purchasing them is not worth the extra cost, as their price is often double that of similar non-eco-labeled products (TG26:545). They expressed a similar attitude towards ready-made meals. If they have to pay three times more for a healthy meal than for "junk food", they prefer to eat fast food (TG28:148). Participants indicated that often it is not a matter of choice, but a necessity, to buy cheaper products (TG36:158).

4.3.2. Associations

Among the frequently mentioned opinions regarding health issues that can be classified as having a negative emotional temperature were those belonging to the category of "Associations". It contained 14 such statements. Among them, a larger proportion (8 statements) consisted of opinions that could be classified into the environmental quality group. Participants pointed out that modern times are unhealthy because the entire environment is contaminated. For example, they cited the problem of most food products being sold in plastic packaging, resulting in them containing microplastics and heavy metals hazardous to health (TG6:97). Despite attempts to introduce EU regulations regulating chemical content in products, spraying still contaminates groundwater and soil (TG38:98). Participants also expressed opinions such as "I can't heal the whole world" (TG15:200).

Another group of statements referring to health issues concerned "knowledge". Dominant among them were opinions about the lack of awareness and knowledge in the current society about the chemicals contained in sold fruits and vegetables (TG25:294). Some participants clearly stated that they see shelves of organic food in stores but are not particularly interested in the subject (TG31:113). Preparing healthier food requires more involvement, searching for recipes, and experimenting, so their dietary monotony is a result of a fast-paced lifestyle, although they declare that it bothers them (TG33:151).

4.3.3. Oppositions

Among the opinions regarding health issues that can be classified as having a negative emotional temperature were also those belonging to the category of "Oppositions". It contained six such statements. Among them, five statements could be classified into the "Eating Habits" group. Among the participants, those who identified unhealthy eating habits as being associated with a specific period of their lives stood out. It consisted of relying on fast-food dishes and a fast-paced lifestyle (TG37:114). This broader issue was developed in statements that explained the cause of such an unhealthy lifestyle, i.e., in the "Actions towards the subject" category.

One of the statements classified into the "Oppositions" category relates to motivation to participate in the project. One of the respondents clearly emphasized that healthy food is not the reason why they would want to grow it. For this participant, participating in the project is not only fun, but also a form of escape from city life, a glimpse of the possibility of returning to work on the land, a slice of land in the city (TG26:346).

5. Discussion

Among the interviewed respondents, the early adopters who expressed a willingness to participate in an innovative experiment aimed at growing their own vegetables and herbs using hydroponic cabins placed in the corridors of their apartment block, three main groups of people can be distinguished. The first group is composed of individuals who are very positively inclined towards health-related issues. They declare a high level of commitment to nutritional matters. Their preferences may result from a general increase in awareness of the benefits of such a lifestyle [28]. On the one hand, they take active steps to prepare and consume balanced and healthy meals in their daily diet. Their efforts are focused not only on preparing meals themselves, but also on sourcing ingredients from smaller local suppliers. Through participation in the project, these participants aspire to enjoy similar access to fresh and healthy vegetables and herbs as users of traditional urban gardens [20]. This access is ensured by independent growth control, which eliminates the harmful heavy metals and pesticides found in commonly available produce [21].

The diffusion of innovations and the formation of environmentally conscious urban communities are processes that are greatly influenced by education, so issues related to the learning of future experimental participants were of interest to the study. Findings indicate that education plays an important role in the lives of individuals in the first group. They emphasized that they dedicate a lot of time to reading, watching programs, listening to broadcasts about nutritional components, optimal food combinations for health, seeking information on balanced and varied diets tailored to their individual needs, as well as health news. This confirms the relationship whereby conscious education has a positive impact on self-care and the environment [29]. Participation in the project has the potential to allow one to deepen their knowledge of food, nutrition, and health topics, as well as acquiring additional related skills that they can implement in their daily practice. Of particular importance to them was the aspect of intergenerational social learning, namely, the opportunity to instill positive habits in their children and peer learning through neighborhood integration for the sake of caring for a shared quality of life and health.

From the perspective of the diffusion of innovations theory, their existing knowledge can be a valuable input for peer learning. Through conversations with others, which are intensified through participation in the intervention, there will be a deeper process of sharing knowledge and experiences [23]. As individuals who are particularly sensitive to health issues and concerned about ensuring a variety of nutrients in their diet, they can have a positive influence on their neighbors' behavior in this regard. Furthermore, they can encourage not only the consumption of a more balanced diet, but also the cultivation of a variety of plants that are less common or less commonly available in shops, but richer in nutrients. One respondent cited watercress as an example of such a less-common plant that could be cultivated.

The second group consists of individuals who have changed their dietary habits under the influence of other people or factors. For some, it was a suggestion from a doctor or partner, for others, a specific illness necessitating a particular diet, or simply concern for the state of our planet. The third group consists of individuals who, due to their lifestyle, do not attach great importance to health issues. This is most often due to a lack of time, which is also confirmed by other studies [30]. Representatives of this group buy unhealthy products for the sake of convenience, or consume unhealthy meals that are easy and quick to prepare. The intention of these individuals is to increase motivation and opportunities to acquire knowledge about healthy eating through participation in the project.

Representatives of each group were critical of the quality of products available in stores. Available products in large chains contain enhancers, carcinogenic substances, antibiotics, or heavy metals [21]. In their opinion, these products spoil relatively quickly, which increases food wastage. Participation in the project may therefore be a source of healthy food that is unavailable to them on a daily basis. A very important issue with a negative emotional temperature, recurring in the statements of participants, is the high cost of products prepared or grown in ecological conditions. It is the main barrier to consuming these products in their daily diet. For some participants, healthy products are clearly inaccessible due to their price, resulting in them replacing them with unhealthy alternatives, including fast-food dishes. Access to healthy products is a clear factor that influenced the decision to participate in the project.

6. Conclusions

The main contribution of this study is in helping us to better understand the health-related motivations, attitudes, intentions, and expectations of participants in an interdisciplinary project aimed at the self-production of food in urban settings. Through a unique educational social experiment, residents of a selected block in Warsaw have the opportunity for the hydroponic cultivation of vegetables and herbs in the corridors of their apartment block. The qualitative study revealed the individual profiles of project participants, individuals with a clearly pro-health lifestyle, individuals for whom health issues are the result of the actions of other people or factors, and busy individuals who declare a lack of time to care for their health. For each of these groups, the opportunity to access healthy products and educational benefits were factors that influenced the decision to participate in the project.

This study indicates that, despite the difficulties in conducting a social experiment, city residents are willing to participate in such innovative activities. It is therefore worthwhile to continue seeking ways to finance unconventional educational interventions utilizing the latest technological solutions. Through them, not only do residents' access to healthy, nutritious products increase, but it also has the potential to motivate them to lifelong learning, influencing their environmental literacy. The findings of the study indicate that a significant proportion of urban dwellers have limited access to healthy and nutritious fruits and vegetables. This is due to a number of factors, including restrictions related to urbanization and the displacement of local suppliers, as well as lifestyle and the fast pace of urban life. The dissemination of innovative solutions could help to enhance awareness, prompting reflection on healthy habits and strengthening motivation to change eating habits.

However, the study is not without limitations. What on the one hand undoubtedly constitutes a strong point of the project—the uniqueness of the experiment—also represents a research limitation, due to the sample size and the deterministic nature of the study—qualitative interviews, the results of which cannot be generalized. On the other hand, the study aims to understand the profiles of individuals who by their nature constitute a small part of the community—early adopters in the process of technological innovation diffusion; therefore, the size of this group is significantly limited, and quantitative studies would not have a clear justification. Future research could be expanded to include a comparative aspect, comparing different groups of individuals who undertake the testing of similar technological solutions in other geographic locations.

This paper presents the results from the initial phase of the project, prior to the participants being included in the experimental phase. Consequently, the attitudes and intentions of the initial users were expressed prior to the innovation testing period. Further research will be conducted on a number of related issues, including the learning process during the adoption of an innovation, the productivity of urban hydroponic farming, and the sharing of food with neighbors, family, and friends. These findings will be presented in subsequent papers.

The results of the study can serve not only other researchers interested in understanding issues related to healthy eating or implementing technological innovations, but also educators interested in promoting a positive attitude towards urban gardening, as well as food safety, diverse, balanced nutrition, and health.

Funding: This research leading to the presented results and the APC was funded by the Norway Grants 2014–2021 and the state budget of Poland through the National Centre for Research and Development, grant number NOR/IdeaLab/SmartFood/0005/2020.

Institutional Review Board Statement: The study was conducted in accordance with the Declaration of Helsinki, and approved by the foreign external experts committee evaluating the proposal and monitoring the project's ongoing progress, approval number DWM/IdeaLab/232/2020 decision of 28 October 2020.

Informed Consent Statement: Informed consent was obtained from all subjects involved in the study.

Data Availability Statement: The data presented in this study are available on reasonable request from the corresponding author.

Conflicts of Interest: The author declares no conflicts of interest. The funders had no role in the design of the study; in the collection, analyses, or interpretation of data; in the writing of the manuscript; or in the decision to publish the results.

References

1. Artmann, M.; Sartison, K.; Ives, C.D. Urban gardening as a means for fostering embodied urban human–food connection? A case study on urban vegetable gardens in Germany. *Sustain. Sci.* **2021**, *16*, 967–981. [CrossRef]
2. Ruiz-Mallén, I.; Satorras, M.; March, H.; Baró, F. Community climate resilience and environmental education: Opportunities and challenges for transformative learning. *Environ. Educ. Res.* **2022**, *28*, 1088–1107. [CrossRef]
3. Knobloch, N. An Introduction: Teaching and Learning in Urban Agricultural Community Contexts. In *Teaching and Learning in Urban Agricultural Community Contexts*; Springer: Berlin/Heidelberg, Germany, 2021; pp. 1–11.
4. Laage-Thomsen, J.; Blok, A. Varieties of green: On aesthetic contestations over urban sustainability pathways in a Copenhagen community garden. *Environ. Plan. E Nat. Space* **2021**, *4*, 275–295. [CrossRef]
5. Dubová, L.; Macháč, J.; Vacková, A. Food provision, social interaction or relaxation: Which drivers are vital to being a member of community gardens in Czech cities? *Sustainability* **2020**, *12*, 9588. [CrossRef]
6. Ramirez-Andreotta, M.D.; Tapper, A.; Clough, D.; Carrera, J.S.; Sandhaus, S. Understanding the Intrinsic and Extrinsic Motivations Associated with Community Gardening to Improve Environmental Public Health Prevention and Intervention. *Int. J. Environ. Res. Public Health* **2019**, *16*, 494. [CrossRef] [PubMed]
7. Koay, W.I.; Dillon, D. Community Gardening: Stress, Well-Being, and Resilience Potentials. *Int. J. Environ. Res. Public Health* **2020**, *17*, 6740. [CrossRef] [PubMed]
8. Tharrey, M.; Darmon, N. Urban collective garden participation and health: A systematic literature review of potential benefits for free-living adults. *Nutr. Rev.* **2022**, *80*, 6–21. [CrossRef] [PubMed]
9. Lampert, T.; Costa, J.; Santos, O.; Sousa, J.; Ribeiro, T.; Freire, E. Evidence on the contribution of community gardens to promote physical and mental health and well-being of non-institutionalized individuals: A systematic review. *PLoS ONE* **2021**, *16*, e0255621. [CrossRef] [PubMed]
10. Pombo, C. Food Sustainability for the Underprivileged: A Comparison of Non-Profit Group Activities in Four U.S. Cities. In *Environmental Philosophy, Politics, and Policy*; Duerk, J.A., Ed.; Lexington Books: London, UK, 2021; pp. 105–120.
11. Sooriyaarachchi, P.; Francis, T.V.; Jayawardena, R. Fruit and vegetable consumption during the COVID-19 lockdown in Sri Lanka: An online survey. *Nutrire* **2022**, *47*, 12. [CrossRef] [PubMed]
12. Aboubakar, A.; El Hajjaji, S.; Douaik, A.; Mfopou Mewouo, Y.C.; Birang a Madong, R.C.; Dahchour, A.; Mabrouki, J.; Labjar, N. Heavy metal concentrations in soils and two vegetable crops (*Corchorus olitorius* and *Solanum nigrum* L.), their transfer from soil to

vegetables and potential human health risks assessment at selected urban market gardens of Yaoundé, Cameroon. *Int. J. Environ. Anal. Chem.* **2023**, *103*, 3522–3543. [CrossRef]
13. Feldmann, F.; Vogler, U. Towards sustainable performance of urban horticulture: Ten challenging fields of action for modern integrated pest management in cities. *J. Plant Dis. Prot.* **2021**, *128*, 55–66. [CrossRef] [PubMed]
14. Oral, H.V.; Carvalho, P.; Gajewska, M.; Ursino, N.; Masi, F.; Hullebusch, E.D.V. A review of nature-based solutions for urban water management in European circular cities: A critical assessment based on case studies and literature. *Blue-Green Syst.* **2020**, *2*, 112–136. [CrossRef]
15. Resh, H.M. *Hydroponic Food Production: A Definitive Guidebook for the Advanced Home Gardener and the Commercial Hydroponic Grower*; CRC Press: Boca Raton, FL, USA, 2022.
16. Verner, D.; Vellani, S.; Goodman, E.; Love, D.C. Frontier Agriculture: Climate-Smart and Water-Saving Agriculture Technologies for Livelihoods and Food Security. In *New Forms of Urban Agriculture: An Urban Ecology Perspective*; Springer Nature: Singapore, 2022; pp. 159–186.
17. Shrestha, S.B. Food Green Cities: A Pathway to Sustainable Urban Development of Nepal. *Nepal J. Sci. Technol.* **2021**, *20*, 147–159. [CrossRef]
18. Pennisi, G.; Pistillo, A.; Appolloni, E.; Orsini, F.; Gianquinto, G. Advanced hydroponics design for plant cultivation in cities. In *Advances in Horticultural Soilless Culture*; Burleigh Dodds Science Publishing: Cambridge, UK, 2021; pp. 303–319.
19. Ashok, A.; Sujitha, E. Hydroponic vegetable cultivation. *Int. J. Chem. Stud.* **2020**, *8*, 1207–1213. [CrossRef]
20. Ghosh, S. Growing health in local food gardens: Case studies of community, school, and home gardens. In *Cultivated Therapeutic Landscapes*; Marsh, P., Williams, A., Eds.; Routledge: London, UK, 2023; pp. 52–82.
21. Verzone, C.; Woods, C. *Food Urbanism: Typologies, Strategies, Case Studies*; Birkhäuser: Basel, Switzerland, 2021.
22. Cepic, S.; Tomicevic-Dubljevic, J.; Zivojinovic, I. Is there a demand for collective urban gardens? Needs and motivations of potential gardeners in Belgrade. *Urban For. Urban Green.* **2020**, *53*, 126716. [CrossRef]
23. Garnett, T.; Mathewson, S.; Angelides, P.; Borthwick, F. Policies and actions to shift eating patterns: What works. *Foresight* **2015**, *515*, 518–522.
24. Rogers, E.M. . *Diffusion of Innovations*, 3rd ed.; A Division of Macmillan Publishing Co., Inc.: New York, NY, USA, 1983.
25. Duda, E.; Gontar, Ł.; Kochański, M.; Korsbrekke, M.H. Urban Living Lab Enhanced by a Mobile Application as a New Way to Educate Towards Green and Inclusive Cities. In Proceedings of the 31st International Conference on Computers in Education. Asia-Pacific Society for Computers in Education, Shimane, Japan, 4–8 December 2023; Volume 2, pp. 970–972.
26. Robin, R. Badanie pól semantycznych: Doświadczenia Ośrodka Leksykologii Politycznej w Saint-Cloud. In *Język i Społeczeństwo*; Głowiński, M., Ed.; Czytelnik: Warsaw, Poland, 1980; pp. 252–281.
27. Fatyga, B. (Ed.) *Praktyki Badawcze*; Instytut Stosowanych Nauk Społecznych UW: Warsaw, Poland, 2015.
28. Muth, A.-K.; Vermeer, A.L.; Terenzi, D.; Park, S.Q. The impact of diet and lifestyle on wellbeing in adults during COVID-19 lockdown. *Front. Nutr.* **2022**, *9*, 993180. [CrossRef] [PubMed]
29. De Almeida, R.; Da Silva Carvalho, P.G. Healthy people living on a healthy planet—The role of education of consciousness for integration as an instrument of health promotion. In *Lifelong Learning and Education in Healthy and Sustainable Cities*; Springer: Berlin/Heidelberg, Germany, 2018; pp. 299–326.
30. Jonsson, L.; Larsson, C.; Berg, C.; Korp, P.; Lindgren, E.C. What undermines healthy habits with regard to physical activity and food? Voices of adolescents in a disadvantaged community. *Int. J. Qual. Stud. Health Well-Being* **2017**, *12* (Suppl. 2), 1333901. [CrossRef] [PubMed]

Disclaimer/Publisher's Note: The statements, opinions and data contained in all publications are solely those of the individual author(s) and contributor(s) and not of MDPI and/or the editor(s). MDPI and/or the editor(s) disclaim responsibility for any injury to people or property resulting from any ideas, methods, instructions or products referred to in the content.

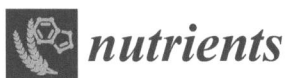

Article

Urban–Rural Disparities in Food Insecurity and Weight Status among Children in the United States

Jayna M. Dave [1,*], Tzuan A. Chen [2,3], Alexandra N. Castro [1], Mamie A. White [1], Elizabeth A. Onugha [4,5], Sloane Zimmerman [6] and Debbe Thompson [1]

1. USDA/ARS Children's Nutrition Research Center, Department of Pediatrics, Baylor College of Medicine, 1100 Bates Avenue, Houston, TX 77030, USA; alexandra.castro@bcm.edu (A.N.C.); mawhite@bcm.edu (M.A.W.); dit@bcm.edu (D.T.)
2. Department of Psychological, Health, and Learning Sciences, University of Houston, 3657 Cullen Boulevard, Houston, TX 77204, USA; tchen3@central.uh.edu
3. HEALTH Research Institute, University of Houston, 4349 Martin Luther King Boulevard, Houston, TX 77204, USA
4. Renal Services, Texas Children's Hospital, 1102 Bates Avenue, Houston, TX 77030, USA; eaonugha@texaschildrens.org
5. Department of Pediatrics—Nephrology, Baylor College of Medicine, 1102 Bates Avenue, Houston, TX 77030, USA
6. Department of Pediatrics—Gastroenterology, Baylor College of Medicine, One Baylor Plaza, Houston, TX 77030, USA; sloane.zimmerman@bcm.edu
* Correspondence: jmdave@bcm.edu

Abstract: Place of residence (urban versus rural) is a contextual determinant of health that has received less attention in the food insecurity literature. The purpose of this study was to assess the urban–rural disparity in the prevalence of food insecurity and weight status among US children. Using data from the National Health and Nutrition Examination Survey (NHANES) 2013–2016 with three age groups of children (2–5, 6–11, and 12–17 years old), the associations of weight status and child and household food security status by urban–rural residence were examined using Rao–Scott Chi-square tests. Statistical significance was set at $p < 0.05$. Children living in urban areas were significantly more likely to experience household food insecurity (29.15%) compared to their rural counterparts (19.10%), among those aged 6–11 years. The associations between children's weight status and child and household food security status were significant for children living in urban areas overall and different age groups but not for children living in rural areas. These trends were more pronounced in older age groups. Given the link between food insecurity and higher obesity rates, particularly among urban children, this study highlights the importance of incorporating food security interventions into future obesity prevention programs.

Keywords: food insecurity; weight status; urban–rural differences; children; NHANES

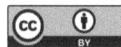

1. Introduction

Childhood obesity is a complex issue with far-reaching consequences. Identifying the behavioral, social, and environmental factors that contribute to it, such as access to healthy foods and the influence of marketing, is essential for designing effective prevention and treatment strategies [1,2]. Living in rural areas may be a risk factor associated with childhood obesity. A meta-analysis of 10 studies found that children in rural areas had a 26% greater risk of obesity than urban children [3]. Similar findings were observed in children and adolescents, with one study reporting greater odds of obesity in rural/nonmetropolitan areas compared to urban/metropolitan areas [4–6].

Prior research consistently shows a high prevalence of overweight and obesity among children living in rural communities in the US. A study in Mississippi found that 54%

of middle school children exceed healthy weight ranges [7]. Similarly, a study in Appalachian Kentucky reported that 33% of elementary school children had a BMI over the 85th percentile [8], indicating a risk of obesity. These findings align with studies on African American children from rural South Carolina [9] and fourth-graders in rural Iowa [10]. While these studies show a consistent pattern, they often focus on specific regions or populations. To gain a broader understanding, data from nationally representative samples of both urban and rural children obtained simultaneously are crucial. Data from the National Survey of Children's Health support the observed pattern and reveal a higher prevalence of overweight and obesity among children living in rural areas than their urban counterparts (35% vs. 30%) [11]. Additionally, two studies utilizing nationally representative samples [6,12] found significantly higher obesity rates among rural children compared to urban children. These findings strengthen the association between rural residency and childhood obesity.

While the link between rural residency and childhood obesity appears clear, the picture becomes more complex when considering food insecurity, which is the limited or uncertain availability of nutritionally adequate and safe foods and is strongly related to poverty [13]. The overall rates of food insecurity in the United States (US) in 2022 were significantly higher than the national average (12.8%) for households with children (17.3%) and households in principal cities (urban—15.3%) and rural areas (14.7%) [13]. Among the 17.3% of the food-insecure households with children, 8.6% of adults experienced food insecurity, while the children themselves were food-secure [13]. In a concerning 8.8% of the households, both children and adults suffered food insecurity at some point during the year [13]. Very low food security, the most severe level, affected both children and adults in approximately 1% (381,000 households) of US households with children [13]. Moreover, rates of food insecurity are highest in urban cities (15.3%), followed by rural areas (14.7%), and are lowest in suburban areas (10.5%) [13].

Research on the association between food insecurity and obesity in low-income children has yielded mixed results. Some studies, including one with a national sample of low-income children 8–17 years of age and another with young preschoolers (predominantly Hispanic) receiving Woman, Infants, and Children (WIC) services, found no association between overweight/obesity and household food insecurity [14,15]. However, other studies, such as one with a national sample of children 12–18 years of age and a longitudinal study of low-income preschool children in the Massachusetts WIC program, reported that children from food-insecure households were significantly more likely to be overweight than their counterparts from food-secure households [16]. These contrasting findings highlight the complexity of the relationship between food insecurity and obesity, particularly among low-income children.

With the increasing rates of both obesity and food insecurity in the US [13,17,18], examining the association between these issues among children is necessary. Thus, the purpose of this study was to investigate how food insecurity and weight status vary between urban and rural areas among US children, utilizing a nationally representative sample. This ongoing research will be crucial for developing effective interventions that address the diverse challenges faced by children across different geographic locations.

2. Materials and Methods

2.1. Participants

This study analyzed data from the National Health and Nutrition Examination Survey (NHANES) conducted between 2013 and 2016. Because the data were publicly available, they were determined to be exempt from review by the Baylor College of Medicine's Institutional Review Board. NHANES, a cross-sectional survey representing the civilian non-institutionalized US population, is conducted by the National Center for Health Statistics (NCHS) of the Centers for Disease Control and Prevention (CDC). Information about the survey methodology and sampling design is available from other sources [19]. We used data from two survey cycles (2013–2014 and 2015–2016) that included information on food security and weight status to increase the reliability and stability of estimates across subgroups [19]. The study focused on children aged 2 to 17 with reported food security status. Children with missing data on key variables were excluded from the analysis. A total of 6403 children were included, with children categorized into three age groups: 2–5 years old; 6–11 years old, and 12–17 years old. Following approval by the US CDC's National Center for Health Statistics (NCHS) Ethics Review Board and after obtaining written informed consent from participants, the NHANES protocols ensured ethical data collection.

2.2. Measures

2.2.1. Sociodemographic Variables

The NHANES gathered information on participants' backgrounds through in-home interviews using a computerized system. Individuals 16 years old or older and those considered legally independent (emancipated minors) were interviewed directly. For children under 16, a designated person (proxy) familiar with their situation provided the information. The interviews captured details on age, gender, race/ethnicity, parent's marital and education status, and household income. Data on participation in federal nutrition assistance programs such as the Supplemental Nutrition Assistance Program (SNAP), WIC, School Breakfast Program (SBP), National School Lunch Program (NSLP), and Summer Food Service Program (SFSP) were also collected.

To understand participants' living environments, NHANES assigned a rural–urban status based on their county of residence. This classification relied on the Urban Influence Code (UIC), established by the United States Department of Agriculture (USDA)'s Economic Research Service (ERS). The 2013 Area Resource File, a comprehensive database of all 2142 US counties, was used to select the county codes for this study. Counties with UICs of 1 or 2 were categorized as urban. The USDA ERS designates all other codes (3–12) as nonmetropolitan codes, which were classified as rural in this study [20,21]. It is important to note that county-level urban–rural status is considered restricted data in NHANES. Access to these data was granted by the NCHS Research Data Center (RDC).

2.2.2. Food Security Status

The standardized 18-item US Household Food Security Survey Module was used during the NHANES in-home interview to assess food security status [22]. An adult in the household answered 10 general questions about the entire household. If children under 18 were present, the adult also answered an additional 8 questions specifically about the children's experiences. Focusing on the past 12-month period, the survey included questions on food security status (household and child level), with responses coded using the USDA's coding guide. A score of 0–18 was calculated by adding the affirmative responses. Higher scores indicate greater food insecurity. Following established guidelines [23], children in the household were classified as food-insecure if the adult answered with two or more affirmative responses to the child-specific questions. NHANES categorizes food security into four levels: high, marginal, low, and very low [24]. For this study, we combined "high" and "marginal" into one category of food security; similarly, "low" and "very low" were combined into one category of food insecurity.

2.2.3. Weight Status

As part of NHANES, height and weight data for the participating children were also collected using standardized procedures [25]. We used body mass index (BMI) to assess weight status in the children included in this study. BMI is a common method that calculates weight in kilograms divided by height in meters squared (kg/m^2). Following the CDC's 2000 sex-specific BMI-for-age growth charts [26], weight status was categorized as underweight (below 5th percentile), normal weight (5th to <85th percentile), overweight (85th to 95th percentile), and obese ($\geq$95th percentile). It is important to note that due to the small sample size for underweight children, this study combined their data with those of the normal-weight group for analysis.

2.3. Data Analysis

The descriptive statistics of the participants' characteristics were calculated for three age groups (2–5, 6–11, and 12–17 years old) representing early childhood, childhood, and adolescence. We examined the associations between participant characteristics and age groups. For continuous variables, we employed ANOVA, while Rao–Scott Chi-square tests were used for categorical variables. To account for the NHANES complex survey design, including non-response, and stratification adjustments, sample weights were incorporated into the analyses.

To ensure that national representative estimates will be generated, the SAS SURVEYFREQ procedure, which accounts for the complex, stratified, multistage probability cluster sampling design, was used, as specified in the instructions for using NHANES data [27]. The associations of weight status and child/household food security status by different urban–rural residence and age groups were examined using Rao–Scott Chi-square tests. All analyses were performed using SAS 9.4. Statistical significance was set at $p < 0.05$.

3. Results

The overall sample of 6403 children included a balanced distribution of age groups—27.33% were 2–5 years old, 40.43% were 6–11 years old, and 32.23% were 12–17 years old (Table 1). Just over half (51%) of the children were male, and the remaining 49% were females, with a slight majority of Hispanic children (30.97–33.80%). The majority of children were classified as normal weight (59.03–71.95%) across each of the age groups. High participation rates in federal nutrition assistance programs were observed (~89% in SNAP and ~90% in school meals programs including SBP and NSLP).

Table 1. Descriptive statistics of participant characteristics by age groups.

	All n = 6403	2–5 Years Old n = 1750	6–11 Years Old n = 2589	12–17 Years Old n = 2064
	Mean ± SD			
Age	7.51 ± 5.25	3.38 ± 1.14	8.44 ± 1.72	14.44 ± 1.68
BMI Percentile	19.81 ± 5.44	16.49 ± 1.85	18.79 ± 4.31	23.84 ± 6.19
	n (%)			
Gender				
Male	3266 (51.01)	903 (51.60)	1311 (50.64)	1052 (50.97)
Female	3137 (48.99)	847 (48.40)	1278 (49.36)	1012 (49.03)
Weight Status				
Normal weight	3893 (63.70)	1172 (71.95)	1547 (62.05)	1174 (59.02)
Overweight	1048 (17.15)	250 (15.35)	431 (17.29)	367 (18.45)
Obese	1170 (19.15)	207 (12.71)	515 (20.66)	448 (22.52)
Ethnicity				
Non-Hispanic White	1730 (27.02)	486 (27.77)	698 (26.96)	546 (26.45)
Non-Hispanic Black	1556 (24.30)	432 (24.69)	632 (24.41)	492 (23.84)
Hispanic	2111 (32.97)	542 (30.97)	875 (33.80)	694 (33.62)
Others	1006 (15.71)	290 (16.57)	384 (14.83)	332 (16.08)
Child Food Security Status				
Child food security	5480 (87.08)	1552 (90.34)	2202 (86.35)	1726 (85.23)
Child food insecurity	813 (12.92)	166 (9.66)	348 (13.65)	299 (14.76)
Household Food Security Status				
Household food security	4535 (72.04)	1268 (73.81)	1837 (72.01)	1430 (70.58)
Household food insecurity	1760 (27.96)	450 (26.19)	714 (27.99)	596 (29.42)

Table 1. Cont.

	All n = 6403	2–5 Years Old n = 1750	6–11 Years Old n = 2589	12–17 Years Old n = 2064
Participation in Federal Nutrition Assistance Programs				
SNAP	2129 (89.68)	673 (90.21)	875 (89.74)	581 (88.97)
WIC	479 (49.33)	479 (49.33)	NA	NA
SBP	2143 (92.57)	187 (94.92)	1253 (92.95)	703 (91.30)
NSLP	2606 (87.66)	218 (92.77)	1407 (88.60)	981 (85.30)
SFSP	640 (34.32)	49 (35.51)	354 (34.40)	237 (33.95)
Any of the FNAP	3722 (72.60)	938 (77.78)	1619 (71.83)	1165 (69.89)

SD: standard deviation; BMI: body mass index; SNAP: Supplemental Nutrition Assistance Program; WIC: Special Supplemental Nutrition Program for Women, Infants, and Children; SBP: School Breakfast Program; NSLP: National School Lunch Program; SFSP: Summer Food Service Program; FNAP: Federal Nutrition Assistance Program.

Children aged 2–5 years old experienced the lowest rates of food insecurity (9.66%) compared to older age groups, which rose to 14.77% among 12–17-year-olds; household food insecurity ranged from 26.19% among 2–5-year-olds to 29.42% in 12–17-year-olds. These can be categorized as moderate rates of food insecurity.

The associations between children's weight status and child food security status were significant for children living in urban areas overall and for different age groups ($p < 0.05$) (Table 2). However, the associations were not significant for children living in rural areas. Underweight/normal-weight children from urban areas were more likely to report experiencing food security; however, overweight or obese children from urban areas were more likely to be in households with food insecurity. These trends were more pronounced in older age groups of children. Similar significant trends were also found for household food security among children in urban areas (Table 3). Children living in rural areas also showed similar non-significant trends in child and household food insecurity by age group.

Table 2. Urban–rural differences in child food security status by weight status of children in different age groups.

Age Group	Urban			Rural		
	Food-Secure	Food-Insecure	p-Value	Food-Secure	Food-Insecure	p-Value
	Weighted %			Weighted %		
All			<0.0001			0.5475
Underweight/Normal weight	59.91	6.05		55.51	6.78	
Overweight	14.23	1.88		17.12	1.52	
Obese	15.08	2.83		16.54	2.53	
2–5 years old			0.0005			0.401
Underweight/Normal weight	68.44	5.36		69.13	5.82	
Overweight	12.82	1.49		13.62	0.51	
Obese	10.09	1.79		10.57	0.35	
6–11 years old			0.0478			0.5357
Underweight/Normal weight	58.21	6.94		57.45	6.72	
Overweight	14.11	2.22		15.58	0.83	
Obese	15.81	2.69		17.41	1.99	
12–17 years old			0.0001			0.7415
Underweight/Normal weight	56.21	5.62		47.76	7.25	
Overweight	15.24	1.80		19.94	2.52	
Obese	17.51	3.63		18.57	3.95	

Table 3. Urban–rural differences in household food security status by weight status of children in different age groups.

Age Group	Urban			Rural		
	Food-Secure	Food-Insecure		Food-Secure	Food-Insecure	
	Weighted %		p-Value	Weighted %		p-Value
All			<0.0001			0.3003
Underweight/Normal weight	52.23	13.74		50.82	11.47	
Overweight	11.89	4.22		15.77	2.87	
Obese	12.32	5.60		14.42	4.65	
2–5 years old			0.0059			0.8454
Underweight/Normal weight	58.44	15.37		62.12	12.83	
Overweight	10.34	3.97		12.15	1.98	
Obese	8.40	3.48		9.53	1.38	
6–11 years old			<0.0001			0.5152
Underweight/Normal weight	51.192	13.96		54.19	9.98	
Overweight	12.377	3.96		14.20	2.22	
Obese	12.697	5.81		14.85	4.55	
12–17 years old			<0.0001			0.4422
Underweight/Normal weight	49.346	12.50		42.98	12.03	
Overweight	12.384	4.64		18.67	3.79	
Obese	14.414	6.72		16.30	6.21	

4. Discussion

This study addresses a critical gap by examining the complex interplay between children's weight status, food security, and their residential environment (urban vs. rural) across different age groups. It delves deeper into exploring these associations across different age groups, a unique contribution compared to previous research.

For the overall sample, the child and household food insecurity rates were categorized as moderate. While these rates may seem statistically moderate, it is crucial to remember that food insecurity exists on a spectrum. Even moderate levels can negatively impact children's health and well-being through nutrient deficiencies, impaired cognitive development, and an increased risk of chronic diseases like obesity and diabetes [28,29]. By acknowledging the multifaceted consequences of even moderate food insecurity, we can emphasize the importance of addressing this issue and ensuring all children have access to a safe and reliable food supply.

This study identified a noteworthy urban paradox. Children 6–11 years old reported higher household food insecurity compared to their rural counterparts. Moreover, in urban areas, significant associations emerged between weight status and both child and household food security for all age groups of children. Underweight and normal-weight children were more likely to be food-secure, while their overweight or obese counterparts faced a higher likelihood of food insecurity. This aligns with some studies suggesting limited access to healthy and affordable food options in urban areas, particularly low-income neighborhoods [30–32]. Children in these situations might experience food insecurity while simultaneously having easier access to calorie-dense, less nutritious options, contributing to obesity.

The observation that these trends strengthened with increasing age suggests a cumulative effect of unhealthy food environments. As children in urban areas age, the challenges associated with accessing healthy food and navigating unhealthy food marketing may become more pronounced, potentially leading to a stronger association between weight status and food insecurity. These results highlight the unique challenges faced by urban children in achieving optimal nutrition. Similar observations on the cumulative effect of unhealthy food marketing exposure in urban environments have been documented in other studies [33–37]. Conversely, no significant associations were observed in rural settings.

There are several explanations for these findings. Urban environments, particularly low-income areas with limited access to healthy foods, often grapple with higher poverty rates [32,38–41]. This translates to increased food insecurity and childhood obesity rates in urban areas [42]. Additionally, exposure to unhealthy food marketing in urban environments may contribute to unhealthy consumption patterns, ultimately leading to weight gain and obesity [35,36]. Moreover, there are social and cultural factors that contribute to the association between food insecurity and childhood obesity in urban areas [43–45]. For example, children living in neighborhoods with a high prevalence of obesity may be more susceptible to social norms that encourage unhealthy eating habits.

The associations observed in urban areas were not significant in rural settings. This disparity suggests that factors influencing children's weight status and food security may differ substantially between rural and urban environments [46]. While urban areas may experience disparities related to socioeconomic status, access to food resources, and dietary behaviors, these disparities may manifest differently or to a lesser extent in rural areas. Understanding these differences is crucial for developing effective and targeted strategies to promote child nutrition and food security across diverse geographic locations.

These findings have important implications for public health and policy efforts. Tailored interventions are required to address the specific challenges associated with childhood obesity and food insecurity in urban areas. These initiatives should consider age-specific dynamics, as the age-food security link strengthens with age. Potential interventions could include educational programs on nutrition, cooking classes, and increased opportunities for physical activity in schools and communities. In contrast, rural areas may require a different approach, recognizing the unique factors that influence child weight status and food security in those settings. The findings also suggest that there is a need to focus on improving access to healthy and affordable foods in urban areas, potentially through initiatives like farmers' markets and community gardens. Policy efforts in urban environments could also focus on regulating unhealthy food marketing and advertising directed toward children.

Further research is needed to gain a deeper understanding of the complex relationship between food security and weight status in children, particularly within urban settings. Future research should (i) focus on identifying the specific factors driving the association between food insecurity and childhood obesity in urban areas, which will be essential for informing the development of targeted interventions; (ii) investigate the long-term health and well-being impacts of food insecurity and childhood obesity; and (iii) further explore the social and cultural factors influencing the weight–food security link in urban environments. This would help to raise awareness of the importance of addressing these issues for a child's overall health and development. This awareness can lead to stronger advocacy efforts and the allocation of resources for programs that address these critical issues for children's nutritional well-being in diverse communities.

This study benefits from several strengths. First, it utilizes a large, nationally representative sample from the US population. This robust sample size allows for reliable conclusions to be drawn about the associations between child weight status, food security (both child and household), and residential environment (urban vs. rural). Second, this study leverages the strengths of NHANES, which employs well-established and reliable measures for anthropometric data (weight and height) through standardized protocols. One limitation of this study is its cross-sectional design. While it can identify associations between variables, it cannot establish cause-and-effect relationships. Other limitations are that this study did not explore potential sex or race differences in the associations of interest and did not control for participants' characteristics such as gender, race/ethnicity, parent's marital status and education status, household income, etc. Also, levels of physical activity were not investigated. This study categorized locations as urban or rural, but future research could benefit from further stratification within urban areas, such as distinguishing between central cities and suburbs, to capture potentially finer-grained variations in food insecurity and weight status. These are important factors that can influence both food security and weight status, and future research should explore how these demographics may influence the observed relationships. Lastly, the use of NHANES 2013–2016 data, while appropriate for investigating the core relationships of interest, represents a timeframe nearing ten years. Future research utilizing more recent NHANES cycles could provide valuable insights into potential changes in prevalence and how these associations may evolve over time.

5. Conclusions

This study reveals a critical urban–rural disparity in how children's weight status relates to their experience with food insecurity. We observed a concerning trend in urban areas, where children experiencing food insecurity were more likely to be overweight or obese across all age groups. Notably, the strength of the association and how it varies by age were unique to urban environments. These findings highlight the need for tailored interventions and policies that consider both geographic location and age to effectively address children's nutritional well-being and food security. In contrast, rural settings displayed no significant associations. This disparity highlights the importance of geographically specific strategies to address the distinct challenges faced by children in different environments. Further research is crucial to identify the underlying factors contributing to these disparities in urban areas. By understanding these factors, we can develop targeted interventions to mitigate the negative effects of food insecurity on children's weight status. Ultimately, such research can inform the creation of programs and policies that promote healthy eating habits, improve access to nutritious food, and ensure food security for all children, regardless of their location or age.

Author Contributions: Conceptualization, J.M.D.; methodology, J.M.D.; validation, J.M.D. and T.A.C.; formal analysis, T.A.C.; writing—original draft preparation, J.M.D.; writing—review and editing, J.M.D., T.A.C., A.N.C., M.A.W., E.A.O., S.Z. and D.T.; visualization, J.M.D.; supervision, J.M.D.; project administration, J.M.D. and T.A.C.; funding acquisition, J.M.D. All authors have read and agreed to the published version of the manuscript.

Funding: This work is a publication of the United States Department of Agriculture/Agricultural Research Service (USDA/ARS) Children's Nutrition Research Center, Department of Pediatrics, Baylor College of Medicine, Houston, Texas, and is funded in part with federal funds from the USDA/ARS under Cooperative Agreement no. 58-3092-0-001 (J.M.D.). The contents of this publication do not necessarily reflect the views or policies of the USDA, nor does mention of trade names, commercial products, or organizations imply endorsement from the US government. This research was also supported by an internal grant funded by the Division of Research, University of Houston awarded to T.A.C.

Institutional Review Board Statement: Data collection for NHANES was approved by the NCHS Research Ethics Review Board (ERB). Analysis of de-identified data from the survey is exempt from the federal regulations for the protection of human research participants. Analysis of restricted data through the NCHS Research Data Center is also approved by the NCHS ERB.

Informed Consent Statement: Not applicable.

Data Availability Statement: For data analysis, we used publicly available data, which can be accessed at https://wwwn.cdc.gov/nchs/nhanes/continuousnhanes/default.aspx?BeginYear=2013 (accessed on 31 January 2019).

Conflicts of Interest: The authors declare no conflicts of interest. The findings and conclusions in this paper are those of the author(s) and do not necessarily represent the views of the Research Data Center, the NCHS, or the CDC.

References

1. Smith, J.D.; Fu, E.; Kobayashi, M.A. Prevention and management of childhood obesity and its psychological and health comorbidities. *Annu. Rev. Clin. Psychol.* **2020**, *16*, 351–378. [CrossRef]
2. Karnik, S.; Kanekar, A. Childhood obesity: A global public health crisis. *Int. J. Prev. Med.* **2012**, *3*, 1–7. [PubMed]
3. Johnson, J.A., III; Johnson, A.M. Urban-rural differences in childhood and adolescent obesity in the United States: A systematic review and meta-analysis. *Child. Obes.* **2015**, *11*, 233–241. [CrossRef] [PubMed]
4. Liu, J.; Bennett, K.J.; Harun, N.; Probst, J.C. Urban-rural differences in overweight status and physical inactivity among US children aged 10-17 years. *J. Rural. Health* **2008**, *24*, 407–415. [CrossRef] [PubMed]
5. Singh, G.K.; Kogan, M.D.; Van Dyck, P.C.; Siahpush, M. Racial/ethnic, socioeconomic, and behavioral determinants of childhood and adolescent obesity in the United States: Analyzing independent and joint associations. *Ann. Epidemiol.* **2008**, *18*, 682–695. [CrossRef] [PubMed]
6. Crouch, E.; Abshire, D.A.; Wirth, M.D.; Hung, P.; Benavidez, G.A. Rural-urban differences in overweight and obesity, physical activity, and food security among children and adolescents. *Prev. Chronic Dis.* **2023**, *20*, E92. [CrossRef] [PubMed]
7. Davy, B.M.; Harrell, K.; Stewart, J.; King, D.S. Body weight status, dietary habits, and physical activity levels of middle school-aged children in rural Mississippi. *South. Med. J.* **2004**, *97*, 571–577. [CrossRef]
8. Crooks, D.L. Food consumption, activity, and overweight among elementary school children in an Appalachian Kentucky community. *Am. J. Phys. Anthropol.* **2000**, *112*, 159–170. [CrossRef]
9. Felton, G.M.; Pate, R.R.; Parsons, M.A.; Ward, D.S.; Saunders, R.P.; Trost, S.; Dowda, M. Health risk behaviors of rural sixth graders. *Res. Nurs. Health* **1998**, *21*, 475–485. [CrossRef]
10. Gustafson-Larson, A.M.; Terry, R.D. Weight-related behaviors and concerns of fourth-grade children. *J. Am. Diet. Assoc.* **1992**, *92*, 818–822. [CrossRef]
11. U.S. Department of Health and Human Services; Health Resources and Services Administration; Maternal and Child Health Bureau. *The Health and Well-Being of Children in Rural Areas: A Portrait of the Nation, 2011–2012*; U.S. Department of Health and Human Services: Rockville, MD, USA, 2015. Available online: https://mchb.hrsa.gov/sites/default/files/mchb/data-research/nsch-health-well-child-rural-04-2015.pdf (accessed on 1 July 2024).
12. Davis, A.M.; Bennett, K.J.; Befort, C.; Nollen, N. Obesity and related health behaviors among urban and rural children in the United States: Data from the National Health And Nutrition Examination Survey 2003–2004 and 2005–2006. *J. Pediatr. Psychol.* **2011**, *36*, 669–676. [CrossRef] [PubMed]
13. Rabbitt, M.P.; Hales, L.J.; Burke, M.P.; Coleman-Jensen, A. Household Food Security in the United States in 2022, ERR-325. Available online: https://www.ers.usda.gov/webdocs/publications/107703/err-325.pdf?v=5285 (accessed on 1 July 2024).
14. Gundersen, C.; Garasky, S.; Lohman, B.J. Food insecurity is not associated with childhood obesity as assessed using multiple measures of obesity. *J. Nutr.* **2009**, *139*, 1173–1178. [CrossRef] [PubMed]
15. Trapp, C.M.; Burke, G.; Gorin, A.A.; Wiley, J.F.; Hernandez, D.; Crowell, R.E.; Grant, A.; Beaulieu, A.; Cloutier, M.M. The relationship between dietary patterns, body mass index percentile, and household food security in young urban children. *Child. Obes.* **2015**, *11*, 148–155. [CrossRef] [PubMed]
16. Holben, D.H.; Taylor, C.A. Food insecurity and its association with central obesity and other markers of metabolic syndrome among persons aged 12 to 18 years in the United States. *J. Am. Osteopath. Assoc.* **2015**, *115*, 536–543. [CrossRef] [PubMed]
17. Centers for Disease Control and Prevention. Childhood Obesity Facts. Available online: https://www.cdc.gov/obesity/php/data-research/childhood-obesity-facts.html (accessed on 1 July 2024).
18. Dyer, O. Obesity in US children increased at an unprecedented rate during the pandemic. *Br. Med. J.* **2021**, *374*, n2332. [CrossRef] [PubMed]
19. Curtin, L.R.; Mohadjer, L.K.; Dohrmann, S.M.; Kruszon-Moran, D.; Mirel, L.B.; Carroll, M.D.; Hirsch, R.; Burt, V.L.; Johnson, C.L. National Health and Nutrition Examination Survey: Sample Design, 2007–2010. Vital and Health Statistics. Series 2, Number 160. Available online: http://www.cdc.gov/nchs/data/series/sr_02/sr02_160.pdf (accessed on 31 May 2024).
20. U.S. Department of Agriculture—Economic Research Service. Urban Influence Codes. Available online: https://www.ers.usda.gov/data-products/urban-influence-codes/ (accessed on 31 May 2024).
21. Centers for Disease Control and Prevention. National Health and Nutrition Examination Survey 1999–2018 Data Documentation, Codebook, and Frequencies: Appendix 1. 1999–2018 GCP Match Census 2010. Available online: https://wwwn.cdc.gov/Nchs/Nhanes/limited_access/GEO_2010.htm#Appendix_1._1999-2018_GCP_Match_Census_2010 (accessed on 31 May 2024).
22. Bickel, G.; Nord, M.; Price, C.; Hamilton, W.; Cook, J. Guide to Measuring Household Food Security, Revised 2000. Available online: https://fns-prod.azureedge.us/sites/default/files/FSGuide.pdf (accessed on 31 May 2024).
23. Gundersen, C.; Lohman, B.J.; Garasky, S.; Stewart, S.; Eisenmann, J. Food security, maternal stressors, and overweight among low-income US children: Results from the National Health and Nutrition Examination Survey (1999–2002). *Pediatrics* **2008**, *122*, e529-40. [CrossRef]
24. National Center for Health Statistics. National Health and Nutrition Examination Survey 2015–2016 Data Documentation, Codebook, and Frequencies. Available online: https://wwwn.cdc.gov/Nchs/Nhanes/2015-2016/FSQ_I.htm (accessed on 31 May 2024).

25. Zipf, G.; Chiappa, M.; Porter, K.S.; Ostchega, Y.; Lewis, B.G.; Dostal, J. *National Health and Nutrition Examination Survey: Plan and operations, 1999–2010*; Vital Health Stat 1 2013; United States Department of Health and Human Services: Washington, DC, USA, 2013; pp. 1–37.
26. Centers for Disease Control and Prevention. NHANES National Youth Fitness Survey, NNYFS 2012 Data Documentation, Codebook, and Frequencies—Weight Status Classifications. Available online: https://wwwn.cdc.gov/Nchs/Nnyfs/Y_BMX.htm#:~:text=Weight%20status%20classification:%20BMI,%20expressed,criteria%20for%20children%20and%20adolescents (accessed on 31 May 2024).
27. Centers for Disease Control and Prevention; National Center for Health Statistics. About the National Health and Nutrition Examination Survey. Available online: https://www.cdc.gov/nchs/nhanes/about_nhanes.htm (accessed on 1 July 2024).
28. Thomas, M.M.C.; Miller, D.P.; Morrissey, T.W. Food insecurity and child health. *Pediatrics* **2019**, *144*, e20190397. [CrossRef] [PubMed]
29. Ke, J.; Ford-Jones, E.L. Food insecurity and hunger: A review of the effects on children's health and behaviour. *Paediatr. Child. Health* **2015**, *20*, 89–91. [CrossRef]
30. Ohri-Vachaspati, P.; DeWeese, R.S.; Acciai, F.; DeLia, D.; Tulloch, D.; Tong, D.; Lorts, C.; Yedidia, M. Healthy food access in low-income high-minority communities: A longitudinal assessment-2009–2017. *Int. J. Environ. Res. Public Health* **2019**, *16*, 2354. [CrossRef]
31. Hilmers, A.; Hilmers, D.C.; Dave, J. Neighborhood disparities in access to healthy foods and their effects on environmental justice. *Am. J. Public Health* **2012**, *102*, 1644–1654. [CrossRef]
32. Ver Ploeg, M. Access to Affordable, Nutritious Food Is Limited in "Food Deserts". Available online: https://www.ers.usda.gov/amber-waves/2010/march/access-to-affordable-nutritious-food-is-limited-in-food-deserts/ (accessed on 31 May 2024).
33. Cairns, G.; Angus, K.; Hastings, G.; Caraher, M. Systematic reviews of the evidence on the nature, extent and effects of food marketing to children. A retrospective summary. *Appetite* **2013**, *62*, 209–215. [CrossRef] [PubMed]
34. Story, M.; French, S. Food advertising and marketing directed at children and adolescents in the US. *Int. J. Behav. Nutr. Phys. Act.* **2004**, *1*, 3. [CrossRef] [PubMed]
35. Harris, J.L.; Pomeranz, J.L.; Lobstein, T.; Brownell, K.D. A crisis in the marketplace: How food marketing contributes to childhood obesity and what can be done. *Annu. Rev. Public Health* **2009**, *30*, 211–225. [CrossRef] [PubMed]
36. Sadeghirad, B.; Duhaney, T.; Motaghipisheh, S.; Campbell, N.R.; Johnston, B.C. Influence of unhealthy food and beverage marketing on children's dietary intake and preference: A systematic review and meta-analysis of randomized trials. *Obes. Rev.* **2016**, *17*, 945–959. [CrossRef] [PubMed]
37. Kraak, V.I.; Story, M.; Wartella, E.A.; Ginter, J. Industry progress to market a healthful diet to American children and adolescents. *Am. J. Prev. Med.* **2011**, *41*, 322–333. [CrossRef]
38. United Nations Development Programme. *Sustainable Urbanization Strategy: UNDP's Support to Sustainable, Inclusive and Resilient Cities in the Developing World*; United Nations Development Programme: New York, NY, USA, 2016.
39. Ver Ploeg, M.; Breneman, V.; Farrigan, T.; Hamrick, K.; Hopkins, D.; Kaufman, P.; Lin, B.H.; Nord, M.; Smith, T.A.; Williams, R.; et al. Access to Affordable and Nutritious Food: Measuring and Understanding Food Deserts and Their Consequences. Report to Congress. Available online: https://www.ers.usda.gov/webdocs/publications/42711/12716_ap036_1_.pdf (accessed on 31 May 2024).
40. Vilar-Compte, M.; Burrola-Méndez, S.; Lozano-Marrufo, A.; Ferré-Eguiluz, I.; Flores, D.; Gaitán-Rossi, P.; Teruel, G.; Pérez-Escamilla, R. Urban poverty and nutrition challenges associated with accessibility to a healthy diet: A global systematic literature review. *Int. J. Equity Health* **2021**, *20*, 40. [CrossRef] [PubMed]
41. Ruel, M.T.; Garrett, J.L. Features of urban food and nutrition security and considerations for successful urban programming. *eJADE Electron. J. Agric. Dev. Econ.* **2004**, *1*, 242–271.
42. Tester, J.M.; Rosas, L.G.; Leung, C.W. Food insecurity and pediatric obesity: A double whammy in the era of COVID-19. *Curr. Obes. Rep.* **2020**, *9*, 442–450. [CrossRef]
43. Lee, A.; Cardel, M.; Donahoo, W.T. Social and environmental factors influencing obesity. In *Endotext*; Feingold, K.R., Anawalt, B., Blackman, M.R., Boyce, A., Chrousos, G., Corpas, E., de Herder, W.W., Dhatariya, K., Dungan, K., Hofland, J., et al., Eds.; MDText.com, Inc.: South Dartmouth, MA, USA, 2000.
44. Ayala, G.X.; Monge-Rojas, R.; King, A.C.; Hunter, R.; Berge, J.M. The social environment and childhood obesity: Implications for research and practice in the United States and countries in Latin America. *Obes. Rev.* **2021**, *22* (Suppl. S3), e13246. [CrossRef]
45. Vargas, C.M.; Stines, E.M.; Granado, H.S. Health-equity issues related to childhood obesity: A scoping review. *J. Public Health Dent.* **2017**, *77* (Suppl. 1), S32–S42. [CrossRef]
46. Lee, G.Y.; Um, Y.J. Factors affecting obesity in urban and rural adolescents: Demographic, socioeconomic characteristics, health behavior and health education. *Int. J. Environ. Res. Public Health* **2021**, *18*, 2405. [CrossRef]

Disclaimer/Publisher's Note: The statements, opinions and data contained in all publications are solely those of the individual author(s) and contributor(s) and not of MDPI and/or the editor(s). MDPI and/or the editor(s) disclaim responsibility for any injury to people or property resulting from any ideas, methods, instructions or products referred to in the content.

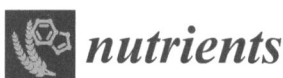

Article

Political Economy of Maternal Child Malnutrition: Experiences about Water, Food, and Nutrition Policies in Pakistan

Farooq Ahmed [1,*], Najma Iqbal Malik [2], Shamshad Bashir [3], Nazia Noureen [4], Jam Bilal Ahmad [5] and Kun Tang [6,*]

1. Department of Anthropology, The Islamia University of Bahawalpur, Bahawalpur 63100, Pakistan
2. Department of Psychology, University of Sargodha, Sargodha 40100, Pakistan; najma.iqbal@uos.edu.pk
3. Department of Psychology, Lahore Garrison University, Lahore 54920, Pakistan; shamshadbashir@lgu.edu.pk
4. Department of Psychology, Foundation University Rawalpindi Campus, Rawalpindi 58001, Pakistan; nazia.ch88@gmail.com
5. Taxila Institute of Asian Studies, Quaid-i-Azam University, Islamabad 45320, Pakistan; jam_bilal@hotmail.com
6. Vanke School of Public Health, Tsinghua University, Beijing 100084, China
* Correspondence: farooq.ahmed@iub.edu.pk (F.A.); tangk@tsinghua.edu.cn (K.T.)

Abstract: This study examined access to water, food, and nutrition programs among marginalized communities in Southern Punjab, Pakistan, and their effects on nutrition. Both qualitative and quantitative data were used in this study. We held two focus group discussions (one with 10 males and one with 10 females) and conducted in-depth interviews with 15 key stakeholders, including 20 mothers and 10 healthcare providers. A survey of 235 households was carried out to evaluate water and food insecurity, with the data analyzed using Wilcoxon's rank-sum test, t-test, and Pearson's chi-square test. The results revealed that 90% of households experienced moderate-to-severe water insecurity, and 73% faced moderate-to-severe food insecurity. Household water and food insecurity were positively correlated with each other (correlation coefficient = 0.205; $p = 0.004$). Greater household water ($p = 0.028$) and food insecurity ($p < 0.001$) were both associated with higher perceived stress. Furthermore, lower socioeconomic status was strongly related to higher levels of water ($p < 0.001$) and food insecurity ($p < 0.001$). Qualitative findings highlight the impact of colonial and post-colonial policies, which have resulted in water injustice, supply issues, and corruption in water administration. Women face significant challenges in fetching water, including stigma, harassment, and gender vulnerabilities, leading to conflicts and injuries. Water scarcity and poor quality adversely affect sanitation, hygiene, and breastfeeding practices among lactating mothers. Structural adjustment policies have exacerbated inflation and reduced purchasing power. Respondents reported a widespread lack of dietary diversity and food quality. Nutrition programs face obstacles such as the exclusion of people with low social and cultural capital, underfunding, weak monitoring, health sector corruption, and the influence of formula milk companies allied with the medical community and bureaucracy. This study concludes that addressing the macro-political and economic causes of undernutrition should be prioritized to improve nutrition security in Pakistan.

Keywords: political economics; water insecurity experiences; food insecurity experiences; nutrition policies; social exclusion; mix-methods; Pakistan

Citation: Ahmed, F.; Malik, N.I.; Bashir, S.; Noureen, N.; Ahmad, J.B.; Tang, K. Political Economy of Maternal Child Malnutrition: Experiences about Water, Food, and Nutrition Policies in Pakistan. *Nutrients* 2024, *16*, 2642. https://doi.org/10.3390/nu16162642

Academic Editors: Ariana Saraiva and António Raposo

Received: 5 July 2024
Revised: 7 August 2024
Accepted: 8 August 2024
Published: 10 August 2024

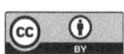

Copyright: © 2024 by the authors. Licensee MDPI, Basel, Switzerland. This article is an open access article distributed under the terms and conditions of the Creative Commons Attribution (CC BY) license (https://creativecommons.org/licenses/by/4.0/).

1. Introduction

Globally, malnutrition accounts for fifty percent of child mortality cases each year, with Severe Acute Malnutrition (SAM) causing the death of one in every three affected children [1]. The highest rates of underweight and stunting are found in Sub-Saharan Africa and South Asia, with 78% of wasted children residing in Bangladesh, India, and Pakistan [2–5]. However, Pakistan has a higher ratio of child malnutrition cases compared to its South Asian counterparts [6,7]. The Pakistan Demographic and Health Survey 2018 indicates that mortality is highest among the most deprived sections of the population [8].

Under-nutrition among children under five is more prevalent in the poorest and most rural areas compared to wealthiest quintiles and urban regions [9]. In rural areas, 44% of children suffer from stunting, 32% are underweight, and 19% experience wasting. In contrast, urban areas report lower rates: 35% stunting, 24% underweight, and 17% wasting [9]. Southern Pakistan regions, such as Sindh, Baluchistan, and South Punjab, have stunting rates between 45–48%, higher than the KP, ICT, and national averages of 35–40%. Within Punjab, South Punjab shows a significantly higher rate of underweight children (26.4%) compared to the rest of Punjab (18.7%), with the highest prevalence in the districts of Rajanpur (34%), Rahim Yar Khan (33%), and D.G. Khan (32%) [10].

Recent systematic reviews in developing countries reveal that multiple social, economic, and political factors indirectly or directly influence the nutritional status of children [11], for example, antenatal care [12], higher fertility [13], maternal illiteracy [14], maternal stress, breastfeeding frequency [15], low caste or class [16], poverty [17], lack of food intake owing to a decline in production [18], and area of residence [19]. These factors can act separately or in combination. In addition, the connection between water, food, and nutrition is well recognized [20]. Water is essential for maintaining a healthy environment. Effective water management is crucial for mitigating water and food insecurity at the household level [21]. Furthermore, effective public nutrition programs are crucial for reducing malnutrition rates [22]. In Pakistan, development programs have been unsuccessful in addressing malnutrition because they have overlooked the entrenched social structures of inequality. The Benazir Income Support Program (BISP), proposed by the World Bank and the world's largest social protection initiative in Pakistan post-2010, proved less effective in improving the status of poor women, ensuring food security, and alleviating hunger due to its disregard for socio-cultural power dynamics. Also, the Community Management of Acute Malnutrition (CMAM), a temporary therapeutic program targeting SAM, was implemented in impoverished southern districts; however, these interventions failed to consider ongoing power dynamics and ignored unequal social relationships [23].

This study contends that malnutrition stems from unequal access to various essential resources. People's access to fundamental nutritional resources, market commodities, and development programs is influenced by their social, economic, and cultural capital. Social groups from remote, rural areas and those belonging to lower castes, classes, and capital are often deprived [24]. Critical medical anthropologists assert that development and biomedical approaches typically focus on curing the "individual body" rather than addressing the "social body". They argue that these approaches fail to consider humans and their experiences of insecurity, illness, and suffering from a holistic perspective [25]. Political economics is essential for understanding the formulation and implementation of public policies and their broader impacts on the economy and social systems. Prominent programs and policies such as the "Green Revolution" and "Structural Adjustments", which shaped the lives of people in developing countries, underscore the significant influence of neoliberal hegemony [26,27].

Politico-economic factors such as colonial history, political instability, structural adjustments, privatization, inadequate market regulation, and foreign debt policies have led to a lack of comprehensive social welfare and unmet governance promises [28–31]. As a result, the state has struggled to manage inflation and provide equitable health and nutrition services. In their most critical periods, mothers and children require diverse social determinants for their well-being [32]. However, in developing countries such as Pakistan, low trade, a fragile economy, and corruption hinder the provision of quality services. Consequently, various groups, including those in the southern regions, face marginalized and insecure living conditions due to their limited access to resources in a privatized, market-driven economy. Previous public health research on malnutrition in Pakistan has often overlooked these broader structural issues, instead attributing problems to local cultures under the influence of neoliberalism [23].

Malnutrition rates are highest in Africa and South Asia, regions that were once colonized. In Pakistan, malnutrition can be seen as a significant postcolonial and post-development challenge. The social, cultural, and economic engineering during colonial and postcolonial periods contributed to the current high prevalence of malnutrition in low-priority areas [25,26]. Resource control was designed and managed to replace indigenous knowledge and practices, reinforce hierarchical inequalities, and foster dependency on external assistance. Interventions to combat malnutrition have often disregarded local socio-cultural contexts, leading to failures in providing equitable access to essential resources.

The impact of political economy has seldom been considered in understanding how colonial, neo-colonial, and neoliberal influences and regional disparities are linked to structural vulnerability. To address this gap, the present study deconstructs the politico-economic factors that adversely affect potential nutritional resources, including water, food, and community-level nutrition programs. This study aims to investigate how experiences of resource insecurity contribute to malnutrition in Southern Pakistan. We hypothesized that household water insecurity is positively correlated with household food insecurity. We further hypothesize that households' lower socioeconomic status and higher perceived stress levels are strongly associated with increased household water and food insecurity.

2. Materials and Methods

2.1. Data Collection and Analysis

The conceptual framework developed by UNICEF (1990) showed mortality and malnutrition as a collective outcome of immediate, underlying, and basic causes. The immediate causes (illness) depend on the underlying causes (inadequate access to food, care, and a healthy environment). Inadequate access is, however, shaped by the following basic causes: political, economic, institutional, ideologies, and policies. The conceptual framework provided below has been adjusted to fit the local context and specific needs. We explore, examine, and interpret experiences about the lack of access to potential resources, particularly water security, food security, public health nutrition programs, and care. We describe how the lack of social and cultural capital affects access to nutritional-specific and sensitive programs controlled by power institutions such as bureaucracy (Figure 1).

Critical medical-nutritional anthropologists frequently suggest examining the political and economic context of local food and water insecurity. This involves conducting in-depth interviews alongside household surveys to better understand and address the nuances of these issues [33]. Therefore, for this study, both qualitative and quantitative methods were employed. First, using snowball sampling, we gathered data from five key informants who had profound knowledge about the area, history, and geography. With the help of these key informants, two focus group discussions (one with males and one with females) were conducted in the most water-insecure areas. In each focus group, which lasted nearly two hours, a maximum of 10 participants were allowed to participate. The group discussions and key informant interviews covered topics such as water justice and the coping strategies of marginalized communities, issues related to water fetching and gender sensitivities, and impacts on agriculture, livestock, Water, Sanitation, and Hygiene (WASH), and Infant and Young Child Feeding (IYCF). Questions also addressed food insecurity, focusing on food affordability, quality versus quantity, and food diversity.

Next, using purposive sampling methods, we started in-depth interviews with key stakeholders, focusing first on healthcare providers (supply side) and then on the mothers of malnourished children (demand side) who were registered and enrolled in the therapeutic program. As interviews were conducted first with healthcare providers, nutrition experts, and key officials from the Health Department (n = 10), it helped identify 30 mothers of severely malnourished children. However, we could obtain consent from only 20 mothers after navigating the gatekeepers (Table 1).

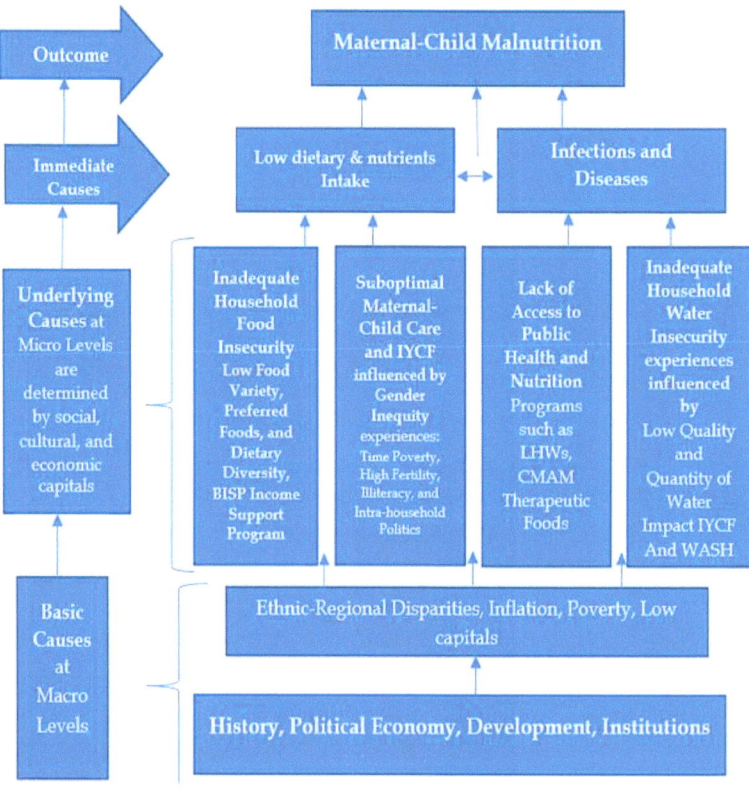

Figure 1. Conceptual framework showing causes of malnutrition.

Table 1. Details about the Respondents.

Details about Discussion and Interviews of This Study	No of Respondents (n)
2 FGDs (1 with males and 1 with Females)	20
Key Informant Interviews in the Community	5
Key Informant Interviews with Healthcare Providers	5
Key Informant Interviews Officers in Nutrition Stabilization Centers	5
In-depth Interviews of local mothers availing Nutrition Programs	20

An interview guide was created to explore the significant structural challenges and barriers faced by women during treatment and therapeutic coverage. This guide was pilot-tested with a few mothers. To ensure comfort and engagement, interviews were conducted at the local residences of the participants. Mothers were queried about their access to healthcare, nutrition-specific and sensitive programs, nutrition stabilization centers, and lady health workers, as well as the obstacles and challenges they face in gaining access to these services. Face-to-face semi-structured interviews were conducted in the participants' local Seraiki language, allowing for a flexible format that lasted between 1–2 h. The sociodemographic characteristics of these mother are given in Table 2.

Table 2. Characteristics of Mothers (*n* = 20).

Indicator	Frequency	Percentage
Mothers' Age		
18 to 24	6	(30%)
25 to 29	5	(25%)
30 to 34	5	(25%)
34 to 40	4	(20%)
Literacy of Mothers		
Illiterate	16	(80%)
~5th–8th	3	(15%)
~10th	1	(5%)
15 to 20	2	(10%)
Occupation of Mothers		
Agriculture	11	(55%)
Domestic labour	7	(35%)
Other	2	(10%)
Income of Household per Month		
~10 K PKR (~90 USD)	10	(50%)
~15 K PKR (~135 USD)	7	(35%)
≥16 K PKR (~150 USD)	3	(15%)

All raw qualitative data and field notes gathered during focus groups, KII, and IDI were carefully reviewed and translated verbatim into English. Key texts and narratives were coded and organized based on common meanings and categories by two researchers. Then, we congregated similar codes to produce wider classifications. Next, narratives were authenticated, inconsistencies were removed, categories were reassessed, and frequently visible subthemes began evolving from the whole data. Both inductive and deductive methods were used by these researchers to identify potential themes and sub-themes from the qualitative data analysis. In the end, three major themes and multiple sub-themes emerged from qualitative data, which have been arranged in three parts in the diagram given below (Figure 2).

Secondly, this study utilized data from a small-scale survey (*n* = 235) conducted in 2018 in water-insecure districts of South Punjab to assess experiences related to water and food insecurity. The FGDs we mentioned earlier were instrumental in determining the survey areas. Additionally, the individuals involved in both the FGDs and the survey were from the same group and communities. The first author (F.A.), a co-investigator from Pakistan and collaborator with an international water consortium, helped develop the Household Water InSecurity Experiences (HWISE) Scale. This scale, used across various cultural settings in 23 low- and middle-income countries, assessed household water insecurity through 34 items covering water attainment, usage, and storage, as well as food insecurity. After applying item-response theories and classical-test methods, 12 items were retained for analysis. Factor analyses demonstrated that these items were unidimensional and reliable (Cronbach's alpha 0.832), and the scale established construct, predictive, convergent, and discriminant validity [34]. The questionnaire was translated from English into Urdu and Seraiki by the first author and adapted for use in South Punjab.

Based on previous area information and key informants' knowledge, households from water insecure clusters were selected through cluster sampling (selection of insecure clusters) and Simple Random Sampling (WHO walk every 3rd HHD) techniques. Enumerators, selected for their experience in survey implementation, familiarity with the area, and fluency in local languages, underwent a 1- to 2-day training. Each day, at the end of the interviews, these surveyors were debriefed, and detailed field notes were extracted. In addition to the items on water insecurity described earlier, data were collected on socio-demographic characteristics, household food insecurity using the Household Food Insecurity Access Scale, and perceived stress using a modified 4-item perceived stress scale.

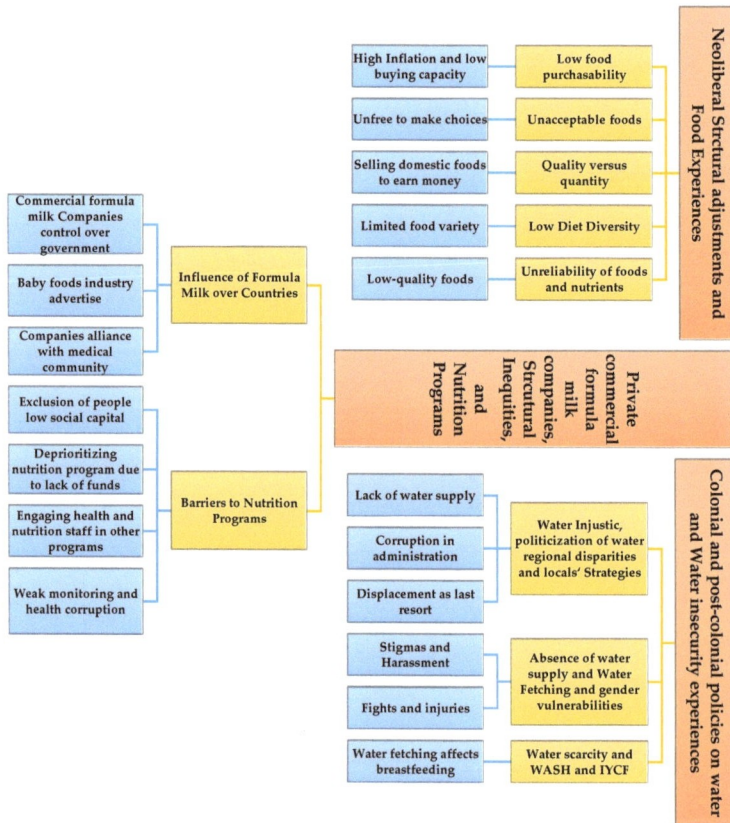

Figure 2. Graphic abstract showing insecurity experiences about water, food, and nutrition programs.

Household Food Insecurity Access Scale (HFIAS) scores and associated indicators, as well as Household Water Insecurity Experiences (HWISE) Scale scores and associated indicators, were calculated using a standardized methodology. Briefly, responses (0 = "never", 1 = "rarely", 2 = "sometimes", 3 = "often" or "always") to each of the 12 items were summed [34]. For all items, responses of "do not know" or "not applicable" were coded as missing, except for the question about water interruptions, for which "not applicable" was recoded as zero. Households were classified as having no-to-marginal (HWISE Scale scores of 0–2), low (3–11), moderate (12–23), or high (24–36). Basic descriptive statistics (Wilcoxon's rank-sum test, t-test, and Pearson's chi-square test) were used to assess whether sociodemographic characteristics, perceived stress, and experiences with resource insecurity varied by water or food insecurity status. We also examined whether continuous food and water insecurity scores were correlated with each other (see Figure 3). Analyses were completed using Stata (v18).

Of a total of 235, 42.55% were male and 57.45% were female. The majority belonged to the occupations of agriculture (<50%) and labor (~22%). The primary monthly income of the majority of participants was less than RS. 20,000 PKR (<100 USD), see Table 3.

Water insecurity
(n=207)

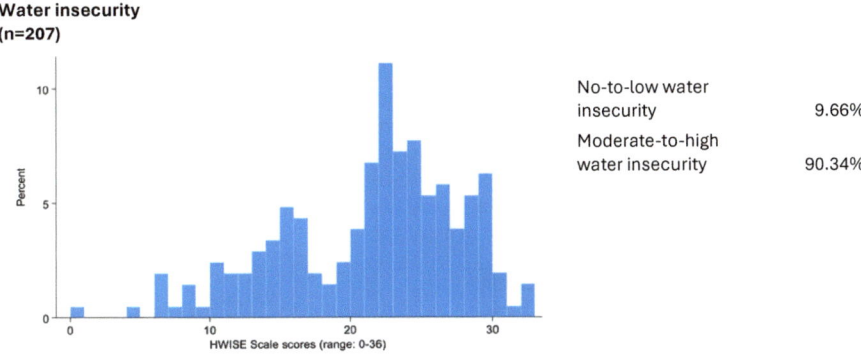

No-to-low water insecurity	9.66%
Moderate-to-high water insecurity	90.34%

Food insecurity
(n=219)

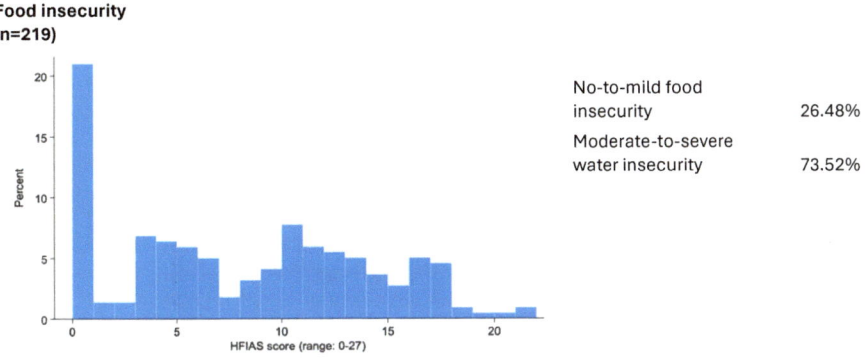

No-to-mild food insecurity	26.48%
Moderate-to-severe water insecurity	73.52%

Correlation (n=198) 0.205 (p=0.004)

Figure 3. Correlation between continuous food and water insecurity scores.

Table 3. Sociodemographic Characteristics of Participants (n = 235).

Indicator	Frequency	Percentage
Sex of Participants		
Female	135	57.45%
Male	100	42.55%
Occupation of Household Head		
Cultivation	110	46.80%
Laborers	52	22.12%
Small business	30	12.76%
Basic subsistence	28	11.91%
Salaried	13	5.53%
Monthly Income of Household		
≤Rs. 10,000 (~90 USD)	135	57.45%
≤Rs. 20,000 (~180 USD)	56	23.82%
≥Rs. 21,000 (~200 USD)	44	18.72%

Source: Household Water and Food Insecurity Survey 2018.

2.2. Ethical Consideration

The Advanced Studies and Research Board of Quaid-i-Azam University Islamabad provided approval for this study. Along with obtaining oral consent from the local population, the purpose and nature of this research were communicated to the participants. In addition, this research strictly adheres to the well-versed approval, confidentiality, privacy, and anonymity of all the study respondents. To seek their formal consent, we informed all these mothers about the kind of research. Respondents' places were deliberately chosen so they could not feel uncomfortable during probing. We also did not use audio recorders due to the cultural sensitivity of local norms.

2.3. Strength and Limitation

The methodology has some limitations. First, translating questionnaires from English to the local language and then back to English may have impacted the accuracy of the meanings. Second, a few respondents showed feelings of mistrust or evasion regarding the survey. Additionally, conducting two separate investigations—focus groups and the survey—in the same community at different times presents a methodological limitation. Nevertheless, using qualitative methods alongside the structured survey offers triangulation, which strengthens this study by validating the results.

3. Results

3.1. Quantitative Water and Food Insecurity Experiences

The hypothesis that a positive correlation exists between continuous food and water insecurity scores was confirmed by the statistical analysis, with a p-value of 0.004, indicating statistical significance between HWISE and HFIAS scores (Figure 3).

The interpretation of our results in Table 4 is as follows: (1) greater number of children in the household associated with greater water insecurity; (2) lower monthly income associated with greater water insecurity ($p < 0.001$); (3) lower perceived SES associated with greater water insecurity ($p < 0.001$); (4) greater access to a basic drinking water source (relative to a less-than-basic water source) associated with greater water insecurity; (5) drinking water thought to be unsafe in the prior month associated with greater water insecurity; (6) borrowing water from others in the prior month associated with greater water insecurity ($p < 0.001$); (7) higher perceived stress associated with greater water insecurity ($p = 0.028$); (8) greater percentage of households with high water insecurity experience severe food insecurity relative to households with no-to-low or moderate water insecurity.

Table 4. Household water characteristics in South Punjab, Pakistan ($n = 207$).

	No-to-Low Water Insecurity	Moderate Water Insecurity	High Water Insecurity	
	(N = 20)	(N = 108)	(N = 79)	p
Woman household head	5.0%	10.2%	11.4%	0.699
Respondent age (years), mean ± SD	35.3 ± 8.5	34.3 ± 9.6	36.0 ± 9.7	0.471
Number of children living in household, mean ± SD	3.0 ± 1.8	3.6 ± 2.0	4.8 ± 2.2	<0.001
Monthly income (USD), median (IQR)	99 (47–180)	90 (59–180)	63 (45–99)	<0.001
Perceived SES standing (1 = best, 10 = worst), mean ± SD	6.3 ± 1.5	7.3 ± 1.5	8.0 ± 1.1	<0.001
Basic drinking water source	73.7%	92.4%	94.9%	0.010
Drank water thought to be unsafe	80.0%	98.1%	100.0%	<0.001
Borrowed water from others	57.9%	84.8%	96.2%	<0.001

Table 4. Cont.

	No-to-Low Water Insecurity	Moderate Water Insecurity	High Water Insecurity	
	(N = 20)	(N = 108)	(N = 79)	p
Perceived Stress Score (range: 0–16), median (IQR)	4 (2–5)	5 (4–9)	7 (3–10)	0.028
HFIAS score (range: 0–27), median (IQR)	5 (0–9)	7 (3–12)	8 (0–14)	0.201
Food insecurity category				
No-to-mild	33.3%	23.5%	30.8%	0.041
Moderate	38.9%	43.1%	21.8%	
Severe	27.8%	33.3%	47.4%	

HWISE Data.

The interpretation of our results in Table 5 is as follows: (1) households headed by women are less likely to have severe food insecurity; (2) lower monthly income is associated with greater food insecurity ($p < 0.001$); (3) lower perceived SES is associated with greater food insecurity ($p < 0.001$); and (4) higher perceived stress is associated with greater food insecurity ($p < 0.001$).

Table 5. Household food characteristics in South Punjab, Pakistan ($n = 219$).

	No-to-Mild Food Insecurity	Moderate Food Insecurity	Severe Food Insecurity	
	(N = 58)	(N = 75)	(N = 86)	p
Woman household head	17.2%	5.3%	7.0%	0.041
Respondent age (years), mean ± SD	33.7 ± 8.5	35.7 ± 9.7	36.3 ± 10.1	0.268
Number of children living in household, mean ± SD	4.1 ± 2.3	3.5 ± 2.0	4.3 ± 2.2	0.065
Monthly income (USD), median (IQR)	144 (90–225)	108 (63–180)	63 (45–90)	<0.001
Perceived SES standing (1 = best, 10 = worst), mean ± SD	6.9 ± 1.6	6.8 ± 1.7	8.3 ± 1.0	<0.001
Perceived Stress Score (range: 0–16), median (IQR)	4 (2–4)	4 (4–9)	8 (6–10)	<0.001

HWISE Data.

Our other hypotheses that lower socioeconomic status and high stress are associated with greater water insecurity and food insecurity are established by the statistical analysis, with the *p*-values demonstrating positive statistical significance as shown in Tables 4 and 5.

3.2. Qualitative Water and Food Insecurity Experiences

Inadequate, unsafe, and low-quality water and food, combined with limited access to healthcare and nutrition programs, negatively impact community health and nutrition. Marginalized communities' experiences with these vital resources need to be explored at deeper levels to link with the high malnutrition prevalence in southern regions.

3.2.1. Water Insecurity Experiences at the Community Level

Water security is an essential component of human health and nutrition. Water insecurity experiences at the community level can help us understand the major causes of the problem and the associated implications for the health of mothers and children. The following major themes and sub-themes emerged from qualitative data (Table 6).

Table 6. Water Insecurity Experiences.

Theme	Sub-Theme	Narratives
Water injustice and communities' coping strategies	Absence of water supply and availability of bad-quality water	"In the past, water distribution was much better, but now it primarily benefits large landlords and people in power. Small landholders in the South frequently experience water shortages. This change began after colonization and land control, and the situation worsened when landlords started profiting from cash crops in the 1960s". (KII, Male, 48) "Canal water distribution in the South Punjab region is unfair, as water is available for less than six months. The canals are controlled by bureaucracy. In many areas of the D.G. Khan division, floodwater is collected in ditches because the underground water is heavy and salty. There is no water supply available here, so water supply schemes are essential. People rely solely on rain or floodwater and pray for rain in the Suleiman Mountains. The responsibility of carrying water primarily falls on women and children". (KII, Male, 45) "The public water supply is consistently unreliable, and the available water is unclean. We have no choice but to use this poor-quality water. The government supports foreign private companies in selling water, but we can't afford bottled water, so we are forced to drink the unclean water". (FGD, Mother, 34)
	Corruption in administration	"The canal's width is narrow, and powerful individuals illegally divert water by creating cuts due to corruption in the irrigation department. As a result, the water level at the tail end is reduced, leaving insufficient water for crops". (KII, Male, 57)
	Displacement as a last resort	"People often have to migrate when the water supply runs out. During their journey, they frequently become homeless and lack access to food, water, and toilets". (FGD, Male, 53)
Water fetching and gender vulnerabilities	Stigmas and harassment	"People may provide water, but they demand something difficult in return. Harassment and even rape are common occurrences while fetching water. (KII, Female, 53)
	Fetching water difficulties	"Fetching water is exhausting; it takes children and women an hour, and in the summer, it becomes even greater challenge". (FGD, Mother, 27)
	Fights and injuries	"Fetching water results in health problems, injuries, and conflicts".
Water scarcity, WASH and IYCF	Feeding requires safe water	"Dirty and muddy water often makes our young children sick and contaminates our food. Doctors recommend mineral water from private companies for sick children, but it is too expensive for most poor and rural mothers to afford". (FGD, Female, 26)
	Fetching affects breastfeeding behaviors	"During the summer months of June, July, and August, the water situation causes significant stress for mothers, leading to increased maternal stress. Consequently, infants suffer due to reduced breastfeeding". (FGD, Female, 19)
Water-food nexus	Low agricultural production	"We can't grow crops during water shortages, which causes our lands to dry up. As hunger increases, we are forced to sell our land at low prices and migrate to earn money for survival". (KII, Female, 53)
	Less milk production	"Our cattle have stopped producing milk due to a lack of food. When our livestock drink less water, their milk production decreases significantly". (FGD, Male, 40)

Source: Field data.

3.2.2. Food Insecurity Experiences at Community Level

Food insecurity and malnutrition are inseparable. Understanding our experiences with food insecurity can help us determine the underlying causes of maternal-child malnutrition. The following major themes and subthemes emerged from qualitative data (Table 7).

Table 7. Food Insecurity Experiences.

Themes	Sub-Themes	Narratives
Diet quality vs. quantity	Daily diet or staple food	"The government historically supported profitable crops like tobacco, sugar, cotton, and wheat, which significantly reduced the cultivation of fruits and vegetables". (KII, 45) "While a variety of items are available in the market, wheat remains the staple diet for most people here. The poor mainly eat wheat bread with a mixture of mint, green chili, and onion". (KII, 38)
	Inflation reduces buying capacity	"Inflation has made our lives very difficult; we dilute a liter of milk with water to stretch its quantity. Meat and fruit are rare in our diet because they are too expensive. Everyone seems worried and mentally stressed due to the rampant inflation". (FGD, Mother, 34)
Preferred vs. disliked food	Unable to make choices freely	"Highly marginalized household domestic workers often collect expired or leftover food from the homes where they work. To manage the smell, we heat the food because we can't afford to buy fresh items". (IDI, Domestic household servant, 29)
Food availability and accessibility	Selling domestic food items to earn a little money	"Poor rural people often sell milk, eggs, or chickens in the local market to earn a little money, but their children often go hungry. They are compelled to sell these items, especially when they are ill or need money for medical treatment. One day at the market, I saw two young children selling a chicken. I asked how much they were selling it for, and the older boy said '400 rupees.' After I paid and took the chicken, the younger child began to cry. I asked him why he was crying, and his older brother said, 'There is nothing.' I was puzzled and asked the older brother to explain. The older boy tearfully revealed that the chicken belonged to his younger brother, who had also eaten its eggs. They were selling it out of necessity because their mother was very sick, and they needed the money for her treatment. The younger brother was distressed because he didn't want to part with the chicken he loved". (KII, Journalist)
Food diversity	Limited food variety and hidden hunger	"Poor mothers and their children can only fill their stomachs with potatoes, peas, and wheat. A diverse and nutritious diet is also crucial". (KII, Nutrition expert from the community)
	All is good for the poor	"Only the names of desirable foods can be mentioned, but they cannot be eaten. For the poor and hungry, anything that is available and accessible is acceptable". (IDI, Mother, 33)
Reliability of food and governance	Commercialization of low-quality junk food	"In the past, people were healthier and happier, free from many diseases. Now, everything is becoming expensive and of poor quality due to a lack of regulation. Milk, medicine, cooking oil—everything is substandard, and there is no one to enforce price and quality controls". (IDI, Local traditional pharmacist)

Source: Field data.

3.2.3. Experiences with Nutritional Programs and Policies

Nutrition-specific and sensitive programs are supposed to facilitate malnourished mothers and children. Poor and marginalized mothers' experiences of negotiating these programs can better explain the real situation on the ground. Table 8 explores the structural barriers, inequities, and governmentality mothers face at the community level.

Table 8. Experiences with Nutrition Programs, Policies, and Access.

Themes	Sub-Themes	Narratives
Global impact of private sector and formula milk companies on countries	Formula milk companies hunt for clients in healthcare settings	"Multinational formula milk representatives are allowed to operate in healthcare centers and promote formula milk to parents of malnourished children. After children recover from SAM with the use of formula 75 or 100 and then Ready-to-Use Therapeutic Food (RUTF), mothers are encouraged by doctors and these representatives to continue using their products". (KII, Nutrition Stabilization Center staff)
	Formula milk companies 'control over the government	"The deliberate lack of oversight or restrictions on the free movement of formula milk company representatives in hospitals indicates a strong influence of these companies over government institutions and bureaucracy". (KII)
	Baby food industry advertisement	"The baby food industry frequently misleads and deceives parents about their products. They use labeling to enhance their messaging and boost sales, but restrictions are seldom imposed". (KII)
	Pakistan Medical Association promotes MNCs	"On what basis is the Pakistan Medical Association running advertisements against open milk? Is it driven by public concern or the funding from multinational companies (MNCs)? Poor farmers sell cow or buffalo milk to these companies at low rates (50–60 rupees), which is then processed into products. In the village, we used to consume open milk and everyone was healthy. The government should investigate these ads and uncover the hidden interests behind them, with the support of the Punjab Food Authority, to ensure transparency and ease in the delivery of open milk". (KII, journalist)
	Formula milk companies in alliance with the medical community	"Although legislation exists to restrict formula milk, companies bribe medical doctors to promote their products. As of now, a federal board and provincial sub-committees to oversee this issue have not yet been established". (KII, Health Official)
Barriers to nutrition-specific and sensitive programs	Lack of a sustainable nutrition policy	Historically, the country has lacked a consistent nutrition policy. Policies have frequently shifted, ranging from food distribution and card-based rationing to cash transfers like BISP, and programs such as Safe Motherhood, CMAM, EPI, MNCH, School Health and Nutrition Program, Tawana Pakistan Project, Sasti Roti Scheme, and the recent "No One Sleeps Hungry" initiative. Each government introduces its policies and programs, highlighting the need for a sustainable and consistent approach". (KII, Nutrition expert)
	Social exclusion of people with low social capital and bureaucratic red-tapism	"Poor and low-caste women often face challenges accessing health and therapeutic programs, while those who are better-off benefit more easily due to their connections with staff and influential figures. To become beneficiaries of the BISP cash program, some women who were missing documentation went to file a complaint but were stopped by the police at the gate. Those who managed to enter the office were shuffled from one department to another, with staff telling them, 'I can't help you; go talk to someone else' or 'I don't have time, come back next month.' The process is exhausting and frustrating, with the poor having to navigate bureaucratic hurdles for years, while the wealthy can get assistance in just minutes". (IDI, Widow enrolled in BISP Program)
	Sociocultural factors, inadequate care, maternal illiteracy, high fertility, and time poverty	"Poverty, traditional gender roles, social stigma against contraception, preference for male children, and side effects of modern contraceptives are key factors contributing to high fertility rates. Frequent pregnancies and inadequate healthcare lead to maternal malnutrition. The demands of economic activities, caring for the husband and his family, domestic chores, and working in agricultural fields significantly burden mothers". (KII, Population Officer)

Table 8. *Cont.*

Themes	Sub-Themes	Narratives
Barriers to nutrition-specific and sensitive programs	Inadequate funding deprioritizes nutrition by health bureaucracy	"The CMAM program has become less effective as a significant portion of funds are diverted to other public programs, such as the polio eradication initiative. The coverage of nutrition-related projects is limited due to insufficient budgetary allocations". (KII, Nutrition Coordinator)
	Insufficient allocation of resources and a shortage of healthcare staff in remote areas	"In South Punjab, a marginalized and underdeveloped region with low literacy rates, structural issues hinder female health workers from filling their designated roles in remote health units. In Southern Punjab, less than half of the Basic Health Units have successfully appointed Lady Health Workers (LHWs) to fill vacancies. For instance, the Rajanpur District Health Information System reported that out of 900 LHW positions, only 650 were filled, leaving 250 positions still vacant". (KII, Health Official)
	Absenteeism and engaging health workers in non-nutrition programs	"In several remote areas, LHWs are frequently absent. Their excessive involvement in other tasks has led to the deprioritization of nutrition activities within the health department. The workload for LHWs should be reduced, and maternal-child health and nutrition should be given a higher priority on their agenda". (KII, Healthcare Provider)
	Geographical constraints	"Nutritional aid delivery is frequently limited due to logistical challenges faced by rural and marginalized communities".
	Other stakeholders' performance	"Many female school teachers and NGO staff were involved in misusing and selling food that was intended for distribution among girls in rural public schools". (IDI, Mother, 40)
	Left against medical advice (LAMA) cases	"Most cases of SAM were from poor, geographically isolated, and flood-affected areas. Children with SAM were admitted to the Nutrition Stabilization Center for treatment with antibiotics and formula milk 75 or 100 until they recovered. Poor mothers, fathers, or grandmothers often had to stay at the center to care for their severely ill and malnourished children. However, many of them eventually abandoned the treatment because they needed to care for other children at home". (KII, Nutrition stabilization center staff)
	Weak system of data management, monitoring, corruption,	"The system for collecting, monitoring, and evaluating data is weak, making strategic planning difficult. Corruption and unethical sales of therapeutic food require monitoring and fair distribution. These issues hinder the effective implementation of nutrition programs". (KII, Senior Health Official)

Source: Field Data.

4. Discussion

This study examined whether continuous food and water insecurity scores were correlated with each other and assessed whether sociodemographic characteristics, perceived stress, and experiences with resource insecurity varied by water or food insecurity status. The quantitative data analysis validated the first hypothesis, showing a positive correlation between household water insecurity and food insecurity with a significant p-value of 0.004 (Figure 3). Additionally, lower socioeconomic status was linked to higher levels ($p < 0.001$) of both water and food insecurity (Tables 4 and 5 respectively). The hypothesis that higher perceived stress is associated with increased household water and food insecurity was also confirmed, with statistically significant p-values ($p = 0.028$ for water insecurity and $p < 0.001$ for food insecurity). In sub-Saharan Africa, significant links between resource insecurity and psychological health have been observed, with research highlighting strong correlations between stress and limited access to preferred food and water [35]. These results are consistent with recent studies in low- and middle-income settings, which attribute water and food insecurity to structural causes at lower levels. These insecurities are interrelated and contribute to a syndemic relationship with stress and overall well-being [36,37].

The findings indicated that water injustice, by interacting with food insecurity, inadequate WASH and IYCF practices, maternal illness, and low breastfeeding, contributes to both acute and chronic malnutrition at the microlevel. Low-income households have faced reduced dietary diversity and a limited range of foods due to ongoing poverty and inflation. It is generally accepted that economic poverty causes mental distress, but a shortage of food or water can also induce stress [38]. The distress caused by water and food insecurity may be complex, as both are significant contributing factors [39]. Stress can arise from various mechanisms, such as material deprivation, shame or stigma, concerns about health and safety, interpersonal conflict, intimate partner violence, and institutional injustice [40]. Several studies emphasize the links between food and water insecurity, highlighting the importance of advocating for policies and interventions that simultaneously address all resource insecurity issues by governmental and non-governmental organizations [41–43].

4.1. Political Economy of Water Insecurity

Qualitative data reveal that water insecurity in southern Punjab is primarily due to water injustice. Specifically, canal water in this region is available for less than six months a year, unlike the rest of Punjab, where it is accessible year-round. This water insecurity affects maternal and child health through various pathways, including gender inequities and inadequate IYCF and WASH conditions. The southern areas are particularly disadvantaged due to the macro-level water situation. Evidence indicates that micro-level water distribution has been consistently neglected. The current irrigation system, which relies on barrages, weirs, and permanent headworks established during British colonial rule, replaced the traditional system of seasonal canals and disrupted the local harvesting practices that were well-suited to the environment [44]. The primary motivation behind this shift in irrigation in central and southwest Punjab was to develop canal colonies and clusters, creating new socio-cultural and economic structures [45]. During the colonial period from 1885 to 1947, over a million people were relocated to nine canal settlements. This led to the creation of a gravity-based, multi-level canal system, which ultimately resulted in a hierarchically controlled network of sub-canals, disadvantaging tail-end farmers due to issues with village course inlets or the Moga system [46] (p. 30), which is consistent with our findings.

Instead of directly addressing individual or farmer access to water, the distribution was influenced by another irrigation control factor: the amount of land connected to each outlet [47]. Under British rule, land proportions became a tool for water allocation, benefiting landlords and creating a discriminatory land division that hindered fair water distribution in Punjab [48]. Colonial policies reinforced the power of rural elites, perpetuated social stratification and class manipulation, and prevented lower sections of society from fully benefiting from agriculture [49]. The undue advantage given to large landholders exacerbated livelihood insecurity as the concurrent mechanization of agriculture continued to shape the social reality of water access [46].

The Green Revolution primarily benefited large landholders who could afford the costly new machinery, leaving small landholders unable to take advantage of the agricultural advancements. Consequently, between 1960 and 1990, tenant farms decreased by nearly fifty percent, while the rural population without land—working as daily wage laborers—increased by forty percent, leading to heightened livelihood insecurity and urban migration [50]. Additionally, the Punjab Irrigation Department, acting as the sole mediator without police or judicial oversight, often failed to address issues with the Moga system and struggled to ensure fair distribution due to inadequate auditing and checks and balances. Favoritism and nepotism allowed big landlords to secure a disproportionate share of water, resulting in frequent protests by small farmers and peasants. The revenue and water tax (Abiana) are contentious, and the enforcement of agricultural labor laws is problematic.

The lack of accountability and the impunity of powerful landlords cannot be addressed in isolation but require reforms in bureaucracy and politics [46].

4.2. Political Economy of Food Insecurity

Qualitative data analysis reveals that while extreme hunger is not widespread among households, most respondents are dissatisfied with the diversity and affordability of their food, with wheat being the primary staple. Research shows that neoliberal policies have been central to Pakistan's economy. The "Green Revolution" in the 1960s, supported by USAID, mainly benefited landlords rather than peasants. Cash crops such as sugar, wheat, and cotton use more water and dangerous pesticides, ultimately reducing food diversity. By the eighties, Pakistan, once self-sufficient in wheat and rice production, became food-dependent again due to global cuts in food prices, leading to reduced grain demand and a formal decline in the agriculture sector [51].

Although imports increased to 2.5 million tons a decade later, hunger and malnutrition persisted due to unfair resource distribution and weak purchasing power. In 2007, as global food grain prices rose, Pakistan was forced to keep exporting its limited wheat surplus under international financial pressures, extending subsistence challenges. Foreign countries and agribusiness investors began acquiring agricultural lands on long-term leases, with all grains intended for export back to the investing countries [52].

Efforts to combat hunger and malnutrition were undermined by minimal state intervention under neoliberal economic policies, keeping food prices high. Wheat prices rose from PKR 400 to PKR 630 per 40 kg between 2004 and 2008, reaching PKR 1400 per 40 kg in 2019 and PKR 2200 per 40 kg in 2022 [53]. Increased international demand led to wheat smuggling, exacerbating the crisis. Additionally, rising petroleum, gas, and fertilizer prices impacted agricultural production, forcing the government to import wheat at high costs of USD 300 per ton. The consumer price index rose by 25%, and wheat prices increased by 20% [54]. The decline in agricultural investment from 2.1% to 1.1% (1999–2009), low-quality research, poor monitoring and evaluation, weak federal policy coordination, and poor provincial implementation intensified hunger and malnutrition [54].

Policy reform was never seriously undertaken but adhered to the demands of the World Bank and the Asian Development Bank for balance of payment and budgetary support. A comprehensive, long-term approach to agricultural development and poverty reduction is impossible without good governance and political reform. Policymakers' focus on production has undermined the accessibility issue for the poor [51]. Addressing issues such as storage, transportation, irrigation, and agriculture are secondary measures; unequal land distribution is the primary structural issue, as access to land would reduce relative food prices [51]. The World Bank [55] found that from 2000 to 2014, food costs rose by 270%, while non-food item prices increased by 180%. Household-level food security is not supported by cash crops such as cotton and sugarcane [56]. In South Punjab, maternal nutrition issues remain unaddressed due to strict household food budgets, intra-household food distribution, economic decline [50], and gender and social inequities. From 1990 to 2008, the number of malnourished individuals rose from 24 to 45 million nationwide. The prices of key items, from staple crops to cooking oil, increased by almost 20% in early 2010, with uncertainty expected to continue, as indicated by the wholesale price index [48]. In May 2022, food prices surged by over 50%, further weakening the already fragile purchasing power of the poor.

4.3. Political-Economy of Nutrition Programs

Our findings indicated a temporary and unsustainable nutrition policy. It corroborated the historical evidence that shows inconsistent national strategies, including food distribution, card-based rationing, wheat subsidies, and distribution to flood victims in Punjab, along with recent federal cash transfer programs for poor women through BISP [57]. UN agencies (UNICEF, WFP, FAO, and WHO) have led various nutritional programs involving health departments in the past. Evidence shows that the formula milk industry often ignored laws and continued advertising their products unlawfully [58]. This illegal and unethical promotion increased malnutrition by depriving children of their mother's milk. Reports revealed that 80% of mothers were instructed by healthcare providers to give formula milk [59]. In theory only, the Punjab Food Authority (PFA) has had 16 laws approved by the Punjab Assembly, banning the marketing and sampling of infant formula milk in hospitals after consulting with the Formula Milk Association. Authorization for formula milk ingredients and marketing is now required from the PFA scientific panel, and all imported products must be labeled in the national language [60].

The targeting of beneficiaries for cash transfers was flawed, as evidence showed that deserving widows and domestic female servants were excluded [61]. Power dynamics control development and poverty alleviation programs [62,63]. Connections to local politicians are crucial for becoming BISP beneficiaries in Pakistan [61]. Deserving families face not only social-structural hurdles but also technicalities and complexities related to the selection process. Therefore, factors leading to social exclusion should be central to advising on program objectives, beneficiary selection, and nomination [62]. On Pakistani bureaucracy, Hull [63] concluded that "A powerful person can move a 'stuck up' file. Those without influence have to 'put wheels on it. Money or political influence can affect not only the speed but the path as well, diverting a file from its normal trajectory". Although the program aimed to uplift the poor through cash grants of PKR 5000 per month to millions of households, reports indicate previous governments misused taxpayers' money (an annual budget of PKR 100 billion for 5.2 million of the poorest women) for political supporters, depriving genuinely deserving individuals. Profiling of BISP beneficiaries revealed that 1.42 million beneficiaries were government employees, including 2543 in grades 17 to 21; 153,302 had taken overseas trips once; 10,476 traveled more than once; 692 were vehicle owners; and 43,746 spouses owned one or more cars [64].

CMAM is also a temporary remedial strategy, particularly in crisis settings. Yet, the sustainable solution to maternal and child undernutrition lies in the social and economic empowerment and education of women [65]. Empirical data shows that the multisectoral solution strategy seems less effective; thus, social safety nets for poor females necessitate micro-level nutrition-sensitive and nutrition-specific interventions, especially after devolution [56]. However, remote areas remain uncovered, and the government often ignores them except for the better-off, indicating a significant gap between theory and practice. Detached from local socio-cultural realities, the global technical solution under RUTFs and CMAM was implemented "under neoliberal governments and facilitated an increasingly inequitable economy with minimal state involvement in an increasingly individualistic social environment" [65] (p. 16). Therefore, forming the Multi-Sectoral Nutrition Centre (MSNC) in the Planning and Development Department at the provincial level is not a genuine solution.

Findings showed that malnutrition has particularly affected women and children from remote areas, especially those who are water-insecure, unemployed, low-income, daily wage workers, domestic household servants, lower caste individuals, illiterate, and poor mothers with high fertility and work burdens. This suggests that ethnic-regional inequalities at the provincial level, the rural-urban gap, and caste-class stratification at the micro level must be addressed through concrete measures [23,66–68]. Ineffective coverage and managerial inefficiencies are evident, with up to 50% of the population in several rural districts not covered by LHWs, especially in the most remote and poorest areas [69]. This research underscores how overarching political and economic factors—such as neoliberal programs, post-colonial bureaucracy, and regional inequalities—diminish essential resources for southern regions. This creates a harmful cycle of inequality that leads to structural vulnerabilities.

5. Conclusions

This study confirms that water and food insecurity are interconnected, with increased levels of both insecurities linked to lower socioeconomic status and higher perceived stress.

Community experiences with water insecurity, low food diversity, structural challenges to therapeutic coverage, and the unrestricted use of formula milk products suggest that Pakistan has been significantly influenced by colonial and neoliberal policies. Government practices and policies have promoted privatization and biomedical solutions rather than addressing social stratification. Instead of tackling local problems with tailored solutions, the state has relied on global remedies. Policymakers can take specific actions to address these challenges. Ensuring water justice in southern Pakistan is crucial. Implementing land reforms and efficiently using water resources will help alleviate food insecurity. Nutrition-specific and sensitive programs (both therapeutic and social safety nets) must address the underlying issues of social inclusion, caste and class structures, rural-urban disparities, and structural vulnerabilities. Combating corruption and management issues is an important aspect and requires the rule of law and good governance at the macro level.

Author Contributions: Conceptualization, F.A. and J.B.A.; methodology, F.A., N.I.M. and N.N.; formal analysis, F.A.; investigation, F.A.; project administration, F.A.; writing—original draft preparation, F.A.; writing—review and editing, F.A., N.I.M., S.B., N.N., J.B.A. and K.T. All authors have read and agreed to the published version of the manuscript.

Funding: The HWISE survey was supported by the Institute for Policy Research at Northwestern University Evanston, IL, USA. The first author (F.A) is site-PI and a member of HWISE-RCN. https://www.ipr.northwestern.edu/wise-scales/about-the-scales/who-created-the-wise-scales/, accessed on 2 August 2023.

Institutional Review Board Statement: This study was conducted according to the guidelines of the Declaration of Helsinki and approved by the Advance Study and Research Board (ASRB) of Quaid-i-Azam University Islamabad, Pakistan (Number: QAU-ASRB-2016-307-S-I; Date of Approval: 20 October 2016).

Informed Consent Statement: All respondents to this study were well informed about the nature of this research beforehand, and then their formal oral consent was obtained. Keeping this research ethics in view, the privacy, anonymity, and confidentiality of all study participants were strictly ensured.

Data Availability Statement: The original contributions presented in the study are included in the article, further inquiries can be directed to the corresponding authors.

Acknowledgments: We acknowledge the contribution and support of local mothers, LHWs, and other health staff, who provided generous data for this study. Also, we thank Sera Young (Institute of Policy Research Institute at Northwestern University Evanston, IL, USA) for her support in the HWISE survey and Joshua Miller (University of North Carolina at Chapel Hill, NC, USA) for his support in our data analysis.

Conflicts of Interest: The authors declare no conflicts of interest.

References

1. United Nations Children Fund. *Nutrition, for Every Child: UNICEF Nutrition Strategy 2020–2030*; UNICEF: New York, NY, USA, 2020; Available online: https://www.unicef.org/media/92031/file/UNICEF%20Nutrition%20Strategy%202020-2030.pdf (accessed on 2 August 2023).
2. Demissie, S.; Worku, A. Magnitude and factors associated with malnutrition in children 6–59 months of age in pastoral community of Dollo Ado district, Somali region, Ethiopia. *Sci. J. Public Health* **2013**, *1*, 175–183. [CrossRef]
3. United Nations Children Fund. *Tracking Progress on Child and Maternal Nutrition: A Survival and Development Priority*; United Nations Children Fund: New York, NY, USA, 2009.
4. UNICEF; WHO; World Bank. Levels and Trends in Child Malnutrition. In *Joint Child Malnutrition Estimates*; UNICEF: New York, NY, USA; WHO: Geneva, Switzerland; World Bank: Washington, DC, USA, 2012.
5. Gross, R.; Webb, P. Wasting time for wasted children: Severe child undernutrition must be resolved in non-emergency settings. *Lancet* **2006**, *367*, 1209–1211. [CrossRef] [PubMed]
6. Bhutta, Z.A.; Gazdar, H.; Haddad, L. Seeing the unseen: Breaking the logjam of undernutrition in Pakistan. *IDS Bull.* **2013**, *44*, 1–9. [CrossRef]
7. Bhutta, Z.A.; Hafeez, A.; Rizvi, A. Reproductive, maternal, newborn, and child health in Pakistan: Challenges and opportunities. *Lancet* **2013**, *381*, 2207–2218. [CrossRef] [PubMed]

8. *Pakistan Demographic and Health Survey*; Islamabad and Calverton, National Institute of Population Studies and ICF International: MA, USA, 2013. Available online: https://dhsprogram.com/pubs/pdf/FR290/FR290.pdf (accessed on 2 August 2023).
9. Black, R.E.; Victora, C.G.; Walker, S.P.; Bhutta, Z.A.; Christian, P.; de Onis, M.; Ezzati, M.; Grantham-McGregor, S.; Katz, J.; Martorell, R.; et al. Maternal and child undernutrition and overweight in low-income and middle-income countries. *Lancet* **2013**, *382*, 427–451. [CrossRef] [PubMed]
10. Govt of Pakistan; UNICEF. UKAID Pakistan National Nutrition Survey. 2018. Available online: https://www.unicef.org/pakistan/reports/national-nutrition-survey-2018-key-findings-report (accessed on 17 July 2024).
11. Katoch, O.R. Determinants of malnutrition among children: A systematic review. *Nutrition* **2022**, *96*, 111565. [CrossRef]
12. Toma, A.; Talukder, A.; Shirin Khan, S.; Razu, S.R. An assessment of the association between antenatal care and child malnutrition in Bangladesh. *Fam. Med. Prim. Care Rev.* **2018**, *4*, 373–378. [CrossRef]
13. Rahman, M.; Islam, M.J.; Haque, S.E.; Saw, Y.M.; Haque, M.N.; Duc, N.H.; Al-Sobaihi, S.; Saw, T.N.; Mostofa, M.G.; Islam, M.R. Association between high-risk fertility behaviours and the likelihood of chronic undernutrition and anaemia among married Bangladeshi women of reproductive age. *Public Health Nutr.* **2017**, *20*, 305–314. [CrossRef] [PubMed]
14. Shahid, M.; Cao, Y.; Ahmed, F.; Raza, S.; Guo, J.; Malik, N.I.; Rauf, U.; Qureshi, M.G.; Saheed, R.; Maryam, R. Does Mothers' Awareness of Health and Nutrition Matter? A Case Study of Child Malnutrition in Marginalized Rural Community of Punjab, Pakistan. *Front. Public Health* **2022**, *10*, 792164. [CrossRef]
15. Nguyen, P.H.; Saha, K.K.; Ali, D.; Menon, P.; Manohar, S.; Mai, L.T.; Rawat, R.; Ruel, M.T. Maternal mental health is associated with child undernutrition and illness in Bangladesh, Vietnam and Ethiopia. *Public Health Nutr.* **2014**, *17*, 1318–1327. [CrossRef]
16. Mukhopadhyay, S. The intersection of gender, caste and class inequalities in child nutrition in rural India. *Asian Popu Studs.* **2015**, *2*, 17–31. [CrossRef]
17. Shahid, M.; Ahmed, F.; Ameer, W.; Guo, J.; Raza, S.; Fatima, S.; Qureshi, M.G. Prevalence of child malnutrition and household socioeconomic deprivation: A case study of marginalized district in Punjab, Pakistan. *PLoS ONE* **2022**, *17*, e0263470. [CrossRef] [PubMed]
18. Gillespie, S.; Haddad, L.; Mannar, V.; Menon, P.; Nisbett, N. The politics of reducing malnutrition: Building commitment and accelerating progress. *Lancet* **2013**, *10*, 552–569. [CrossRef] [PubMed]
19. Fakir, A.M.S.; Khan, M.W.R. Determinants of malnutrition among urban slum children in Bangladesh. *Health Econ. Rev.* **2015**, *5*, 22. [CrossRef] [PubMed]
20. Choudhary, N.; Schuster, R.; Brewis, A.; Wutich, A. Water insecurity potentially undermines dietary diversity of children aged 6–23 months: Evidence from India. *Matern. Child. Nutri.* **2020**, *16*, e12929. [CrossRef] [PubMed]
21. Sultana, F.; Loftus, A. *Water Politics: Governance, Justice, and the Right to Water*; Routledge: Abingdon, UK; New York, NY, USA, 2020.
22. Puett, C.; Guerrero, S. Barriers to access for severe acute malnutrition treatment services in Pakistan and Ethiopia: A comparative qualitative analysis. *Public Health Nutr.* **2015**, *18*, 1873–1882. [CrossRef] [PubMed]
23. Ahmed, F.; Malik, N.I.; Malik, N.; Qureshi, M.G.; Shahzad, M.; Shahid, M.; Zia, S.; Tang, K. Key challenges to optimal therapeutic coverage and maternal utilization of CMAM Program in rural southern Pakistan: A qualitative exploratory study. *Nutrients* **2022**, *14*, 2612. [CrossRef] [PubMed]
24. Ahmed, F.; Malik, N.I.; Zia, S.; Akbar, A.S.; Li, X.; Shahid, M.; Tang, K. Rural mothers' beliefs and practices about diagnosis, treatment, and management of children health problems: A qualitative study in marginalized Southern Pakistan. *Front. Public Health* **2023**, *10*, 1001668. [CrossRef]
25. Scheper-Hughes, N.; Lock, M. The Mindful Body: A Prolegomenon to Future Work in Medical Anthropology. *Med. Anthro. Quarter* **1987**, *1*, 6–41. [CrossRef]
26. Escobar, A. *Encountering Development: The Making and Unmaking of the Third World*; Princeton University Press: Princeton, NJ, USA, 1995.
27. Ferguson, J. *The Anti-Politics Machine: "Development," Depoliticization and Bureaucratic Power in Lesotho*; Cambridge University Press: Cambridge, UK, 1990.
28. Khan, S.R.; Aftab, S. Sustainable Development Policy Institute. In *Structural Adjustment, Labor and the Poor in Pakistan*; Sustainable Development Policy Institute: Islamabad, Pakistan, 1995.
29. Abbasi, K. The World Bank and world health: Focus on South Asia-II: India and Pakistan. *BMJ* **1999**, *318*, 1132–1135. [CrossRef]
30. Haider, M. Pakistan's Total Debt, Liabilities Rise to Rs35tr. 21 May 2019. Available online: https://www.thenews.com.pk/print/473930-pakistan-s-total-debt-liabilities-rise-to-rs35tr (accessed on 6 March 2020).
31. Younus, U. Pakistan's Debt Policy Has Brought Us to the Brink. Another Five Years of the Same is Unsustainable. DAWN. 30 October 2018. Available online: https://www.dawn.com/news/1442378 (accessed on 16 October 2019).
32. Bhutta, Z.A. Structural adjustments and their impact on health and society: A perspective from Pakistan. *Int. J. Epi.* **2001**, *30*, 712–716. [CrossRef] [PubMed]
33. Himmelgreen, D.; Romero-Daza, N. Anthropological approaches to the global food crisis: Understanding and addressing the "Silent Tsunami". *Napa Bull.* **2009**, *32*, 1–11. [CrossRef]
34. Young, S.L.; Boateng, G.O.; Jamaluddine, Z.; Miller, J.D.; Frongillo, E.A.; Neilands, T.B.; Collins, S.M.; Wutich, A.; Jepson, W.E.; Stoler, J. The Household Water InSecurity Experiences (HWISE) Scale: Development and validation of a household water insecurity measure for low-income and middle-income countries. *BMJ Global Health* **2019**, *4*, e001750. [CrossRef]

35. Workman, C.L.; Ureksoy, H. Water insecurity in a syndemic context: Understanding the psycho-emotional stress of water insecurity in Lesotho, Africa. *Soc. Sci. Med.* **2017**, *179*, 52–60. [CrossRef]
36. Workman, C.L.; Brewis, A.; Wutich, A.; Young, S.; Stoler, J.; Kearns, J. Understanding biopsychosocial health outcomes of syndemic water and food insecurity: Applications for global health. *Am. J. Trop. Med. Hyg.* **2021**, *104*, 8. [CrossRef]
37. Boateng, G.O.; Workman, C.L.; Miller, J.D.; Onono, M.; Neilands, T.B.; Young, S.L. The syndemic effects of food insecurity, water insecurity, and HIV on depressive symptomatology among Kenyan women. *Soc. Sci. Med.* **2022**, *1*, 113043. [CrossRef] [PubMed]
38. Kohrt, B.A.; Mendenhall, E. Social and structural origins of mental illness in global context. In *Global Mental Health: Anthropological Perspectives*; Routledge: New York, NY, USA, 2016; pp. 51–56.
39. Brewis, A.; Choudhary, N.; Wutich, A. Household water insecurity may influence common mental disorders directly and indirectly through multiple pathways: Evidence from Haiti. *Soc. Sci. Med.* **2019**, *1*, 112520. [CrossRef] [PubMed]
40. Wutich, A.; Brewis, A.; Tsai, A. Water and mental health. *Wiley Interdisciplinary Reviews: Water* **2020**, *7*, e1461. [CrossRef]
41. Young, S.; Frongillo, E.; Jamaluddine, Z.; Melgar-Quiñonez, H.; Pérez-Escamilla, R.; Ringler, C.; Rosinger, A. The importance of water security for ensuring food security, good nutrition, and well-being. *Adv. Nutri* **2021**, *1*, 1058–1073. [CrossRef]
42. Ringler, C.; Paulo, D. *Water and nutrition: Harmonizing Actions for the United Nations Decade of Action on Nutrition and the United Nations Water Action Decade*; United Nations System Standing Committee on Nutrition: Rome, Italy, 2020. Available online: https://www.unscn.org/uploads/web/news/document/Water-Paper-EN-WEB-12feb.pdf (accessed on 22 September 2020).
43. Miller, J.D.; Frongillo, E.A.; Weke, E.; Burger, R.; Wekesa, P.; Sheira, L.A.; Mocello, A.R.; Bukusi, E.A.; Otieno, P.; Cohen, C.R.; et al. Household water and food insecurity are positively associated with poor mental and physical health among adults living with HIV in Western Kenya. *J. Nutri.* **2021**, *151*, 1656–1664. [CrossRef]
44. D'Souza, R. Water in British India: The Making of a Colonial Hydrology. *Hist. Compass* **2006**, *4*, 621–628. [CrossRef]
45. Agnihotri, I. Ecology, Land Use and Colonization: The Canal Colonies of Punjab. *Indian Eco. Soc. Hist. Rev.* **1996**, *33*, 37–58. [CrossRef]
46. Mustafa, D.; Gioli, G.; Karner, M.; Khan, I. *Contested Waters: The Sub-National Scale of Water and Conflict in Pakistan*; United States Institute for Peace USIP: Washington, DC, USA, 2017.
47. Gilmartin, D. Water and Waste: Nature, Productivity and Colonialism in the Indus Basin. *Econ. Polit. Wkly.* **2003**, *38*, 5057–5065.
48. Farooqi, H.; Wegerich, K. Institutionalizing Inequities in Land Ownership and Water Allocations during Colonial Times in Punjab, Pakistan. *Water Hist.* **2015**, *7*, 131–146. [CrossRef]
49. Ali, I. Malign Growth? Agricultural Colonization and the Roots of Backwardness in the Punjab. *Past. Present.* **1987**, *114*, 110–132. [CrossRef]
50. Mustafa, D.; Sawas, A. Urbanization and Political Change in Pakistan: Exploring the Known Unknowns. *Third World Q.* **2013**, *34*, 1293–1304. [CrossRef]
51. Gera, N. Food Security under Structural Adjustment in Pakistan. *Asian Surv.* **2004**, *44*, 353–368. [CrossRef]
52. Kugelman, M. Pakistan's Food Insecurity: Roots, Ramifications, and Responses. In *HUNGER PAINS: Pakistan's Food Insecurity*; Kugelman, M., Hathaway, R., Eds.; The Woodrow Wilson International Center for Scholars: Washington, DC, USA, 2010; pp. 13–14.
53. National Planning Commission. Government of Pakistan. Task Force on Food Security Report, 2009. Pakistan. 2009. Available online: https://www.pc.gov.pk/uploads/annualplan/2009-2010.pdf (accessed on 6 May 2017).
54. Malik, S.J. Food Supply Challenges and Implications for Food Security. In *HUNGER PAINS: Pakistan's Food Insecurity*; Kugelman, M., Hathaway, R., Eds.; The Woodrow Wilson International Center for Scholars: Washington, DC, USA, 2010; pp. 13–14.
55. World Bank. 2015. Available online: http://data.worldbank.org/country/pakistan (accessed on 12 June 2016).
56. Di-Cesare, M.; Bhatti, Z.; Soofi, S.B.; Fortunato, L.; Ezzati, M.; Bhutta, Z.A. Geographical and socioeconomic inequalities in women and children's nutritional status in Pakistan in 2011, An analysis of data from a nationally representative survey. *Lancet Glob. Health* **2015**, *3*, e229–e239. [CrossRef] [PubMed]
57. Zaidi, S.; Bhutta, Z.A.; Rashid, A.; Nawaz, G.; Hayat, N.; Mohmand, S.K.; Acosta, A.M. *Nutrition Political Economy, Pakistan*; Province Report; Agha Khan University: Karachi, Pakistan, 2013.
58. Ebrahim, Z. *Bottle vs. Breast if Mothers Milk Is Best Why Use Formula Milk*; Dawn: Karachi, Pakistan, 2015; Available online: https://www.dawn.com/news/1198547 (accessed on 25 February 2020).
59. Wasif, S. Doctors Promoting Formula Milk at the Expense of Babies' Lives. *The Express Tribune*, 5 October 2013. Available online: https://tribune.com.pk/story/613582/doctorspromoting-formula-milk-at-expense-of-babies-lives-islamabad-city/ (accessed on 25 February 2020).
60. The News. Formula Milk Marketing Banned in Hospitals. *The News*, 7 October 2017. Available online: https://www.thenews.com.pk/print/235121-Formula-milk-marketingbanned-in-hospitals (accessed on 26 March 2020).
61. Aziz, A.; Khan, F.A.; Wood, G. Who is excluded and how? An analysis of community spaces for maternal and child health in Pakistan. *Health Res. Policy Syst.* **2015**, *13* (Suppl. S1), 56. [CrossRef]
62. Kwiatkowski, L.M. *Struggling with Development: The Politics of Hunger and Gender in the Philippines*; Westview Press: Boulder, CO, USA, 1998.
63. Hull, M.S. The file: Agency, authority, and autography in an Islamabad bureaucracy. *Lang. Comm.* **2003**, *23*, 287–314. [CrossRef]
64. Maqbool, S. 2543 Govt. Officers among Ineligible BISP Beneficiaries. *The News.* 9 January 2020. Available online: https://www.thenews.com.pk/print/595841-2-543-govt-officers-among-ineligible-bisp-beneficiaries (accessed on 5 March 2020).

65. Nott, J. "How Little Progress"? A Political Economy of Postcolonial Nutrition: "How Little Progress"? A Political Economy of Postcolonial Nutrition. *Popul. Dev. Rev.* **2018**, *44*, 771–791. [CrossRef]
66. Ahmed, F.; Shahid, M. Understanding food insecurity experiences, dietary perceptions and practices in the households facing hunger and malnutrition in Rajanpur District, Punjab Pakistan. *Pak. Perspect.* **2019**, *24*, 115–133.
67. Ahmed, F.; Malik, N.I.; Shahzad, M.; Ahmad, M.; Shahid, M.; Feng, X.L.; Guo, J. Determinants of Infant Young Child Feeding Among Mothers of Malnourished Children in South Punjab, Pakistan: A Qualitative Study. *Front. Public Health* **2022**, *10*, 834089. [CrossRef] [PubMed]
68. Ahmed, F.; Shahid, M.; Cao, Y.; Qureshi, M.G.; Zia, S.; Fatima, S.; Guo, J. A qualitative exploration in causes of water insecurity experiences, and gender and nutritional consequences in South Punjab, Pakistan. *Int. J. Environ. Res. Public Health* **2021**, *18*, 12534. [CrossRef]
69. Bhutta, Z.A.; Hafeez, A. What can Pakistan do to address maternal and child health over the next decade? *Health Res. Policy Sys.* **2015**, *13* (Suppl. S1), S49. [CrossRef]

Disclaimer/Publisher's Note: The statements, opinions and data contained in all publications are solely those of the individual author(s) and contributor(s) and not of MDPI and/or the editor(s). MDPI and/or the editor(s) disclaim responsibility for any injury to people or property resulting from any ideas, methods, instructions or products referred to in the content.

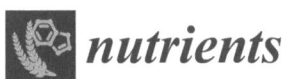

Article

Nutritional Health Risk (Food Security) in Thai Older Adults and Related Factors

Teeranut Harnirattisai [1], Sararud Vuthiarpa [2], Lisa Renee Pawloski [1,3,*], Kevin Michael Curtin [4], Eden Blackwell [3], Jenny Nguyen [5] and Sophia Madeleine Bourgeois [5]

[1] Faculty of Nursing, Thammasat University, Khlong Nueng 12120, Thailand; teeranut@nurse.tu.ac.th
[2] Faculty of Nursing, Rattana Bundit University, Khlong Nueng 12160, Thailand; vsararud@yahoo.com
[3] Department of Anthropology, University of Alabama, Tuscaloosa, AL 35401, USA; beblackwell@crimson.ua.edu
[4] Department of Geography and the Environment, University of Alabama, Tuscaloosa, AL 35401, USA; kmcurtin@ua.edu
[5] Department of Biology, University of Alabama, Tuscaloosa, AL 35401, USA; jtnguyen2@crimson.ua.edu (J.N.); smbourgeois@crimson.ua.edu (S.M.B.)
* Correspondence: lpawloski@ua.edu

Abstract: The older adult population in Thailand has been steadily increasing in recent years, and urbanization has resulted in many older adults living independently, leaving many at nutritional risk. The purpose of this research is to explore food security among Thai older adults using a simple screening tool, the DETERMINE tool, as well as from three surveys which reflect seniors' health and ultimately food security including the mini-mental state examination (MMSE), the self-efficacy for physical activity scale (SEPAS), and the health literacy questionnaire. The DETERMINE tool was used in Thailand for the first time in this study. The findings revealed a moderate risk of food insecurity amongst participants, as most of them claimed to have underlying diseases, eat alone, eat a few nutrient-rich foods, and take medication. The MMSE, SEPAS, and health literacy questionnaire results suggested that food security was found to be negatively correlated with higher cognitive ability, higher physical activity, self-efficacy, and higher health literacy. In conclusion, there appears to be a high risk for malnutrition among older adults in Thailand, particularly in those with low income and underlying diseases.

Keywords: nutritional health risk; food security; Thai older adults

1. Introduction

1.1. Overview of Food Security and Older Adults in Thailand

Nutritional health is an important component of independence and quality of life among older adults. Food security is a nutritional risk factor and necessary for good nutritional heath. Food security is defined by the World Health Organization as "when all people have physical, social, and economic access to sufficient, safe, and nutritious food that meets their dietary needs and food preferences" [1]. Food insecurity occurs when such access and availability is limited and can increase nutritional risk. Vulnerable populations at risk for food include but are not limited to those living in poverty, displaced peoples, children, and older adults. Older adult populations are often faced with limited finances, comorbidities, limited mobility, physiological changes, and other challenges that limit access to sufficient nutrient-dense foods. Thailand is not limited to such risk, particularly as the aging population in Thailand rises, and fewer resources become available to support the complexities of the aging needs. Phulkerd et al. [2] reported that Thailand holds the second highest number of individuals over 60 in the ASEAN member countries, and it has been projected that one in three Thais will be over the age of 60 years by 2040.

1.2. Nutrition and Food Security of Older Adults in Thailand

While obesity has increased dramatically among children and adolescents in Thailand over the past twenty years [3], it has also impacted older adults, increasing risk for chronic disease and disability. However, throughout Thailand there is still a greater risk for undernutrition among older adults, contributing to more complex health-related risks. Nawai et al. (2021) reported that in Chiang Mai Thailand, over 50% of older adults were malnourished (undernourished) or at risk of malnutrition [4]. These findings were greatly affected by socioeconomic status and functional status. Further, Vapattanawong et al. noted from a prospective study that older adults who were obese were actually protected more from mortality [5]. However, more recent literature suggests such protection is changing to a greater risk of obesity-related chronic diseases such as cardiovascular disease and diabetes. Duangjai et al. (2023) [6] recently reported that about 25% of their study population from a group of community-dwelling older adults (over 55 years) had a BMI over 25, and another study by Sukchan et al. (2022) [7] noted the prevalence of obesity among a group of older adults living in Southern Thailand was 35.2%. Obesity can also be associated with micronutrient deficiencies due to an overconsumption of calories but limited intake of nutrient-dense foods. Thus, when determining nutritional risk among older adult populations in Thailand, it is important to consider both under and over nutrition.

While there is growing literature reporting the prevalence and comorbidity relationships of nutritional status in older adults in Thailand, very few studies have examined its determinants, and particularly, the impact of food security on senior populations in Thailand. Much of the literature on the determinants of nutritional status include studies on food consumption patterns and selection and the impact of COVID-19. One recent study revealed that almost 30% of an aging population in Thailand exhibited indicators of food insecurity, which was also associated with financial hardships [8]. As food security is one of the major risk factors affecting nutritional health among older adults all over the world and food security in the Thailand literature is under-represented, particularly in older adults, we present an analysis using a simple tool to examine food insecurity among a population of older adults living in suburban Bangkok, Thailand. The purpose of this research is to explore food security among Thai older adults using a simple screening tool, the DETERMINE tool. In addition, we have presented data correlations with the findings from this tool from three other surveys which reflect senior health and ultimately food security, including cognitive function, physical activity self-efficacy, and health literacy.

1.3. Food Security Screening Tools and Use of DETERMINE Tool

As part of the US Nutrition Screening Initiative, a relatively simple to use, self-assessment tool was developed to determine nutrition and food security risk among older adults. This screening tool, "Determine Your Health Risk", and noted in this paper as the DETERMINE tool, is also known as the Nutrition Screening Initiative checklist (NSI). The tool was developed in collaboration with the American Dietetic Association, the American Academy of Family Physicians, and the National Council on the Ageing [9]. The tool includes a checklist of ten questions to be answered yes or no. Each question is given a different weight that is associated with nutritional risk among the older adults. Nutritional risk includes poor calorie intake (too many or too few) and inadequate macronutrient and micronutrient intake. Nutrition risk can be impacted by food security, which includes access and availability to necessary nutrients. The DETERMINE tool can be helpful in predicting risk in community populations but is not intended to be a clinical diagnostic tool. As it is self-administered, it is helpful in assessing perceived health and nutritional risk; it may also help identify those with nutrient deficiencies [10]. The checklist has been validated in a few studies, and mostly in the U.S., a few studies have noted the tool to provide a weak predictor of mortality, but helpful in predicting nutrition risk [10,11].

In terms of international use, this tool has been used in studies in Denmark [10], Greece [12], and Europe more broadly [13,14], China [15], Singapore [16,17], and Japan [18,19], among others. These studies have shown usefulness in identifying and understanding the determinants of malnutrition and food insecurity among older adults. For example, one study found that food selection was based on foods that were "easy to chew", thus reducing the variety and selection of nutrient-dense foods [20]. Further, one study identified a correlation with nutrient risk and fewer social interactions and food insecurity [12]. Many of these studies are conducted primarily to screen and identify malnourished older adults living in community settings. However, until now, the tool has not been used in Thai populations. Thus, this paper is the first to explore the findings from the DETERMINE tool in a Thai senior population. Here we present our findings on food security risk among Thai older adults using the DETERMINE tool, along with the results of a demographic survey of personal, familial, and basic health information. Those demographic factors that can be associated with higher nutritional health risk are explored vis a vis the cultural nutritional norms in Thailand.

1.4. Food Security in Asia

In Asia, the proportion of elders in the population is rapidly growing, and it is predicted that Asia will be the region with the largest older adult population in the world, exceeding over 4.9 billion (Asian Development Bank 2022). With this growing population, exploring the major issues that an aging society will face may be relevant for developing future interventions and policies. One of these issues is the widespread prevalence of malnutrition in older adult populations. Several studies have been conducted in Asian countries including China, Japan, Singapore, and Taiwan to assess nutritional risk and risk factors among older adults using the DETERMINE tool. Yap et al. (2007) and Sugiura et al. (2016) [17,19] assessed community-dwelling elders in Singapore and Japan, respectively, and found that activity of daily living disabilities and depression were significant indicators of high risk for poor nutrition using the DETERMINE tool. Sugiura [19] also found that declining functional capacity over a 2-year period was linked with higher nutritional risk. While functional disabilities and mental illness affect nutritional risk in elders, financial and educational barriers also play a role. Koo et al. (2013) [16] assessed the nutritional risk of senior recipients of financial assistance aged 55 and found that 50.3% were at risk of malnutrition. Major risk factors included advanced age, financial limitations, and lack of education about subsidized food sources. Understanding the determinants that influence nutritional risk and malnutrition in Asian elders may be beneficial for identifying at-risk populations and implementing the proper policies.

2. Materials and Methods

Study Design and Study Population

This study was a cross-sectional study with the objective of surveying nutritional health risk in Thai older adults and related factors. The population group to be studied consisted of older adults (defined as 60 years of age or over) in the urban areas of two provinces of Thailand (Greater Bangkok Metropolitan Region). The goal was to conduct a representative survey using a multistage, stratified sampling of the Thai population. A demographic and lifestyle survey was used to collect information about the subjects' age and gender, marital status, education, religion, and other family status variables. Information about underlying disease, smoking, and the use of alcohol was collected. The DETERMINE checklist was used as an indicator of nutritional health risk. Additional instruments were used to measure cognitive ability (mini mental state examination MMSE), and self-efficacy for physical activity (SEPAS), along with a health literacy questionnaire. SPSS software program version 22 was used to analyze the data. Statistics included descriptive statistics of the demographic data, with standard deviations noted for the interval ratio data. Frequencies and percentages were determined for the DETERMINE instrument for each item and means and standard deviations were calculated for each of the instruments. Finally, the Pearson Correlation Coefficient with a significance of $p < 0.05$ was used to examine the relationship between the tools.

For this study, the DETERMINE tool, also described earlier, was translated into Thai and back-translated to English with content experts in nutrition, geriatrics, and nursing. The sensitivity, specificity, and positive predictive value of the tool were originally conducted by Posner et al. (1993) [20] who evaluated the effectiveness of the tool and the nutritional risk cut-off points. The authors examined the reliability of the DETERMINE tool in Thailand using a random sampling with 30 participants and found Cronbach alpha of 0.7. The screening tool has been implemented in many Asian countries including Japan and Singapore, but this is the first use in Thailand.

More specifically, the mini-mental state examination test (MMSE-Thai 2002) of the Institute of Geriatric Medicine [21] is a set of questions for screening cognitive functions. This examination is suitable to indicate the presence of cognitive impairment, such as a person with dementia or suffering the effects of a head injury. The MMSE-Thai 2002 consists of 11 questions. Score interpretation is based on educational level. The instrument was validated for content validity by Thai content experts and was not retested. The reliability was validated through a coefficient by testing MMSE on 30 people with similar characteristics of the sample and the correlation coefficient was calculated to be 0.88. The maximum score for the MMSE survey is 30, and a score of 25 or higher is within the normal range. If the score is below 24, it may indicate possible cognitive impairment [22]. The self-efficacy for physical activity scale (SEPAS) has individuals rate their perceived confidence in their ability to perform each specific physical activity (e.g., leisure time activity, household activity, and work-related activity). SEPAS was developed by modifying the Self-Efficacy for Exercise by Resnick & Jenkins, 2000 [23].. It was also based on the Physical Activity Scale for older adults that look at physical activity in terms of leisure time, household tasks, and work-related activities [24]. The SEPAS contains 17 items and employs a semantic differential scale with scores ranging from 0 (no confidence) to 10 (total confidence). This instrument had been approved for content validated by five Thai experts and tested for reliability with 30 Thai older adults, resulting in an Alpha Cronbach of 0.90. Health literacy (knowledge capacity) refers to the ability of individuals to gain access to, understand, and use information in ways which promote and maintain good health for themselves. The health literacy questionnaire for older adults) [25,26] was analyzed in this study and the test for reliability resulted in an Alpha Cronback of 0.96. This questionnaire contains 22 items across 4 sections: (1) access to information (6 items), (2) understanding health information (5 item), (3) evaluating and selecting information (6 items), and (4) applying information (5 items). This questionnaire is a rating scale ranging from 6 (highest) to 1 (lowest).

The appropriate sample size was calculated based on G*Power. The calculation for correlation used alpha = 0.5, with effect size 0.3. The test employed a power of 80%, confidence interval of 95%, and acceptable error of 5%. The required number of participants according to the calculation was 263 cases. With an expectation of a 10% drop-out rate, a minimum of 290 older adults would need to be recruited for this study. A multistage, random sampling method was used for the study sample selection. In the first stage, based on the community characteristics of the two provinces, all 20 districts were divided into two categories of urban and rural areas. Based on the National Statistical Office Report [27], urban refers to municipalities which are inhabited by at least 200 persons per square kilometer, whereas rural indicates any area with a population density lower than 200 persons per square kilometer. According to this definition, there are a total of 12 subdistricts that are considered urban areas. A random selection of health promotion centers in those urban areas was carried out for this study.

At the last stage, the older adult subject population was randomly selected using the criteria described below and invited to participate in the study. The proportion of the samples from urban areas was based on a representative population size in six locations. A total of 302 participants with complete questionnaires were accepted. The inclusion criteria (beyond age and urban area classification) were (1) the respondents must be able to help themselves assessed by Activities of Daily Living (ADL) measurement, and (2) the respondents must have no dementia as assessed by a category test (Set Test). The exclusion criteria were (1) any active health problem or psychiatric condition that interferes with the provision of information, and (2) any problem of hearing, vision, or the ability to communicate in Thai with the researcher. The discontinuation criteria were (1) being unable to provide 100% information, (2) experiencing severe disease symptoms or being admitted to a hospital, and (3) any request to withdraw from the research. A summary of the demographic characteristics of the population is provided in Table 1.

Table 1. Descriptive demographic data of the study sample older adult population ($n = 302$).

Item	Response	#/Avg/%	Item	Response	#/Avg/%
Age	57–87 years	69.05 ± 6.18		Having underlying diseases	272 (90.1%)
Gender	Male	56 (18.5%)		Diabetes mellitus	73 (24.2%)
	Female	246 (81.5%)		Hypertension	157 (52.0%)
				Heart/coronary artery disease	39 (12.9%)
Marital status	Single	40 (13.2%)		Pulmonary disease	5 (1.7%)
	Married	141 (46.7%)		Psychiatric disease	1 (0.3%)
	Divorced/separated	26 (8.6%)		Orthopedic disease	45 (14.9%)
	Widowed	95 (31.5%)		Gastrointestinal disease	10 (3.3%)
				Cerebrovascular disease	7 (2.3%)
Education level	Unlettered	20 (6.6%)	Underlying disease	Dyslipidemia	85 (28.1%)
	Elementary school	158 (52.3%)		Cancer	7 (2.31%)
	Secondary school	74 (24.5%)		Systemic lupus erythematous	2 (0.6%)
	Vocational certificate	15 (5.0%)		Allergic rhinitis	6 (2.0%)
	Bachelor's degree	31 (10.3%)		Thyroid	6 (2.0%)
	Postgraduate	4 (1.3%)		Cataract	3 (1.0%)
				Benign prostate hyperplasia	4 (1.3%)
Religion	Buddhism	296 (98.0%)		Parkinson disease	1 (0.3%)
	Christianity	3 (1.0%)		Chronic kidney disease	4 (1.3%)
	Islam	2 (0.7%)		Rheumatoid arthritis	1 (0.3%)
	Missing	1 (0.3%)		Hepatitis	1 (0.3%)
				Anemia	3 (1.0%)
				Muscle weakness	1 (0.3%)
Occupation	Agriculturist	5 (1.7%)			
	Merchant	45 (14.9%)			
	Officialdom	2 (0.7%)		Often	9 (3.0%)
	Employee	43 (14.2%)		Sometimes	3 (1.0%)
	Company employee	4 (1.3%)	Smoking	Seldom	14 (4.6%)
	Unemployed	174 (57.6%)		Never	270 (89.4%)
	Others	29 (9.6%)		Missing	6 (2.0%)
	Retirement	25 (86.2%)			
	Health volunteer	3 (10.3%)			
	Personal business	1 (3.5%)			
Personal Income	0–100,000	6,522.57 ± 10,159.51	Alcohol consumption	Often	3 (1.0%)
				Sometimes	27 (8.9%)
Family Income	0–200,000	16,549.11 ± 20,686.70		Seldom	21 (7.0%)
				Never	248 (82.1%)
				Missing	3 (1.0%)
Adequate income	Adequate	94 (31.1%)			
	Inadequate	165 (54.7%)			
	Saving	23 (7.6%)	Nutrition health risk score		4.84 ± 3.55
	Dept	20 (6.6%)			
Caregiver	Couples	107 (35.4%)	Nutrition health risk level	Good (0–2 score)	
	Sibling	27 (8.9%)		Moderate risk (3–5 score)	
	Children	168 (55.6%)		High risk (6 or more)	
	Grandchild	36 (11.9%)			
	Neighbor	15 (5.0%)			
	Health volunteer	31 (10.3%)			
	Formal caregiver	1 (0.3%)			
Living	Couples	130 (43.0%)			
	Relative or children	203 (67.3%)			
	Alone	44 (14.6%)			
	Others	3 (1.0%)			

This study was approved by the Human Research Ethics Committee of Thammasat University (Science) (COA No.048/2021 approved on 18 May 2020) prior to data collection. All sub-district health promotion centers responsible for the older adults were also granted approval. The researchers provided information regarding the purpose of the study to the participants, and written informed consent was obtained from all the participants. Data were collected for three months from August 2022 to October 2022. The researchers collaborated with the contact nurses in the sub-district health-promoting centers who helped to coordinate the identification of potential participants for the study. In the data collection at the older adult clubs, the researcher instructed the participants regarding the questionnaires and read aloud each item of the questionnaires and asked the participants to rate each item by themselves. Approximately 45 min were required to complete the questionnaire.

3. Results

Table 1 provides descriptive data of the sample. Most were female (81.5%), married (46.7%), reported as having inadequate income (54.7%), and unemployed (57.6%) or retired (86.2%). Also, few were educated beyond secondary school, and the mean age was 69.05 years. Further, most reported having some kind of underlying disease (90%) of which the majority had hypertension. Very few reported smoking (8%) and most (82%) reported never drinking alcohol. Overall, from the DETERMINE tool, the participants showed an average score of moderate risk (4.84), where 0 to 2 is good, 3–5 is of moderate risk, and 6 and higher is of great risk for food insecurity and malnutrition.

Table 2 presents the individual items for the DETERMINE tool and the frequency and percentage of those who noted those items. From these results, three of the indicators are interesting to highlight, which include the two items with the highest frequencies and the one item with the lowest frequency: (1) I have tooth and mouth problems that makes it difficult to eat. (2) I eat alone most of the time and (3) I drink beer, liquor, or wine three times (almost every day). In terms of frequency of responses, most participants noted issues with tooth and mouth problems (46%) and that they eat alone (52%). Also, the item that received the lowest frequency response was the item asking about drinking alcohol (2.6%). We discuss these three findings in greater detail in the Discussion section as well as address issues related to the other indicators noted. Other items that had high percentages and frequencies included items about eating few fruits and vegetables (33.1%), taking three or more over the counter or prescribed drugs per day (40.7%), and having an illness (45%). Other items that noted low percentages and frequencies included eating fewer than two meals per day (7.6%), not being able to physically shop, cook, and nourish oneself (8.3%), without the need for gaining or losing weight within 6 months (9.3%), and not having enough money to buy food (21.2%).

Table 2. Nutritional health risk indicators among study participants (n = 302).

Item	Frequency	Percent
1. I have an illness or condition that made me change type and/or amount of food I eat	136	45%
2. I eat fewer than 2 meals per day	23	7.6%
3. I eat few fruits, vegetables, or products of milk.	100	33.1%
4. I drink beer, liquor, or wine three times (a day?) almost every day.	8	2.6%
5. I have tooth and mouth problems that makes it difficult to eat.	139	46%
6. I do not always have enough money to buy the food I need.	64	21.2%
7. I eat alone most of the time.	157	52%
8. I take 3 or more prescribed or over-the-counter drugs a day.	123	40.7%
9. Without need, I lose or gain 10 pounds within 6 months.	28	9.3%
10. I am not always physically able to shop, cook, and/or nourish myself.	25	8.3%

Table 3 presents the mean and standard deviations of the items from the MMSE, health literacy, SEPAS, and food security instruments. The MMSE survey resulted in a mean score of 25.4; this falls within the normal range, but is slightly low, noting the maximum score is 30. The results of the health literacy tool resulted in a mean of 4.56, where 6 is the highest possible value. The SEPAS tool resulted in a mean of 7.52, where 10 equates to the highest confidence in perception of physical activity ability. Again, the DETERMINE mean score of 4.84 suggests moderate risk of food insecurity.

Table 4 presents correlation data that examine the relationships between the DETERMINE tool score and three other instruments related to health and wellness among seniors. These instruments measure cognitive ability, physical activity self-efficacy, and health literacy. The significance level is set at 0.05, and the statistical method used was the Pearson correlation coefficient. Food security was negatively correlated with all three measures, indicating that higher cognitive ability, higher physical activity self-efficacy, and higher health literacy are associated with a lower risk of food insecurity.

Table 3. Mean and standard deviation (SD) of key variables among study participants (n = 302).

Variables	Mean ± SD
Cognitive ability (MMSE)	25.40 ± 0.219
Health Literacy	4.56 ± 0.92
SEPAS	7.52 ± 1.53
Food Security	4.84 ± 0.204

Table 4. Correlation between cognitive ability, physical activity self-efficacy, health literacy, and food security risk among older adults (n = 302).

	Cognitive Ability	Physical Activity Self-Efficacy	Health Literacy	Food Security Risk
Cognitive Ability	1	0.186 **	0.124 *	−0.137 *
Physical Activity Self-Efficacy	0.186 **	1	0.219 **	−0.237 *
Health Literacy	0.124 *	0.219 *	1	−0.154 *
Food Security Risk	−0.137 *	−0.237 *	−0.154 *	1

Statistical significance is indicated by asterisks: $p < 0.01$ (**) and $p < 0.05$ (*). The Pearson correlation test was employed to assess the relationships between these variables.

4. Discussion

This is the first study identified through our literature review to use the DETERMINE tool to assess risk for food insecurity and malnutrition among older adults in Thailand. These results show that there is indeed a risk for malnutrition among older adults in Thailand, particularly among those who have limited income and those with underlying diseases. Interestingly, the results highlighted three areas which may be more specific to Thailand and be impacted by Thai culture and values. These include the three items which were selected at higher frequencies: (1) I have tooth and mouth problems that makes it difficult to eat, (2) I eat alone most of the time, and (3) I drink beer, liquor, or wine three times (a day?) almost every day. Each of these factors suggests an interpretation that is rooted in Thai culture, particularly Thai foodways and family dynamics.

Thailand's unique foodways and traditional values related to aging intersect in ways that can have a meaningful impact on the health of older adult Thais. Thailand is well known for its varied cuisine which makes heavy use of herbs and fresh fruits and vegetables with rice and seafood staples [28,29]. Thai food culture has shifted in recent decades to meet the demands of labor market changes and features street food and "public eating" of meals prepared outside the home (which frequently include higher amounts of meats, fat, and sugar) [29,30]. Nonetheless, meal sharing is a culturally valued aspect of eating, particularly within the family [29]. Like much of Asia, Thailand has a strong tradition of filial piety and care of aging elders by younger generations; however, the performance of these obligations is shifting and is largely being met through financial remittances and long-distance communication rather than traditional co-residence in multi-generational households [31,32]. Increasingly, older Thais are finding themselves living and eating alone or without their adult children, with consequences for their diet and wellbeing [2,33]. In a study of elder happiness in Thailand, Phulkerd et al. [2] found that older adults who reported having all their meals with family members had the highest probability of happiness of adults who shared fewer meals with family.

Thai healthcare is widely available due to long-standing national healthcare provision programs. This suggests that those with persistent tooth and mouth problems may be at such a disadvantage that they cannot access even the most widely available healthcare. Analysis of the Thai National Oral Health Survey by Kaewkamnerdpong et al. [34] showed that the leading cause of mouth problems was tooth loss and too few occlusal pairs (pairs of teeth that make contact when chewing). More than half (60.6%) of Thai adults between

60 and 74 reported difficulty chewing food. Hyposalivation, or dry mouth, while it is not specified in the DETERMINE "mouth problems" item, is common in older age and has been linked to poor oral health, altered taste of food, and malnutrition [35]. Tooth loss and dry mouth contribute to poor chewing ability which frequently lead to avoiding certain foods, eating less, and ultimately poor diet. As noted above, adults in this study frequently reported low consumption of fruits and vegetables which require chewing or additional preparation to make them easier to consume for people with compromised ability to chew or swallow.

With regard to eating alone, although in rural populations there has been an increasing incidence of older people living alone while other, younger family members migrate to larger cities for employment opportunities, this is less prevalent in the urban and suburban areas where this study was conducted. Our study population reflects the national statistics in living arrangements for older adults in that most are aging at home with a spouse or other relatives, usually their adult children [36]. Therefore, this factor again suggests that those with greater health risk are the most vulnerable given their unusual lack of a familial support system. Further, Thai-specific values of intergenerational co-residence and psychological wellbeing are important to consider with using the DETERMINE tool in Thailand as loneliness and depression could drive poor eating and limited dietary diversity. Nawai [4] identified living alone as one of several factors associated with nutrition risk among older adults in Thailand. Older adults living alone were found to have decreased dietary diversity [33]. In an earlier study focusing on community-dwelling older people, Chalermsri et al. [37] found loneliness to be an important determinant of food choice which is related to nutrient intake. Research has also shown negative psychological effects of frequent (four times or more per week) eating alone where commensal eating is valued. Mikami et al. [18] found an association between frequent eating alone and poor appetite among older adults in Japan. In both China and Thailand, researchers have found associations between eating alone and depression or unhappiness, particularly among women [15,38]. Yiengprugsawan et al. [38] suggest these outcomes are linked to a departure from cultural norms.

Finally, the use of alcohol in anything other than moderation is not widely culturally acceptable among Thais. Men in Thailand are far more likely to drink than women who are considered "culturally protected" from related outcomes; the sample here is heavily skewed towards women, so the low report of alcohol consumption might be a factor of gender [39,40]. However, as Knodel and Pothisiri [41] found, the likelihood of drinking decreased for both men and women 60 and older who lived with family. While there are conflicting data on how Thailand compares against regional averages in alcohol consumption, rates of drinking have increased in recent decades with links to related increases in risks of Non-Communicable Diseases (NCDs) and poor diet [40]. This provides another piece of evidence that those with the highest nutritional health risk are often among those furthest from the core of Thai cultural norms. It may also be important to note that the DETERMINE criteria for alcohol consumption reflect daily drinking behaviors. Increased risks for poor diet (decreased fruits and vegetables and increased fried foods) and NCDs were found among Thai adults who engaged in non-daily binge drinking (four or more drinks per occasion according). Binge-drinking behaviors that threaten food security may be missed by the DETERMINE tool [40].

The other indicators having high frequencies included eating few fruits and vegetables, having an illness, and taking three or more over the counter or prescribed drugs per day. Eating few fruits and vegetables can be related to one of the highlighted indicators, tooth decay as well as ability to breakdown fibrous foods, common in Thai cuisine [42]. As noted earlier, cuisine in Thailand has become more public and there are fewer fruits and vegetables included. Nawai et al. [4] have shown that it is common in Thailand to see illnesses or conditions which lead to changes in eating habits in Thai elders, particularly dyslipidemias and osteoarthritis as well as severe changes in mental and physical health and limitations that these chronic illnesses cause. Those that take three or more over the counter drugs may lead to nutritional risk as medications may impact the appetite due to nausea, changes in taste, or nutrient interactions. While healthcare costs are relatively low in Thailand, medications may come at an extra cost that may impact the ability to purchase food for some with very low incomes. This is particularly a concern in the U.S. context.

Other indicators having lower frequency responses in this population included eating fewer than two meals per day, not being able to physically shop, cook, and nourish oneself, without the need for gaining or losing weight, and not having enough money to buy food. Food is widely available and accessible in Thailand, again, now in public settings. Thus, the availability and accessibility to have fewer than two meals a day might not be as common. Family and social support are also important in Thailand and while the necessities to cook are not always available due to transportation, mobility, etc., many social supports are available to assist with those who have physical limitations. The indicator related to losing or gaining weight without need would need to be explored more, but the low-response percentage may be due to the lack of access to scales and regular weight screening, one limitation which was noted in the development of a protein energy malnutrition screening tool in residential homes in Thailand [43]. Lastly, the indicator concerning not having enough money to buy food was noted by 21% of the participants, a lower frequency, but not low enough to ignore. While food is relatively inexpensive, available, and accessible, in Thailand, older adults concerned about medications and not bringing in income can be more greatly impacted economically. Further analyses in this population should be carried out to understand who is at most risk.

The correlations with the tools concerning cognitive ability, physical activity self-efficacy, and health literacy revealed expected results such that those with poorer cognitive ability, confidence in physical activity, and health literacy are at higher risk for food security. One importance of including these tools in these analyses was to add important components which the DETERMINE tool does not include or focus on, but are known determinants of poor senior health. Earlier literature has shown that poor health literacy is associated with poor physical activity and nutritional status [44].

These tools in addition to the DETERMINE tool are quite helpful in understanding determinants of health among senior populations. These results also suggest that the DETERMINE tool may be useful on its own when needing a fairly fast and simple screening tool to assess nutritional risk among senior populations in Thailand. The other tools for understanding senior health more comprehensively are more complex and take much longer to administer.

The DETERMINE screening tool may also assist health nurses and healthcare professionals to understand what focus of health education may be needed in order to decrease nutritional health risk and improve health status. Nurses play an important role in health education emphasizing on dental care, self-care for their chronic illness, eating with friends and family, and choices of foods that are specific for older adults. However, it is also important that nurses and health professional are aware of the impact of social determinants as well as health literacy, cognitive ability, and confidence in physical activity when providing health education.

5. Limitations and Implications for Practice

There are several limitations of this study. First, this study was conducted in a limited geographic area of two provinces that are largely urban or suburban. These findings cannot be immediately extended to rural populations without further investigation. Moreover, each of the provinces in this study are in the greater Metropolitan Bangkok region of Thailand. The results may vary in other regions of Thailand, particularly where there are variations in cultural institutions (e.g., ethnicity, religion). Further, the use of the DETERMINE tool may not entirely capture the local cultural and dietary characteristics that affect food security and nutrition among Thai older adults.

One challenge of using tools such as DETERMINE in different cultures and settings is to ensure that the items being used have an impact and to understand that certain items may have a greater impact or weight in the analyses. While this tool has been shown to be easily administered and useful in its simplicity as well as helpful in identifying at risk older adults, it is important to note that use in different cultures and settings may impact the overall score or selection of its items.

One additional limitation, regarding all the surveys, includes the use of self-reported data, which can be subject to bias. In this study, participants may have different perceptions regarding their dietary habits, health conditions, or the frequency of medication use.

Despite these limitations, the clear findings outlined above regarding the factors associated with higher health risk clearly suggest some potential practical approaches that may alleviate nutritional insecurity. Given that older adults living alone, and those who consume alcohol regularly are at greatest risk, individuals with these characteristics can be identified during any routine health screening and provided with nutritional support, education regarding nutritional choices, or references to community support agencies that can ameliorate nutritional risks.

As the DETERMINE tool is a useful and simple tool for Thai populations, it is critical that the next steps include validity analyses to better weigh individuals items in the DETERMINE screening tool. The tool's applicability and relevance in the Thai context need further validation to ensure its accuracy and reliability. Further research would include exploring the causal relationships with the results from the other surveys to best understand senior health and the use of these instruments. Also important would include confounding factors, such as social support systems, economic status, and access to healthcare services, which might also play significant roles. And lastly, additional analyses on the oral health of older adults would be helpful to better understand the nutritional risk of this population.

6. Conclusions

This article explores results from the DETERMINE screening tool among a group of older adults in urban and semi-urban Thailand. It also explores the relationship with these findings and other health indicators among older adults. The findings revealed that there is a high risk for malnutrition among older adults in Thailand, particularly in those with low-income and underlying diseases. While the tool is useful and simple, more research is needed to explore its applicability and relevance within the Thai context.

Author Contributions: T.H.: conception and design, data collection, revising critically, final approval to be published; S.V.: conception and design, data collection, revising critically, final approval to be published; L.R.P.: conception, literature review, drafting of paper, revising critically, final approval to be published; E.B.: drafting of paper, literature review; J.N.: drafting of paper, literature review; S.M.B.: drafting of paper and revisions; K.M.C.: analysis and interpretation of the data, drafting of the paper, revising critically, final approval to be published. All authors have read and agreed to the published version of the manuscript.

Funding: This research was funded by the Thammasat University Bualuang ASEAN Chair Professorship Grant and the U.S. Fulbright Foundation/Fulbright Thailand.

Institutional Review Board Statement: The study was conducted in accordance with the Declaration of Helsinki, and approved by the Institutional Review Board of Thammasat This study was approved by the Human Research Ethics Committee of Thammasat University (Science), COA No.048/2021 approved on 18 May 2020.

Informed Consent Statement: Written informed consent has been obtained from the participants to publish this paper.

Data Availability Statement: The raw data supporting the conclusions of this article will be made available by the authors on request.

Conflicts of Interest: The authors declare no conflict of interest.

References

1. Food Security & Nutrition: Essential Ingredients to Build Back Better. Available online: https://www.who.int/news-room/events/detail/2022/10/18/default-calendar/food-security-nutrition-essential-ingredients-to-build-back-better (accessed on 12 February 2024).
2. Phulkerd, S.; Gray, R.S.; Chamratrithirong, A.; Pattaravanich, U.; Thapsuwan, S. Financial satisfaction, food security, and shared meals are foundations of happiness among older persons in Thailand. *BMC Geriatr.* **2023**, *23*, 690. [CrossRef] [PubMed]
3. Pawloski, L.R.; Harnirattisai, T.; Vuthiarpa, S.; Curtin, K.M.; Nguyen, J.T. Gender-Based Determinants of Obesity among Thai Adolescent Boys and Girls. *Adolescents* **2023**, *3*, 457–466. [CrossRef]

4. Nawai, A.; Phongphanngam, S.; Khumrungsee, M.; Leveille, S.G. Factors associated with nutrition risk among community-dwelling older adults in Thailand. *Geriatr. Nur.* **2021**, *42*, 1048–1055. [CrossRef] [PubMed]
5. Vapattanawong, P.; Aekplakorn, W.; Rakchanyaban, U.; Prasartkul, P.; Porapakkham, Y. Obesity and mortality among older Thais: A four year follow up study. *BMC Public Health* **2010**, *10*, 604. [CrossRef] [PubMed]
6. Duangjai, A.; Phanthurat, N.; Sajjapong, W.; Ontawong, A.; Pengnet, S.; Yosboonruang, A.; Jongsomchai, K.; Thatsanasuwan, N. Association of abdominal obesity and systolic blood pressure indices with cardiovascular disease risk prediction among community-dwelling older adults. *Electron. J. Gen. Med.* **2023**, *20*, em458. [CrossRef] [PubMed]
7. Sukchan, P.; Wamae, D.; Chemoh, W. Prevalence and Risk Factors of Overweight and Obesity and Physical Activity Patterns among Elderly Individuals in Southern Thailand: A Community Cross-Sectional Study. *J. Med. Assoc. Thail. Chotmaihet Thangphaet* **2022**, *105*, 861–871. [CrossRef]
8. Phulkerd, S.; Thapsuwan, S.; Chamratrithirong, A.; Gray, R.S.; Pattaravanich, U.; Ungchusak, C.; Saonuam, P. Financial Hardship on Food Security in Ageing Populations. *Int. J. Public Health* **2023**, *68*, 1605755. [CrossRef] [PubMed]
9. Barrocas, A.; White, J.V.; Gomez, C.; Smithwick, L. Assessing Health Status in the Elderly: The Nutrition Screening Initiative. *J. Health Care Poor Underserved* **1996**, *7*, 210–218. [CrossRef] [PubMed]
10. Beck, A.M.; Ovesen, L.; Osler, M. The 'Mini Nutritional Assessment' (MNA) and the 'Determine Your Nutritional Health' Checklist (NSI Checklist) as predictors of morbidity and mortality in an elderly Danish population. *Br. J. Nutr.* **1999**, *81*, 31–36. [CrossRef]
11. Sahyoun, N.R. Usefulness of Nutrition Screening of the Elderly. *Nutr. Clin. Care* **1999**, *2*, 155–163. [CrossRef]
12. Katsas, K.; Mamalaki, E.; Kontogianni, M.D.; Anastasiou, C.A.; Kosmidis, M.H.; Varlamis, I.; Hadjigeorgiou, G.M.; Dardiotis, E.; Sakka, P.; Scarmeas, N.; et al. Malnutrition in older adults: Correlations with social, diet-related, and neuropsychological factors. *Nutr. Burbank Los Angel. Cty. Calif* **2020**, *71*, 110640. [CrossRef]
13. De Groot, L.; Beck, A.M.; Schroll, M.; van Staveren, W.A. Evaluating the DETERMINE Your Nutritional Health Checklist and the Mini Nutritional Assessment as tools to identify nutritional problems in elderly Europeans. *Eur. J. Clin. Nutr.* **1998**, *52*, 877–883. [CrossRef] [PubMed]
14. De Morais, C.; Oliveira, B.; Afonso, C.; Lumbers, M.; Raats, M.; de Almeida, M.D.V. Nutritional risk of European elderly. *Eur. J. Clin. Nutr.* **2013**, *67*, 1215–1219. [CrossRef] [PubMed]
15. Wang, X.; Shen, W.; Wang, C.; Zhang, X.; Xiao, Y.; He, F.; Zhai, Y.; Li, F.; Shang, X.; Lin, J. Association between eating alone and depressive symptom in elders: A cross-sectional study. *BMC Geriatr.* **2016**, *16*, 19. [CrossRef] [PubMed]
16. Koo, Y.X.; Kang, M.L.; Auyong, A.; Liau, G.Z.; Hoe, J.; Long, M.; Koh, A.; Koh, F.; Liu, R.; Koh, G. Malnutrition in older adults on financial assistance in an urban Asian country: A mixed methods study. *Public Health Nutr.* **2014**, *17*, 2834–2843. [CrossRef] [PubMed]
17. Yap, K.B.; Niti, M.; Ng, T.P. Nutrition screening among community-dwelling older adults in Singapore. *Singapore Med. J.* **2007**, *48*, 911–916. [PubMed]
18. Mikami, Y.; Motokawa, K.; Shirobe, M.; Edahiro, A.; Ohara, Y.; Iwasaki, M.; Hayakawa, M.; Watanabe, Y.; Inagaki, H.; Kim, H.; et al. Relationship between Eating Alone and Poor Appetite Using the Simplified Nutritional Appetite Questionnaire. *Nutrients* **2022**, *14*, 337. [CrossRef] [PubMed]
19. Sugiura, Y.; Tanimoto, Y.; Imbe, A.; Inaba, Y.; Sakai, S.; Shishikura, K.; Tanimoto, K.; Hanafusa, T. Association between Functional Capacity Decline and Nutritional Status Based on the Nutrition Screening Initiative Checklist: A 2-Year Cohort Study of Japanese Community-Dwelling Elderly. *PLoS ONE* **2016**, *11*, e0166037. [CrossRef]
20. Posner, B.M.; Jette, A.M.; Smith, K.W.; Miller, D.R. Nutrition and health risks in the elderly: The nutrition screening initiative. *Am. J. Public Health* **1993**, *83*, 972–978. [CrossRef]
21. Thailand Ministry of Public Health, Department of Medical Services, Institute of Geriatric Medicine. *Medical Technology Assessment: A Comparison of Mini-Mental State Examination-Thai (MMSEThai) 2002 and Thai Mini Mental State Examination (TMSE) for Screening Older Persons with Dementia Nonthaburi: Institute of Geriatric Medicine*; Thai Institute for Geriatric Medicine: Nonthaburi, Thailand, 2008.
22. Kurlowicz, L.; Wallace, M. The Mini-Mental State Examination (MMSE). *J. Gerontol. Nurs.* **1999**, *25*, 8–9. [CrossRef]
23. Resnick, B.; Jenkins, L.S. Testing the reliability and validity of the Self-Efficacy for Exercise scale. *Nurs. Res.* **2000**, *49*, 154–159. [CrossRef] [PubMed]
24. Allison, M.J.; Keller, C.; Hutchinson, P.L. Selection of an instrument to measure the physical activity of elderly people in rural areas. *Rehabil. Nurs. Off. J. Assoc. Rehabil. Nurses* **1998**, *23*, 309–314. [CrossRef] [PubMed]
25. Srisaeng, P.; DeeNamnam, W. Health knowledge in taking care of oneself to be healthy of people. Elderly in Bangkok Development and quality checking of tests. *J. R. Thai Army Nurses* **2019**, *20*, 340–350.
26. Deechum, W.; Srisang, P. Knowledge of health in self-care for good health among the elderly in Bangkok: A case study of enhancement of health knowledge in the elderly. *Urban Med.* **2019**, *63*, 74–82.
27. Statistical Yearbook Thailand 2020 | SEADELT. Available online: https://seadelt.net/Documents/?ID=519 (accessed on 9 November 2023).
28. Seubsman, S.; Kelly, M.; Yuthapornpinit, P.; Sleigh, A. Cultural Resistance to Fast-Food Consumption? A Study of Youth in North Eastern Thailand. *Int. J. Consum. Stud.* **2009**, *33*, 669–675. [CrossRef] [PubMed]
29. Watanasin, R. Thai Food: A Gateway to Cultural Understanding. *J. R. Inst. Thail.* **2012**, *IV*, 145–154.
30. Yasmeen, G. Not 'From Scratch': Thai food systems and 'public eating'. *J. Intercult. Stud.* **2000**, *21*, 341–352. [CrossRef]
31. Knodel, J.; Kespichayawattana, J.; Wivatvanit, S.; Saengtienchai, C. The Future of Family Support for Thai Elderly: Views of the Populace. *J. Popul. Soc. Stud.* **2013**, *21*, 110–132.

32. Knodel, J.; Teerawichitchainan, B.P. *Family Support for Older Persons in Thailand: Challenges and Opportunities*; Research Collection School of Social Sciences; Singapore Management University: Singapore, 2017.
33. Chalermsri, C.; Rahman, S.M.; Ekström, E.-C.; Muangpaisan, W.; Ackplakorn, W.; Satheannopakao, W.; Ziaei, S. Sociodemographic characteristics associated with the dietary diversity of Thai community-dwelling older people: Results from the national health examination survey. *BMC Public Health* **2022**, *22*, 377. [CrossRef]
34. Kaewkamnerdpong, I.; Harirugsakul, P.; Prasertsom, P.; Vejvithee, W.; Niyomsilp, K.; Gururatana, O. Oral status is associated with chewing difficulty in Thai older adults: Data from a National Oral Health Survey. *BMC Oral Health* **2023**, *23*, 35. [CrossRef]
35. Samnieng, P. Association of hyposalivation with oral function, nutrition and oral health in community-dwelling elderly Thai. *Community Dent. Health* **2012**, 117–123. [CrossRef]
36. Bandaogo, M.; Van Doorn, R. *Labor Markets and Social Policy in a Rapidly Transforming and Aging Thailand: The Macroeconomic and Fiscal Impact of Aging in Thailand*; World Bank: Washington, DC, USA, 2021.
37. Chalermsri, C.; Herzig van Wees, S.; Ziaei, S.; Ekström, E.-C.; Muangpaisan, W.; Rahman, S.M. Exploring the Experience and Determinants of the Food Choices and Eating Practices of Elderly Thai People: A Qualitative Study. *Nutrients* **2020**, *12*, 3497. [CrossRef] [PubMed]
38. Yiengprugsawan, V.; Banwell, C.; Takeda, W.; Dixon, J.; Seubsman, S.-A.; Sleigh, A.C. Health, happiness and eating together: What can a large Thai cohort study tell us? *Glob. J. Health Sci.* **2015**, *7*, 270–277. [CrossRef] [PubMed]
39. Assanangkornchai, S.; Sam-Angsri, N.; Rerngpongpan, S.; Lertnakorn, A. Patterns of Alcohol Consumption in the Thai Population: Results of the National Household Survey of 2007. *Alcohol Alcohol.* **2010**, *45*, 278–285. [CrossRef] [PubMed]
40. Wakabayashi, M.; McKetin, R.; Banwell, C.; Yiengprugsawan, V.; Kelly, M.; Seubsman, S.; Iso, H.; Sleigh, A. Thai Cohort Study Team Alcohol consumption patterns in Thailand and their relationship with non-communicable disease. *BMC Public Health* **2015**, *15*, 1297. [CrossRef] [PubMed]
41. Knodel, J.; Pothisiri, W. Smoking and Drinking Behaviors among Older Adults: A Comparative Analysis of Three Southeast Asian Countries. *J. Cross-Cult. Gerontol.* **2021**, *36*, 369–386. [CrossRef] [PubMed]
42. Teerawattananon, Y.; Luz, A. *Obesity in Thailand and Its Economic Cost Estimation*; Asian Development Bank: Bangkok, Thailand, 2017.
43. Phodhichai, T.; Satheannoppakao, W.; Tipayamongkholgul, M.; Hutchinson, C.; Sasat, S. Development of a protein energy malnutrition screening tool for older Thais in public residential homes. *Public Health Nutr.* **2022**, *25*, 565–577. [CrossRef]
44. Geboers, B.; de Winter, A.F.; Luten, K.A.; Jansen, C.J.M.; Reijneveld, S.A. The association of health literacy with physical activity and nutritional behavior in older adults, and its social cognitive mediators. *J. Health Commun.* **2014**, *19* (Suppl. 2), 61–76. [CrossRef]

Disclaimer/Publisher's Note: The statements, opinions and data contained in all publications are solely those of the individual author(s) and contributor(s) and not of MDPI and/or the editor(s). MDPI and/or the editor(s) disclaim responsibility for any injury to people or property resulting from any ideas, methods, instructions or products referred to in the content.

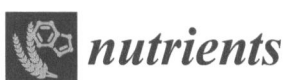

Article

Using Household Dietary Diversity Score and Spatial Analysis to Inform Food Governance in Chile

Martín del Valle M [1,*], Kirsteen Shields [1] and Sofía Boza [2]

[1] Global Academy of Agriculture and Food Systems, The University of Edinburgh, Edinburgh EH8 9YL, UK; kirsteen.shields@ed.ac.uk

[2] Department of Management and Rural Innovation, Faculty of Agricultural Sciences, University of Chile, Santiago 8330111, Chile; sofiaboza@uchile.cl

* Correspondence: martin.delvalle@ed.ac.uk

Abstract: This study explores how the Household Dietary Diversity Score (HDDS) and spatial visualization can inform food governance in Chile, focusing on socio-demographic and geographical determinants affecting food consumption patterns. A national household database (n = 4047), including households from 2019 (n = 3967; 98.02%) and 2020 (n = 80; 1.98%), provided by the "Family Support Program of Food Self-Sufficiency" (FSPFS) of the Ministry of Social Development and Family, was analyzed. The findings revealed that Chilean vulnerable households were led mostly by women (86.6%), with an age average of 55.9 ± 15.6 years old, versus 68.9 ± 12.9 years in the case of men. The intake frequency analysis showed that dairy, fruits, and vegetables were below the recommended values in at least half of the households, and that fats and sugars were above recommended levels. Regarding the HDDS (0–189), the national average was 91.4 ± 20.6 and was significantly influenced by the number of minors in the households, water access, food access issues, and residing in the Zona Sur. Finally, the spatial visualization showed that the Zona Central had higher consumption of fruits and vegetables, while the extreme zones Norte Grande and Zona Austral showed higher intakes of fats and sugars. These findings emphasize the importance of leveraging data insights like the HDDS and spatial visualization to enhance food security and inform food governance strategies.

Keywords: Chile; food security; food governance; Household Dietary Diversity Score; spatial visualization

Citation: del Valle M, M.; Shields, K.; Boza, S. Using Household Dietary Diversity Score and Spatial Analysis to Inform Food Governance in Chile. *Nutrients* **2024**, *16*, 2937. https://doi.org/10.3390/nu16172937

Academic Editors: Ariana Saraiva and António Raposo

Received: 16 August 2024
Revised: 27 August 2024
Accepted: 28 August 2024
Published: 2 September 2024

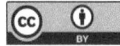

Copyright: © 2024 by the authors. Licensee MDPI, Basel, Switzerland. This article is an open access article distributed under the terms and conditions of the Creative Commons Attribution (CC BY) license (https://creativecommons.org/licenses/by/4.0/).

1. Introduction

1.1. Household Dietary Diversity as an Indicator of Food Security

Household dietary diversity is commonly defined as a qualitative measure of food consumption at the household level that reflects access to a variety of foods and serves as a proxy for nutrient adequacy (Refs. [1–3]) and micronutrient adequacy in resource-poor settings [4], and encompasses a range of methodologies provided by different approaches related to the number of food groups and to whom they are directed. For example, ref. [1] highlights the Household Dietary Diversity Score (HDDS), Child Dietary Diversity Score (CDDS), and Women Dietary Diversity Score (WDDS). Refs. [2,4] introduced the Minimum Dietary Diversity for Women (MDD-W) score, which is based on the consumption of 10 specific food groups. Refs. [5,6] provided the Household Dietary Diversity Score (HDDS), focusing on 12 food groups for assessment. Ref. [7] adapted the MDD-W methodology by using 10 food groups as a basis for their measurement. The Food and Agriculture Organization suggests a dietary diversity questionnaire underlining the importance of considering various food groups to gauge the extent of dietary diversity in individuals or households [3].

The HDDS can be assessed through various indicators and components, each shedding light on the variety and quality of foods consumed within a household. Ref. [8] indicate that these methodologies need to be simple to better predict micronutrient adequacy. According to [1], the Household Dietary Diversity Score (HDDS) is a commonly utilized indicator, calculated based on the number of food groups consumed by the household over specific timeframes, typically within either 24 h or 7 days. This score has proven to be a reliable predictor of nutrient adequacy in the diet and typically consists of 12 food groups, including cereals, vegetables, fruits, meat, poultry, eggs, legumes, milk, oils, sweets, spices, and beverages. Another approach, highlighted by [6], involves assessing the number of different food groups or types of food consumed by household members over a specified period. The Household Dietary Diversity Score (HDDS) is a valuable tool in this regard, ranging from 0 to 15, reflecting the number of food groups consumed. Households are categorized based on their dietary diversity, generally classifying those consuming at least four different food groups (DDS $\geq$ 4) as having medium dietary diversity. Ref. [7] discusses an adapted version of the Minimum Dietary Diversity for Women (MDD-W) methodology, focusing on 10 defined food groups to assess dietary diversity. Respondents recall their food consumption over a 24-h period, and enumerators categorize the foods into these 10 groups, ultimately assigning a dietary diversity score (DDS) out of 10. Similarly, Ref. [2] use the Minimum Dietary Diversity for Women (MDD-W) score, assessing whether women have consumed foods from five or more of the 10 defined food groups in the previous day. These food groups encompass a wide range, including grains, pulses, dairy, meat, poultry, eggs, and various fruits and vegetables. However, these methodologies also present limitations, as stated by [8], like small sample sizes in some data sets and potential underreporting and overreporting of dietary intakes, or food groups misreported when adding foods in small quantities to sauces [9].

A diverse diet that includes a variety of food groups is generally associated with better nutrient intake and overall health (Refs. [9,10]). These chosen dietary diversity indicators, such as the Household Dietary Diversity Score (HDDS) or Dietary Diversity Score (DDS), are intrinsically linked to food security by quantifying the variety and quality of food consumed. Ref. [10] emphasized the vital role of policies and programs aimed at bolstering household dietary diversity to ensure access to a diverse array of foods, ultimately improving food security. Ref. [11] demonstrated positive correlations between dietary diversity indicators and macro/micronutrient adequacy in various age groups. Strategies like enhancing market access for farm produce and generating off-farm employment are recognized as effective means to boost dietary diversity, thus positively impacting food security. Additionally, dietary diversity indicators serve as invaluable monitoring tools to assess the efficacy of food security interventions. Ref. [5] highlighted the practical utility of the HDDS in identifying vulnerable households requiring targeted food security interventions, particularly during crises like the COVID-19 pandemic. Ref. [6] emphasized the role of their DDS in enhancing dietary diversity, which contributes to improved food security and nutrition while also promoting agricultural sustainability through diverse crop cultivation. Ref. [12] showed in Burkina Faso that higher intakes of organ meat, flesh foods, vitamin A- and vitamin C-rich fruits and vegetables, and legumes and nuts were significantly associated with a lower risk of micronutrient inadequacy. Ref. [7] further underscored the connection between dietary diversity and food security, advocating for the incorporation of dietary diversity into policymaking to enhance nutritional quality and overall well-being.

1.2. Spatial Visualization Food Insecurity Warning Systems

Spatial visualization is a crucial tool in addressing food insecurity, providing a geospatial lens to understand its distribution and severity. Refs. [13,14] highlighted the value of spatial visualization in identifying high-risk areas, thereby supporting effective intervention targeting. Similarly, Ref. [15] emphasized the utility of spatial analysis, particularly mapping, in identifying unmet needs, facilitating a comprehensive understanding of the relationship between poverty, population density, and food access. Ref. [16] underscored the practical significance of visualizing food insecurity in prioritizing interventions, as evidenced by their research in Rajasthan, India. These tools enhance the targeting of vulnerable populations, facilitating effective decision-making and resource allocation

(Refs. [13,17,18]). By mapping spatial patterns, these tools offer visual representations of food insecurity across regions (Refs. [13,19]), aiding policymakers in targeting interventions and understanding local geographic influences (Refs. [19,20]). Additionally, these tools reveal spatial disparities, informing sustainable territorial-based agriculture and food security policies [19]. They also highlight significant household and individual-level variations, capturing diverse factors influencing food security and dietary quality [18]. Indeed, these tools prevent oversimplification of food insecurity, enhancing the depth and accuracy of information [20]. The integration of geo-referenced data collection via handheld devices has reduced costs, enabling better data collection and targeted interventions in urban areas (Refs. [13,20]). Finally, spatial visualization tools enable comparison of different geographic resolutions, offering new perspectives for policy research and providing a comprehensive view of deprivation and food insecurity [20]. They aggregate summaries of food stores, food banks, and bus stops, contextualizing the entrenched issues of food insecurity.

There are several successful case studies and applications that showcase the effectiveness of different spatial visualization tools and methodologies in addressing food insecurity. For example, Ref. [13] highlighted the Integrated Food Security Phase Classification (IPC) system by the World Food Programme (WFP), a standardized approach employed in over 30 countries. The IPC system classifies food security outcomes at different geographic levels, allowing for cross-country comparisons and targeted interventions. Ref. [17] described a successful web-based prototype developed in Bogota, Colombia, which integrated diverse data sources such as census, socioeconomic, and accessibility data to visualize community kitchens and food resources. This prototype aided in the spatial exploration of food security challenges in specific neighborhoods. Refs. [18,19] emphasized the use of GIS-based indicators and spatially explicit methodologies for mapping local spatial interactions and identifying geographically deprived areas and clusters with high concentrations of food insecurity hotspots. Furthermore, Ref. [19] discussed the integration of spatially targeted interventions to combat inequalities and improve household livelihoods and welfare, particularly in western Kenya. The application of small area estimation (SAE) was highlighted by [13] as a successful method for estimating food insecurity indicators at the district level in Bangladesh, providing precise and representative estimates that are valuable for resource allocation and policy-making. Additionally, Ref. [18] showcased the efficiency and cost-effectiveness of tablet-based data collection, as demonstrated by [21] in conservation projects, achieving cost reductions of up to 75% compared to traditional paper-based surveys. Finally, Ref. [14] conducted a critical review and mapping of indicators to measure the food access dimension of food security, providing valuable insights for assessing and addressing food insecurity.

Despite the advantages highlighted before, spatial visualization also faces important limitations. One of the main restrictions is the limited availability of high-quality subnational data, especially in low-income countries, which can affect the accuracy of spatial analysis [13]. Additionally, there is the potential for misinterpretation of spatial data, particularly by users unfamiliar with data acquisition methods, and the possibility of spatial bias due to non-representative data or poorly defined spatial units. In addition, spatial visualization tools rely heavily on limited data sources and require continuous updates to maintain their accuracy. These tools are primarily based on census and survey data collected at infrequent intervals, which can restrict the timeliness and precision of the information (Refs. [17,20]). The validity and accuracy of data based on self-reported measures by households, and the need for additional validation through local surveys, highlight significant challenges (Refs. [19,20]). Furthermore, the high costs associated with collecting spatially disaggregated data, especially through in-person surveys using electronic devices, further complicate their implementation, and the complex socio-ecological interactions involved in food insecurity require a precision approach tailored to individual and neighborhood-level factors, which can be challenging to execute [18]. There is also a notable bias towards those with access to the platform originating the observed data and significant difficulty in linking heterogeneous data sources to enhance insights [20].

Also, potential differences in food insecurity experiences between urban and rural areas, driven by the clustering of emergency food assistance and supermarkets around population centers, need to be considered [20]. Lastly, the risk of misinterpretation of maps by policymakers and the need for continuous updates to ensure the accuracy and relevance of spatial information pose further limitations [13].

1.3. Research Rationale and Objectives

The most recent "Report on Food Consumption in Chile" [22] highlighted a concerning trend: all income quintiles are consuming healthy food groups below the recommended levels, with the lowest income quintile being the most affected. In an average household of 3.3 people, monthly consumption includes 23.4 L of sweetened beverages, 17.5 kg of bread, and 5.1 kg of sweets, whereas the intake of fruits, vegetables, and legumes barely reaches 24.7 kg [22]. Furthermore, the latest National Socioeconomic Characterization Survey [23] indicates that 16.3% of Chilean households face moderate food insecurity, with 3.5% experiencing severe food insecurity, largely due to financial constraints. These statistics underscore the pressing challenges faced by vulnerable households, particularly those in the lower income quintile, in achieving the recommended dietary intake. Understanding the dietary diversity, food security status, and geographical location of these households is crucial, as they encounter the most significant barriers to consuming essential food groups such as fruits, vegetables, and legumes.

This research aims to provide a comprehensive assessment of the dietary habits, socio-demographic characteristics, and geographical distributions of these vulnerable households. The insights gained will be vital for informing strategies and interventions to address food insecurity and enhance the well-being of the most marginalized segments of the Chilean population.

Thus, the main objective of this study is "to analyze the interplay between socio-demographic factors, food consumption patterns, and food security in Chile's most vulnerable households, and to develop a spatial visualization information system that visually identifies and warns about areas of food insecurity across different food groups at both national and regional levels". In order to deepen the analysis, the following secondary objectives have been proposed:

- To describe the socio-demographic characteristics of Chile's most vulnerable households, represented by the "Family Support Program of Food Self-Sufficiency (FSPFS)" diagnostic survey.
- To calculate the intake frequency of different food groups in Chile's vulnerable households at the national and macro-zone levels.
- To calculate a national and regional Household Dietary Diversity Score (HDDS) and analyze its association with socio-demographic characteristics, food security determinants, and geographical macro-zones.
- To develop a geospatial warning system based on spatial visualization of food-insecure areas for different food groups.

2. Materials and Methods

The current research received ethical approval from the Human Ethical Review Committee (HERC) of the Royal (Dick) School of Veterinary Studies at the University of Edinburgh, with approval number HERC_2022_148 on 31 October 2022. The approval letter is available in Supplementary Material, and it was granted on the condition that the research is conducted according to the description provided in the application and the assurances made.

The methodological framework for this chapter was designed to dissect the socio-demographic and nutritional contours of Chile's most vulnerable households, based on the work done by [5] focused on the determinants of household food security and dietary diversity during the COVID-19 pandemic in Bangladesh. Segregated into four strategic objectives, this chapter evaluates household composition, dietary intake patterns, the HDDS, and the development of a Spatial Warning System, each section providing a critical lens on different facets of food security. For the purposes of this research, the HDDS methodology was chosen due to its generality over other, more specific methods of measuring dietary diversity in households, such as methodologies focused on women suggested by [1,2], or on children [1]. For the spatial visualization of food security, Ref. [13] was used as a reference; however, spatial clustering analysis was not conducted due to concerns about low representativeness and high sensitivity to small data variations, which could hinder the identification of significant spatial patterns.

Households' information was gathered from a database that contains the results of the diagnostic survey for the Family Support Program of Food Self-Sufficiency (FSPFS) (Programa de apoyo a familias para el autoconsumo) of the Ministry of Social Development and Family of Chile and the Solidary Fund of Social Innovation (FOSIS), which was obtained through a request for transparency and confidentiality agreement to the Secretary of Social Services of said ministry. The households invited to participate in this program are those belonging to the 40% most vulnerable population in Chile, according to the socio-economic characterization survey conducted nationwide. This program seeks to increase the availability of healthy food for vulnerable families, through education and self-provision to supplement their food needs and improve their living conditions. It mainly considers support for production activities (cultivation and breeding of small livestock) and, secondarily, activities aimed at the preservation, processing, and correct preparation of food. It also has an educational component, as it aims to provide information, promote learning, and reinforce knowledge associated with eating habits and, complementarily, with healthy lifestyles. The diagnostic questionnaire is applied to all households that will be part of the program in order to obtain information from three main areas: family group socio-demographic characteristics, general food security determinants, and food diagnosis. We selected the items of each area that best matched this study's aims, as shown in Table 1.

Table 1. Diagnostic questionnaire content.

Area	No of Items	Items
Family group socio-demographic characteristics	11	Region; commune; head of household (Hoh) gender; (Hoh) age; (Hoh) main work activity; 0–5 years old; 6–9 years old; 10–17 years old; 18–64 years old; 65+ years old; total family members.
General food security determinants	4	Food access issues; food availability issues; water access issues; pollution free environment.
Food diagnosis	24	"Weekly intake frequency" and "below recommended/recommended/above recommended" for the following food groups: vegetables, fruits, dairy, white meat, red meat, eggs, legumes, water, bread, cereals, fat, sugar.

Until 2013, the FSPFS was focused on increasing family savings and security through self-production of food. Following an evaluation of the program, it was concluded that the saving capacity was difficult to measure and that it should shift focus to peoples' "right to food", paralleling a broader change of prioritization among those working for food security. Thus, from 2013 onwards, the program focused on safeguarding the consumption and diversity of food in the most vulnerable families in the country through the improvement of the availability of healthy foods and food education.

Each family responds to a specific diagnosis regarding their frequency of consumption for 12 food groups, which then lead to three types of recommendations: "below-recommended", "recommended", and "above-recommended". Although the dietary recommendations for the Chilean population for the year 2009/2010 were taken as a reference, most are the result of the program's own creation. For each of the 12 food groups, a frequency of consumption was defined in order to approximate, over a period of 1 month, dietary intake, and thus determine whether to work on a production technology if the consumption is below what is recommended, or focus on dietary education if consumption is above recommendations. The three categories mentioned above were created based on international standards and the previously mentioned dietary guidelines for the Chilean population and seek to make it easier for the executor, who is the figure that works directly with the families, to perform the job of uploading the information to the centralized system. However, the program recognizes that this type of question never provides information that is 100% accurate, since food guidelines should also be based on the territory, realities, and integrating cultural aspects. A total standardization can, among other things, end up suggesting a culturally or otherwise inappropriate way of asking about culinary or consumption patterns. Finally, one of the most recent modifications of the diagnostic instrument involved adding information on the consumption of the different food groups in terms of "quantity", improving the accuracy provided by the information associated with the frequency of consumption.

In order to add the geographical characteristics to this study, we added to our dataset a column with the five Chilean macro-zones: Norte Grande, Norte Chico, Zona Central, Zona Sur, and Zona Austral, due to climate differences between each macro-zone. We wanted to see if there were territorial differences regarding the intake of the food groups amongst the macro-zones. Thus, each macro-zone groups the following regions, climate type according to the Köppen–Geiger classification, and agricultural production, as shown in Table 2.

Table 2. Chilean regions grouped in macro-zones (adapted from Sarricolea et al., 2017 [24] and Meza et al., 2021 [25]).

Macro-Zone	Regions	Climate Type	Agricultural Production
Norte Grande	Arica y Parinacota, Tarapacá, Antofagasta	Arid and polar climates due to the Atacama Desert and high altitude.	Smallholder farming: horticultural crops (corn, lettuce, tomato, bell pepper). Fruit trees: citrus, mangoes, olives
Norte Chico	Atacama, Coquimbo	Arid but also experiences polar climates at higher elevations.	Table grapes, wine grapes, mandarins, avocados, blueberries.
Zona Central	Valparaíso, Metropolitana, O'Higgins, Maule, Ñuble, Biobío	The primary agricultural zone, where temperate climates cover over 90% of the region.	Export-oriented agriculture: fruits (grapes, apples, berries), vegetables. Large-scale farming systems with diverse crops.
Zona Sur	La Araucanía, Los Lagos, Los Ríos	Temperate climate with minor tundra zones.	Transition to export-oriented fruit trees: walnuts, blueberries, hazelnuts, cherries. Traditional crops: pastures, wheat, barley. Dairy and beef farming.
Zona Austral	Aysén, Magallanes	Mix of polar and temperate climates, reflecting the cold and humid conditions.	Limited agricultural activity. Focus on livestock, mainly sheep, and forestry.

Methods Employed by Objective

Objective 1—Socio-Demographic Analysis of Vulnerable Households: The first step involved a comprehensive analysis of the FSPFS survey, focusing on households identified in 2019 and expanded to include additional data from 2020. The investigation centered around socio-demographic characteristics, such as household headship, gender of the family head, and number of underaged family members. The analysis was further deepened into food security determinants, including food availability issues, food access issues and water access, and territorial determinants, including all macro-zones.

Objective 2—Dietary Intake Frequency Assessment: For the evaluation of dietary habits, a quantitative approach was adopted, which was based on categorizing the intake frequency of n = 12 food groups, listed below, according to national dietary guidelines and intake recommendations.

1. Vegetables
2. Fruits
3. Dairy
4. White meat
5. Red meat
6. Eggs
7. Legumes
8. Water
9. Bread
10. Cereals
11. Fat
12. Sugar

The assessment stratified households based on "below recommended", "recommended" and "above recommended" intake levels, further dissecting consumption patterns into weekly intake frequencies (never [0 times/week]; sometimes [0.5 times/week]; [1–2 times/week]; [3–5 times/week]; every day [7 times/week]) to provide a detailed portrayal of the dietary landscape among Chile's vulnerable populations.

Objective 3—Dietary Diversity Score Calculation and Analysis: The HDDS served as a pivotal metric in this phase, calculated for a sizable cohort to explore correlations with socio-demographic variables, food security determinants, and regional disparities. This objective employed descriptive statistics for a national-level dietary diversity overview, while regional scores were scrutinized to pinpoint macro-zone dietary patterns. Multivariate regression techniques were applied to assess the impact of various socio-demographic and food security factors, alongside geographical considerations, on the HDDS.

The calculation of the HDDS for each household was conducted in several steps utilizing the data on weekly intake frequencies of n = 12 food groups from the FSPFS diagnosis. The methodology employed is outlined as follows:

a. Quantification of Intake Frequencies: The weekly intake frequency of each food group was recorded as $HWFfg_i$ (Household Weekly Frequency), where i represents each of the 12 food groups. The frequency was quantified on a scale based on the reported intake:

- Never [0 times/week] = 0
- Twice per month [0.5 times/week] = 0.5
- 1–2 times/week = 1.5
- 3–5 times/week = 4
- Every day [7 times/week] = 7

b. Weighting of Food Groups: Each $HWFfg_i$ was then multiplied by a weight factor W_i specific to each food group to reflect its importance in the diet, as shown in Table 3. The weight factors W_i were derived from [26] nutritional guidelines that emphasize the relative nutritional contribution of each food group:

$$Weighted\_HWFfg_i = HWFfg_i \times W_i$$

c. Calculation of HDDS: The HDDS for each household was calculated by summing the weighted frequencies of all 12 food groups:

$$HDDS = \sum_{i=1}^{12} Weighted\_HWFfg_i$$

Table 3. Weight factors per food group.

Food Group	Weight Factor
Vegetables	1.0
Fruits	1.0
Dairy	4.0
White meat	4.0
Red meat	4.0
Eggs	4.0
Legumes	3.0
Water	1.0
Bread	2.0
Cereals	2.0
Fat	0.5
Sugar	0.5

The final HDDS is a summative score that indicates the dietary diversity of the household, serving as a proxy for nutritional adequacy. Higher HDDS values suggest greater dietary diversity and, potentially, better household nutritional status.

Using the "lm" function in R, a multilinear regression model with HDDS as the dependent variable was constructed. The model included Head of Household Age, Gender, Underaged family members, Food Access Issues, Food Availability Issues, Water Access, and Macro-zone as independent variables. To assess the collinearity among the variables in the dataset, a Variance Inflation Factor (VIF) test was employed by calculating VIF values for each predictor using the "vif" function from the "car" package. A VIF value exceeding 5 was considered indicative of significant collinearity.

Objective 4—Development of a Spatial Warning System: The data for this objective analysis were extracted from the diagnostic surveys from the FSPFS database. Based on Objective 2 of our preliminary analysis, which identified problematic food group intakes, five critical food groups were selected: fruits, vegetables, dairy products, sugars, and fats. These groups were chosen due to their significant deviation from the recommended intake levels—fruits, vegetables, and dairy intake were typically under the recommended thresholds, while sugars and fats were consumed above the recommended thresholds.

Descriptive statistics were computed for each of the five critical food groups across all macro-zones. For the data analysis, the RStudio environment was utilized with its packages "tidyverse", "chilemapas", "sf", "ggplot2", and "dplyr". The monthly intake averages were calculated to determine the mean number of days each food group was consumed. To capture the variability in consumption patterns, we identified the highest and lowest intake frequencies, along with the corresponding number and percentage of households. The mode representing the most common reported intake frequency was also calculated along with its prevalence among the households. To quantify the degree of intake deficiency, we determined the percentage of households consuming at/below/above the recommended levels for each food group.

The spatial visualization analysis of the five critical food groups' intakes across macro-zones in Chile involved the following steps of data processing and geographical mapping:

a. Conversion of Weekly Intake Frequency to Monthly Frequency:

Since the data provided by the FSPFS diagnosis survey considered a weekly intake, the function $MonthlyIntake(i)$ was defined to convert weekly frequency intake to monthly frequency intake.

$$\begin{cases} 30 \text{ if Everyday} \\ 16 \text{ if } 3-5 \text{ times per week} \\ 6 \text{ if } 1-2 \text{ times per week} \\ 2 \text{ if Sometimes} \\ 0 \text{ if Never} \end{cases}$$

b. Calculation of Commune-Level Averages

For each commune, i.e., the smallest administrative division in Chile, the average monthly frequency intake, defined as $CommuneAverage(i)$ was calculated, by aggregating individual household monthly frequency intakes for a given food group i and then dividing by the total number of households in the commune.

$$CommuneAverage(i) = \frac{\sum MonthlyIntake(i)}{Total\ number\ of\ households\ in\ the\ commune}$$

where n is the number of households in the commune.

Each commune's $CommuneAverage(i)$ was georeferenced using its coordinates provided by the "chilemapas" package in RStudio. This process involved associating the calculated average intake values with their respective spatial locations on the Chilean map.

A Choropleth map was applied to represent the average intake values. Communes with higher average intakes of a particular food group are displayed in darker shades, while those with lower average intakes are shown in lighter shades. This gradient visually represents the distribution of intake frequencies across different communes and macro-zones.

We identified and grouped communes within the macro-zones based on the proportion of households with intake levels below the recommended threshold for fruits, vegetables, and dairy, and above the recommended threshold for fats and sugars. The benchmark for categorization was set at 50% or more of households deviating from the recommended intake levels.

For visual representation, we employed a horizontal barplot with a red gradient fill, where the intensity of the red color corresponded to the proportion of households in each commune with above or below the recommended dietary intake. The gradient provided a visual scale of adherence to dietary recommendations, with darker shades indicating a higher percentage of households not meeting the recommended intake. The analysis was designed to yield both visual and quantitative interpretations of dietary patterns, facilitating the development of targeted nutritional interventions. The formula employed for determining the thresholds was

$$Threshold\ Proportion = \frac{Number\ of\ households\ not\ meeting\ recommendations}{Total\ number\ of\ households\ in\ the\ commune} \times 100 \quad (1)$$

where a proportion equal to or greater than 50% indicated a significant deviation from recommended dietary patterns. The proportion of households not meeting the recommendations per food group in different macro-zones can be found in Supplementary Material.

3. Results

3.1. Socio-Demographic Analysis of Vulnerable Households

3.1.1. Household Composition, Size, and Type

It was found that all necessary data were available for n = 3967 households, from a total of n = 3996 households initially included for 2019, meaning an inclusion rate of 99.3%. In addition, six communes from 2020 were incorporated in the analysis, resulting in a total of n = 4047 households and n = 12,534 individuals. Of these, n = 3505 (86.6%) households had a woman as head, whereas n = 542 households (13.4%) were led by men.

On average, each household had 3.05 members: 3.2 members when the household was led by a woman, and 2.15 members when it was led by a man. When analyzing this variable in the different macro-zones, while in all cases there were more female heads of households, in the Norte Grande, the difference was 77.0% vs. 23.0%, whereas the largest difference was found in the Zona Central, with 89.2% vs. 10.8%. At the national level, it was found that small households were the most frequent, comprising 63.8% of the total, followed by medium-sized households (32.9%), and large households (3.3%). Small households consist of up to 3 members, medium-sized households consist of 4–6 members, and large households consist of 7 or more members. This trend was consistent across all macro-zones, although with variations. For example, in the most extreme zones (i.e., northern and southern regions), Norte Grande and Zona Austral, smaller households accounted for 86.6% and 78.6% of the total, while larger households constituted only 1.7% and 2%, respectively. Refer to Table 4 for detailed statistics on household composition, headship by gender, and size across different macro-zones in Chile.

Table 4. Household composition, headship by gender and size across Chilean macro-zones, 2019–2020 *.

Macro-Zone	Households Analyzed	Households with Female Head	Households with Male Head	Average Household Size	Small Households	Medium-Size Households	Large Households
Norte Grande	178 (4.4%)	137 (77.03%)	41 (23.03%)	3.1	111 (62.36%)	56 (31.46%)	11 (6.18%)
Norte Chico	298 (7.4%)	265 (88.93%)	33 (11.07%)	3.1	180 (60.4%)	105 (35.23%)	13 (4.36%)
Zona Central	1668 (41.2%)	1488 (89.21%)	180 (10.79%)	3.1	1052 (63.07%)	565 (33.87%)	51 (3.06%)
Zona Sur	1805 (44.6%)	1533 (84.93%)	272 (15.07%)	3.1	1163 (64.43%)	585 (32.41%)	57 (3.16%)
Zona Austral	98 (2.3%)	82 (83.67%)	16 (16.33%)	2.5	77 (78.57%)	19 (19.39%)	2 (2.04%)

* Note: Percentages may not sum to 100 due to rounding.

3.1.2. Age and Regional Variations

The national average age for men was 68.9 ± 12.1 years, and for women, it was 55.9 ± 15.6 years, representing a difference of 13 years. The highest average ages were found in the Zona Austral, while the lowest were in the Norte Chico. It is notable that the groups aged 18 to 64, often considered the workforce group, were the most frequent, followed by individuals older than 64 years. Regional variations in age distributions should be noted as well. Refer to Table 5 For detailed information on the average age of household heads by gender and the distribution of age groups across different Chilean macro-zones.

Table 5. Average age of household heads and age group distribution by gender in Chilean macro-zones, 2019–2020 *.

Macro-Zone	Average Age of Male Heads (Years)	Average Age of Female Heads (Years)	Percentage of Workforce Age Group (%)	Percentage of Elderly (65+)
Norte Grande	67.9	51.2	39.6	18.6
Norte Chico	66.5	54.1	50.6	13.7
Zona Central	69.3	55.2	51.1	16.4
Zona Sur	68.5	57	49.5	20.8
Zona Austral	76.5	61.1	42.9	29

* Note: The workforce age group is defined as individuals aged 18 to 64 years.

3.1.3. Employment Status and Main Work Activities

Regarding the employment status of household heads, there was a noticeable difference between households led by women and men. It was found that 25.4% (796 individuals) of women who were household heads were employed, while 37.45% (298 individuals) of men who were household heads were employed. When analyzing the main work activities of the family representative, it was found that, for women, the main activities were homemaker (59.86%), pensioner (12.21%), and farmer/food production (9.64%). In the case of households headed by men, the primary activities were pensioner (42.25%), farmer/food production (29.52%), and other occupations (17.34%). For the purposes of this study, homemaker and unemployed were considered mutually exclusive categories. Refer to Table 6 for more details on occupation according to head of household.

Table 6. Occupation according to head of household, 2019–2020.

Head of Household Gender	Occupation					
	Farmer/Food Production	Homemaker	Pensioner	Unemployed	Other	No Information
Female	338 (9.64%)	2098 (59.86%)	428 (12.21%)	54 (1.54%)	558 (15.92%)	29 (0.83%)
Male	160 (29.52%)	43 (7.93%)	229 (42.25%)	5 (0.92%)	94 (17.34%)	11 (2.03%)

3.2. Dietary Intake Frequency Assessment

Intake of Different Food Groups among Chilean Vulnerable Households at the National Level

When analyzing the intake of different food groups among Chilean vulnerable households according to the "recommendation" categories, it was possible to highlight different tendencies (Table S1) all shown schematized in Figure 1. First, it was found that recommended intake of food groups such as bread, cereals, eggs, legumes, sugar, water, and white meats were each met or exceeded by at least 75% of the households. Secondly, not all food groups had intakes in the "above recommended" category; these food groups included vegetables, fruits, dairy and water. In addition, only in the case of vegetables, fruits and dairy, there were more households with "below recommended" intake in comparison to those with "recommended" and "above recommended" intake. Finally, the only food groups that were regularly overconsumed were fats and sugars.

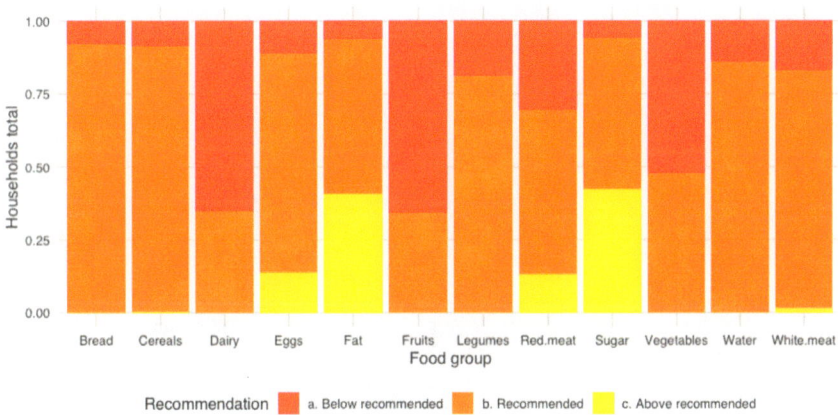

Figure 1. Recommended intake of different food groups in vulnerable Chilean households, 2019–2020.

However, the above describe the proportion of households within each recommendation category and do not give any detail regarding the frequency of intake for the different food groups. Thus, Figure 2 shows this information according to the intake frequency detailed in Supplementary Material. One of the main findings in this analysis is related to the intake of bread, which is consumed daily by 92% of households. It was also found that nearly half of the households consumed vegetables and cereals on a daily basis. Also, fats and sugar were consumed at least once a week by all households. Most households consumed protein at least once per week, mainly through white meat and/or legumes. Finally, most members of households consumed water daily.

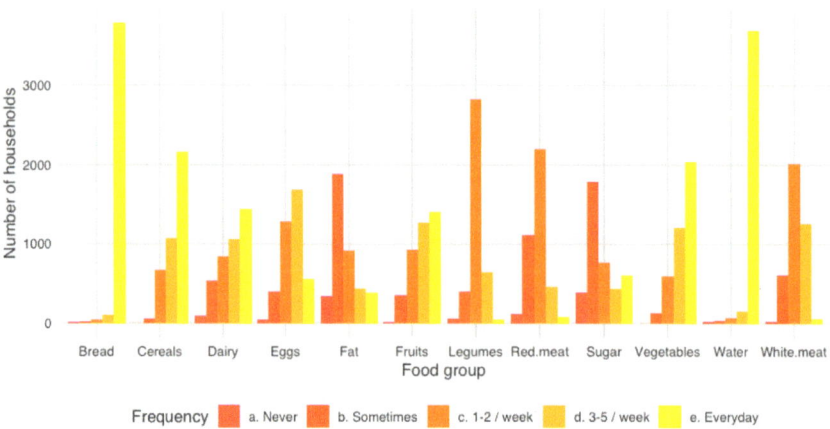

Figure 2. Frequency of intake of different food groups in vulnerable Chilean households, 2019–2020.

3.3. HDDS Calculation and Analysis

3.3.1. Chilean Vulnerable HDDS

National Level

The 4047 observations of the HDDS showed a mean value of 91.4 ± 20.63, indicating a noticeable variability in the dietary diversity across households. The median value of 91.75 closely aligns with the mean, suggesting a symmetric distribution. The range from a minimum score of 20 to a maximum of 163.25 showcases considerable variability in dietary diversity scores. The slight negative skewness of −0.064 indicates that the distribution is slightly skewed to the left, although this skewness is minimal. The HDDS histogram in available in Figure 3.

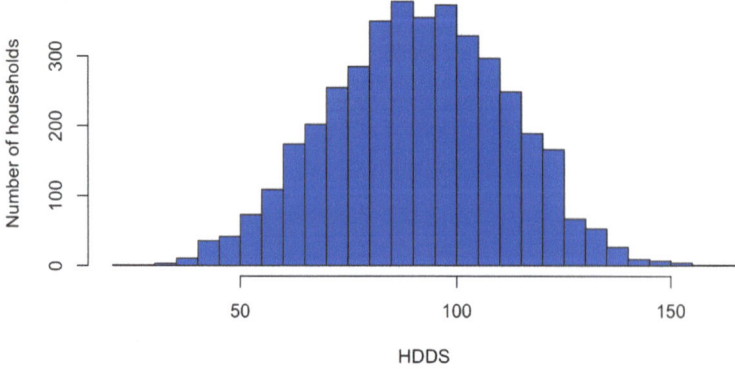

Figure 3. National Household Dietary Diversity Score (HDDS), 2019–2020.

Macro-Zone Level

The HDDS data provide a comprehensive overview of dietary diversity among Chile's macro-zones, as schematized in Figure 4. The mean HDDS indicates moderately diverse diets in Norte Grande (96.07 ± 19.23) and Zona Central (94.15 ± 19.81), while Norte Chico (93.35 ± 19.03) and Zona Austral (91.26 ± 20.56) also exhibit reasonable diversity. Zona Sur shows a somewhat lower mean HDDS at 88.1 ± 21.28, suggesting a somewhat less diverse diet. The standard deviations reflect the variability within these regions. Median values closely align with the means, indicating relatively balanced distributions. Zona Central stands out with a mode of 110, suggesting a substantially greater HDDS. The interquartile range (IQR) demonstrates the spread of data, with Zona Central having the widest range (20.00 to 163.25), while Zona Sur exhibits the narrowest range (30.50 to 158.25). Details for all macro-zones can be found in Table 7.

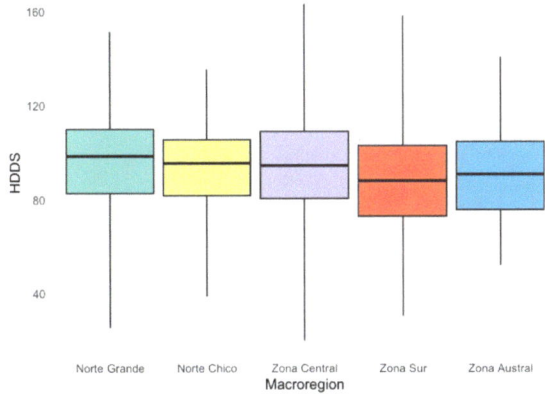

Figure 4. Distribution of HDDS across Chilean macro-zones, 2019–2020.

Table 7. Household Dietary Diversity Score (HDDS) across Chilean macro-zones, 2019–2020.

Macro-Zone	Mean ± SD	Median	Mode	Q25	Q75	Min	Max
Norte Grande	96.07 ± 19.23	98.50	90.0	82.75	110	25.50	151.50
Norte Chico	93.35 ± 19.03	95.50	97.0	81.75	105.5000	38.75	135.50
Zona Central	94.15 ± 19.81	94.50	110.0	80.50	109.0000	20.00	163.25
Zona Sur	88.1 ± 21.28	88.00	95.0	73.00	103	30.50	158.25
Zona Austral	91.26 ± 20.56	90.75	76.5	75.75	104.6875	52.00	140.75

3.3.2. HDDS Association with Household Socio-Demographic Characteristics, Food Security Determinants, and Geographical Determinants

The multiple linear regression analysis conducted to evaluate the relationship between the HDDS and socio-demographic characteristics, food security and geographical determinants showed significance in the overall model (R^2 adjusted = 0.0284, $F_{10,4036}$ = 12.84, $p < 0.001$). The HDDS was positively correlated with number of minors in the household ($\beta = 0.969$, $p = 0.005$) and water access ($\beta = 1.410$, $p = 0.050$). In contrast, having food access issues ($\beta = -2.267$, $p = 0.002$) and residing in the ZS macro-zone, compared to NC as reference ($\beta = -4.976$, $p < 0.001$), were negatively associated with the HDDS. Other variables, namely age, gender, and food availability issues, did not show significant associations (Table 8).

Table 8. HDDS association with household socio-demographic characteristics, food security determinants, and geographical determinants, 2019–2020.

	Variables			n	%	HDDS β	t-Value	p-Value
Socio-demographic	Head of household age			-	-	0.011	41.582	0.672
	Gender of family head		M	542	13.4%	0.896	0.423	0.362
			F	3505	86.6%	-	-	-
	Underaged family members			-	-	0.969	2.791	0.005 *
Food security determinants	Access issues							
			Yes	1943	48.0%	−2.26	−3.080	0.002 *
			No	2104	52.0%	-	-	-
	Availability issues							
			Yes	1805	44.6%	−1.28	−1.714	0.087
			No	2242	55.4%	-	-	-
	Water access							
			Yes	2786	68.8%	1.4	−1.962	0.05 *
			No	1261	31.2%	-	-	-
Geographical determinants	Macro-zone							
		Norte Grande		178	4.4%	3.082	1.592	0.111
		Norte Chico		298	7.4%	-	-	-
		Zona Central		1668	41.2%	0.872	0.682	0.495
		Zona Sur		1805	44.6%	−4.98	−3.874	0.0001 *
		Zona Austral		98	2.4%	−1.90	−0.798	0.425

Note: n: number of households; %: percentage of households of the total; β: regression coefficient. * $p < 0.05$.

The calculated GVIF values, as shown in Table 9, confirm that no variable exhibits significant collinearity, supporting the robustness of the regression model.

Table 9. Variance inflation factor (VIF) analysis for predictor variables, 2019–2020.

Variable	VIF
Head of household age	1.804657
Head of household gender	1.098242
Underaged family members	1.750329
Food access issues	1.323603
Food availability issues	1.352717
Water access	1.083933
Macro-zone	1.111615

3.4. Development of a Spatial Warning System

3.4.1. Food Group Intake in Vulnerable Households According to Geographical Macro-Zones Including "Norte Grande", "Norte Chico", "Zona Central", "Zona Sur", and "Zona Austral"

Fruits

The highest averages for fruit consumption were found in the Zona Central (19.8 ± 10.1) and Norte Chico (18.0 ± 9.7), whereas the lowest were found in the Zona Sur (16.3 ± 10.2) and the Zona Austral (15.9 ± 9.4). Although there was a difference of almost 4 days per month between the macro-zones with the highest and lowest intake, it was found that all macro-zones had, on average, an intake of once every two days. All macro-zones showed a daily intake of fruits in at least one of their communes. However, n = 8 communes in the Zona Central (0.48%), n = 4 (0.2%) communes in the Zona Sur, and n = 5 (5.1%) communes in the Zona Austral showed no intake of fruit during the month. Finally, whereas a daily intake of fruits was found as the more frequent value in the Norte Grande and Zona Central, in the Zona Austral, the most repeated value, representing 28% of the households, was an intake of 6.4 days/month. Regarding the number of households below the recommended fruit intake, the southern macro-zones showed the highest values, with the Zona Austral (n = 81) reaching 82.6% of households under that condition, and Zona Sur (n = 1290) 78.1% of households under the same classification. Details about the values of these indicators for each region and the spatial representation of these differences can be found in Table 10 and Figure 5, respectively.

Table 10. Fruit intake across Chilean geographical macro-zones, 2019–2020.

Fruit	Norte Grande	Norte Chico	Zona Central	Zona Sur	Zona Austral
Monthly intake average (days)	17.5 ± 10.7	18 ± 9.7	19.8 ± 10.2	16.3 ± 10.2	15.9 ± 11
Highest (days)	30	30	30	30	30
n (%) [Households]	64 (36)	98 (32.9)	746 (44.7)	562 (31.1)	31 (31.6)
Lowest (days)	2.1	2.1	0	0	0
n (%) [Households]	25 (14)	16 (5.4)	8 (0.48)	4 (0.2)	5 (5.1)
Mode (days)	30	17.1	30	17.1	6.4
n (%) [Households]	64 (36)	110 (37)	739 (44)	596 (33)	27 (28)
No. of households below recommended * (%)	113 (63.4)	199 (66.8)	938 (55.2)	1290 (78.1)	81 (82.6)

* Details of communes with more than 50% of households below recommended intake can be found in Figure S1.

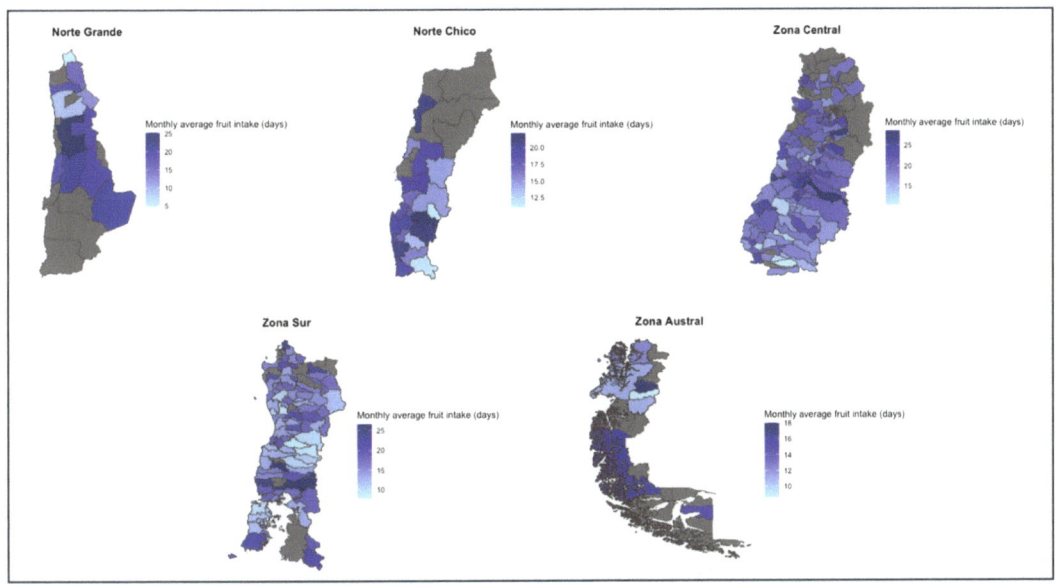

Figure 5. Monthly average fruit intake in days per macro-zone, 2019–2020.

Vegetables

The Zona Central (23.81 ± 8.8) and Norte Grande (21.2 ± 9.5) were the macro-zones with the highest monthly average intake of vegetables per household, whereas the Zona Austral (18.1 ± 8.9) and the Norte Chico (19.9 ± 9.8) were the macro-zones with the lowest monthly average intake. All macro-zones had at least one household with an average intake of vegetables of 30 days/month, with the Zona Central (n = 1058; 63.4%) being the macro-zone with the highest number, and the Zona Austral (n = 29; 29.6%) the macro-zone with the lowest. However, it was only in the Zona Sur where we found households (n = 2; 0.1%) with no consumption of vegetables. Finally, except for the Zona Austral, whose most frequent vegetable intake average was 17.1 days/month in n = 38 (39%) of their households, all other macro-zones had a daily intake of vegetables as their most frequent value, compared to the other intake frequencies. As with fruit intake, the southern macro-zones were those with the greatest proportion of households in the "below recommended" category (Zona Sur: n = 1128 (63.5%); Zona Austral n = 69 (70.4%)). Details about the values of these indicators for each region and the spatial representation of these differences can be found in Table 11 and Figure 6, respectively.

Table 11. Vegetable intake across Chilean geographical macro-zones, 2019–2020.

Vegetables	Norte Grande	Norte Chico	Zona Central	Zona Sur	Zona Austral
Monthly intake average (days)	21.2 ± 9.5	19.8 ± 9.8	23.8 ± 8.8	20.2 ± 9.6	18.1 ± 8.9
Highest (days)	30	30	30	30	30
n (%) [Households]	86 (48.3)	128 (43)	1058 (63.4)	784 (43.4)	29 (29.6)
Lowest (days)	2.1	2.1	2.1	0	6.4
n (%) [Households]	9 (5)	12 (4)	29 (1.7)	2 (0.1)	26 (6.4)
Mode (days)	30	30	30	30	17.1
n (%) [Households]	86 (48)	127 (43)	1053 (63)	767 (42)	38 (39)
No. of households below recommended (%) *	93 (52.2)	175 (58.7)	646 (38)	1128 (63.5)	69 (70.4)

* Details of communes with more than 50% of households below recommended intake can be found in Figure S2.

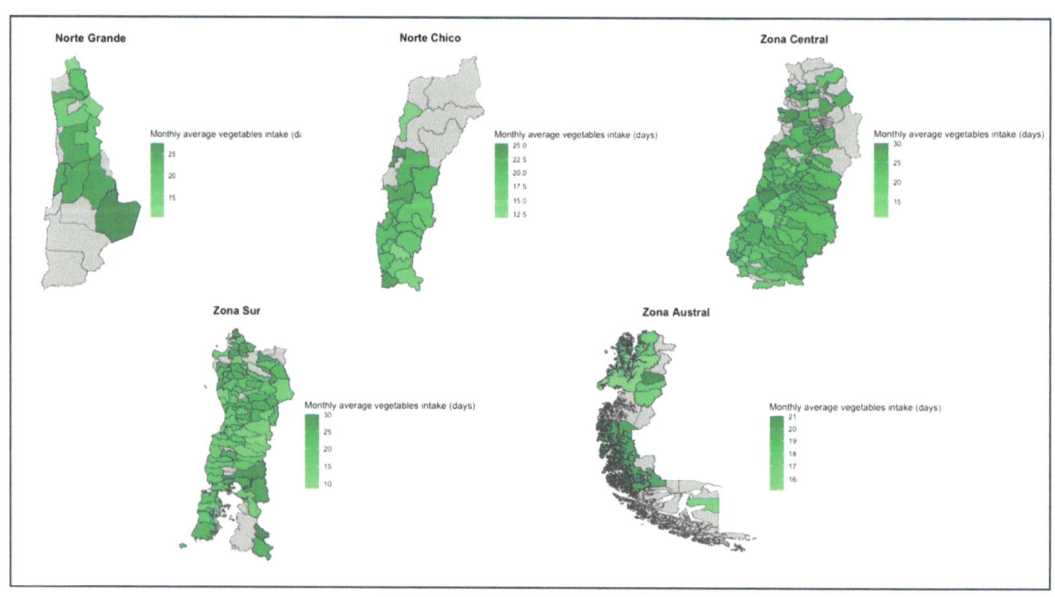

Figure 6. Monthly average vegetable intake in days per macro-zone, 2019–2020.

Dairy

The highest averages for dairy intake per household were found in the Norte Grande (19.2 ± 10.8) and the Zona Central (18.5 ± 10.9), whereas the lowest averages were in the Zona Austral (15.9 ± 11) and the Zona Sur. All macro-zones had at least one household that showed a daily intake of dairy products, with the Norte Grande (44%) and the Zona Central (41.8%) being those with a major proportion. However, all macro-zones had a daily intake of dairy products as their most frequent value. In addition, at least one household in all macro-zones showed a zero intake of dairy products within the monthly period, most commonly in the Zona Central (n = 51; 3.05%) and the Zona Austral (n = 5; 5.1%). For this food group, 72.3% (n = 1284), of Zona Sur households were below the recommended intake of dairy products, whereas 69.4% (n = 68) of households in the Zona Austral fell into this classification. Details about the values of these indicators for each region and the spatial representation of these differences can be found in Table 12 and Figure 7, respectively.

Table 12. Dairy intake across Chilean geographical macro-zones, 2019–2020.

Dairy	Norte Grande	Norte Chico	Zona Central	Zona Sur	Zona Austral
Monthly intake average (days)	19.2 ± 10.8	17.4 ± 10.4	18.5 ± 10.9	15.6 ± 11	15.9 ± 11
Highest (days)	30	30	30	30	30
n (%) [Households]	79 (44.4)	101 (33.9)	697 (41.8)	524 (29)	31 (31.6)
Lowest (days)	0	0	0	0	0
n (%) [Households]	3 (1.7)	2 (0.7)	51 (3.05)	40 (2.2)	5 (5.1)
Mode (days)	30	30	30	30	30
n (%) [Households]	79 (44)	103 (35)	694 (42)	542 (30)	39 (40)
No. of households below recommended (%) *	101 (56.7)	198 (66.4)	988 (58.1)	1284 (72.3)	68 (69.4)

* Details of communes with more than 50% of households below recommended intake can be found in Figure S3.

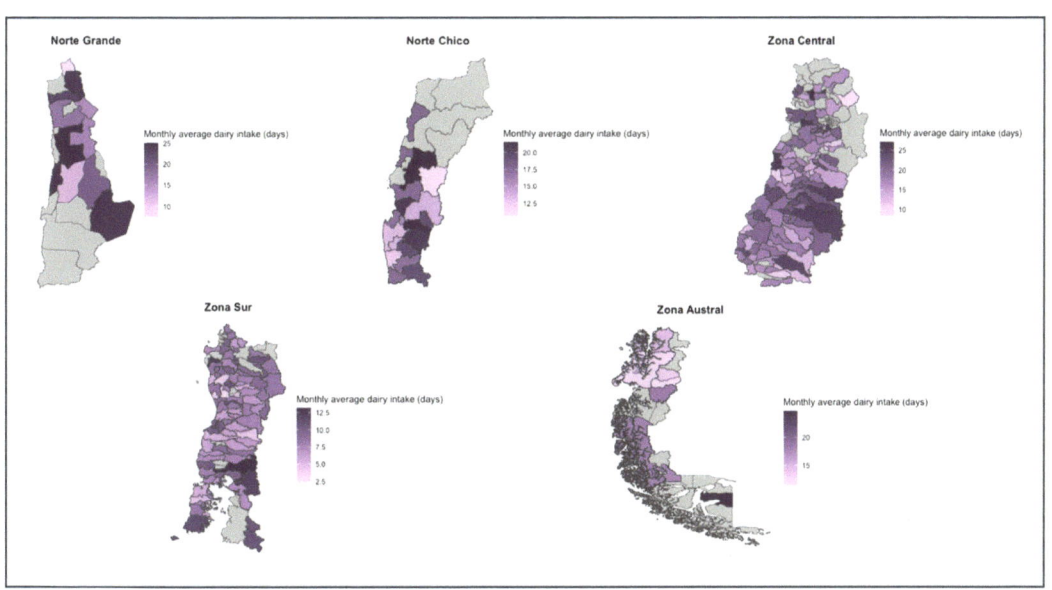

Figure 7. Monthly average dairy intake in days per macro-zone, 2019–2020.

Fat

The Norte Grande (9.8 ± 10.7) and the Norte Chico (10.5 ± 10.2) were the macro-zones with the highest average intake of fat. All macro-zones had at least one household with a daily intake of fat: the Norte Grande (n = 31; 17.4%) and the Norte Chico (n = 46; 15.4%) had the highest values. Similarly, all macro-zones showed at least one household with no intake of fat at all. Of these, the Norte Grande (n = 21; 11.8%) and the Zona Austral (n = 10; 10.2%) were the macro-zones with major representation. Finally, the most frequent value for household fat intake across all macro-zones was 2.1 days/month. The northern macro-zone had the highest values regarding the overconsumption of fat. Thus, the Norte Chico presented 56% (n = 167) of households under this classification, whereas the Norte Grande had a rate of 50.6% (n = 90). Details about the values of these indicators for each region and the spatial representation of these differences can be found in Table 13 and Figure 8, respectively.

Table 13. Fat intake across Chilean geographical macro-zones, 2019–2020.

Fat	Norte Grande	Norte Chico	Zona Central	Zona Sur	Zona Austral
Monthly intake average (days)	9.8 ± 10.7	10.5 ± 10.2	7.9 ± 9.4	6.1 ± 7.6	6.7 ± 8
Highest (days)	30	30	30	30	30
n (%) [Households]	31 (17.4)	46 (15.4)	197 (11.8)	118 (6.5)	7 (7.1)
Lowest (days)	0	0	0	0	0
n (%) [Households]	21 (11.8)	15 (5)	166 (10)	137 (7.6)	10 (10.2)
Mode (days)	2.1	2.1	2.1	2.1	2.1
n (%) [Households]	63 (35)	109 (37)	767 (46)	940 (52)	48 (49)
No. of households above recommended (%) *	90 (50.6)	167 (56)	741 (43.6)	603 (34)	46 (46.9)

* Details of communes with more than 50% of households above recommended intake can be found in Figure S4.

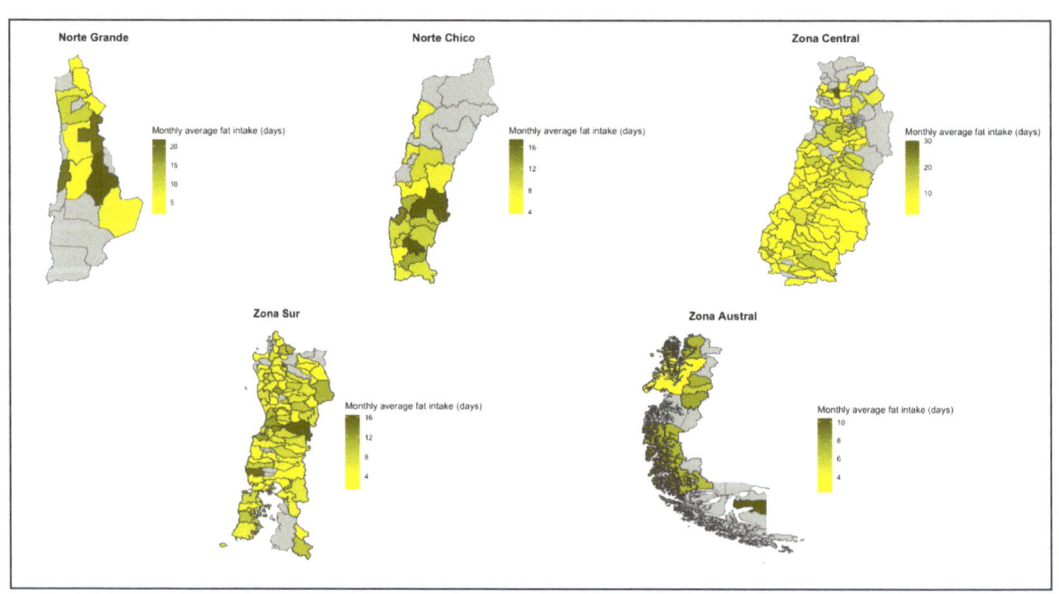

Figure 8. Monthly average fat intake in days per macro-zone, 2019–2020.

Sugar

The macro-zones with the highest average sugar intake were the Norte Grande (10.5 ± 11.1) and the Zona Central (10.5 ± 11.3). All macro-zones had at least one household with a daily intake of sugar, with the Zona Central (n = 363; 21.8%) and the Norte Grande (n = 36; 20.2%) being those with the highest values. Similarly, all macro-zones included some households with no intake of sugar. In this case, the Zona Austral (n = 11; 11.2%) and the Zona Sur (n = 192; 10.1) had the highest values. For all macro-zones, the most frequent household sugar intake was 2.1 days/month. The Norte Grande (n = 88; 49.4%), Norte Chico (n = 149; 50%), and Zona Central (n = 840; 49.5%) presented the highest rates for households with overconsumption of sugar. Details about the values of these indicators for each region and the spatial representation of these differences can be found in Table 14 and Figure 9, respectively.

Table 14. Sugar intake across Chilean geographical macro-zones, 2019–2020.

Sugar	Norte Grande	Norte Chico	Zona Central	Zona Sur	Zona Austral
Monthly intake average (days)	10.5 ± 11.1	9.4 ± 10	10.5 ± 11.3	6.8 ± 8.7	6.3 ± 8.1
Highest (days)	30	30	30	30	30
n (%) [Households]	36 (20.2)	43 (14.4)	363 (21.8)	169 (9.4)	7 (7.1)
Lowest (days)	0	0	0	0	0
n (%) [Households]	15 (8.4)	18 (6)	160 (9.6)	192 (10.1)	11 (11.2)
Mode (days)	2.1	2.1	2.1	2.1	2.1
n (%) [Households]	71 (40)	123 (41)	664 (40)	900 (50)	54 (55)
No. of households above recommended (%) *	88 (49.4)	149 (50)	840 (49.5)	593 (33.4)	38 (38.8)

* Details of communes with more than 50% of households above recommended intake can be found in Figure S5.

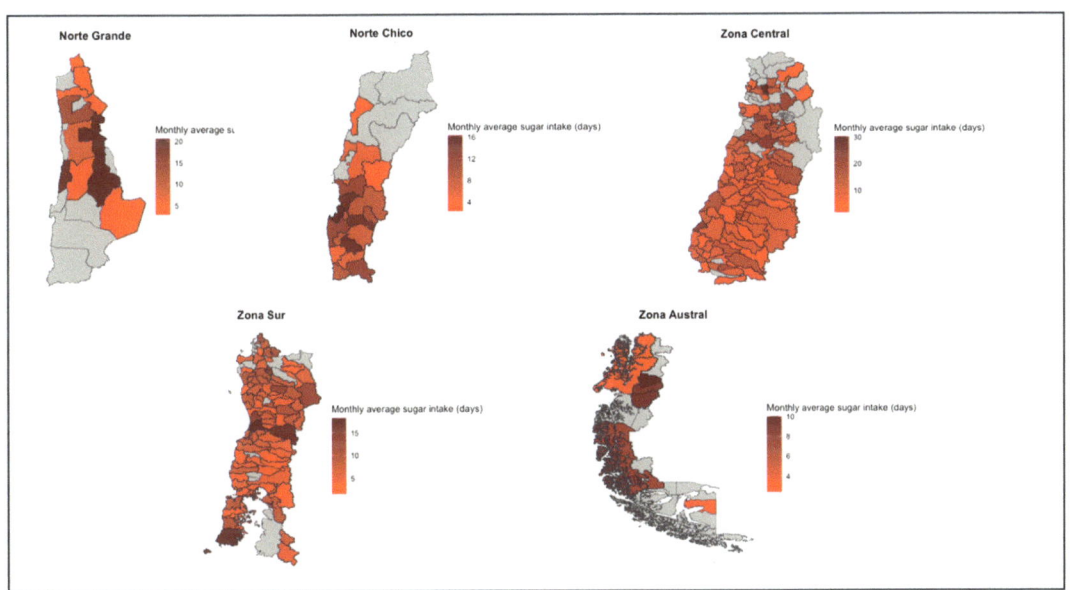

Figure 9. Monthly average sugar intake in days per macro-zone, 2019–2020.

4. Discussion

The results of this research indicate significant differences in the HDDS based on the number of underage family members, access to water, food access issues and residing in the Zona Sur macro-zone. Additionally, although the multivariate regression analysis showed that the gender of the head of household was not significantly related to the HDDS, the reality is that 86.6% of the households in the analyzed sample were led by women. Therefore, there is a need for special attention to how gender-focused food policies are addressed These relationships between socio-demographic factors and dietary diversity in Chile reflect global trends. This is further contextualized by research from Honduras [2], suggesting the unique challenges of female-headed households, a demographic that is prevalent in Chile and that requires targeted interventions. In this sense, these findings could mean a first step to deepen analysis into women's diet quality and micronutrient status in developing countries to better inform interventions and policies, as suggested by [4]. Similarly, in South Africa [27], the link between education level and dietary diversity, as the approach followed by the FSPFS, emphasizes the potential for educational initiatives to enhance food security in Chile. These global insights highlight the importance of contextualized, gender-sensitive, and education-focused strategies to address the dietary diversity and food security nexus within Chilean households.

While the HDDS is a valuable tool for identifying food security and nutritional needs, it is important to note that the model explained approximately 2.84% of the variability in the HDDS. This indicates that other factors not included in the analysis might be influencing household dietary diversity. For example, Ref. [5] noted that the HDDS fails to capture actual food consumption amounts, could be subject to reporting bias, and might not be representative due to its cross-sectional nature. Ref. [6] also pointed to the potential for measurement error given its reliance on self-reported data and its lack of granularity regarding the quantity of food within groups. Ref. [2] echoed this, emphasizing the score's inability to account for the specific nutritional content of foods. Ref. [7] added concerns about potential biases and the lack of empirical evidence linking dietary diversity with energy intake. Lastly, Ref. [27] criticized the HDDS for not considering intra-household food distribution inequalities and the difficulty in comparing HDDSs across different studies due to variations in food groupings. Furthermore, the HDDS is a number that can be reached through different combinations of food group consumption, so it must also be viewed with caution.

The prevalent consumption patterns, particularly the under-consumption of fruits, vegetables, and dairy, and the over-consumption of fats and sugars, have direct implications for the nutritional health of vulnerable populations. The dietary patterns observed in Chile, characterized by the under-consumption and over-consumption of certain food groups, mirror global concerns highlighted in international research. In South Africa, Ref. [27] noted that despite high dietary diversity, there is a lack of micronutrient-rich foods, a pattern that might be reflected in Chile's vulnerable populations, who also demonstrate gaps in essential nutrient intake. This is compounded by the findings from Honduras, which indicate that despite adequate caloric intake, nutrient-rich dietary diversity is lacking [2], a concern that is likely paralleled in Chile. Similarly, Ref. [7] in Myanmar reported low dietary diversity with negative health implications, echoing the potential nutrient deficiencies among the Chilean populace. In Malawi, Ref. [6] suggested that increased dietary diversity correlates with better food security, a strategy that could be beneficial for Chile. Lastly, the socioeconomic factors affecting dietary habits in Bangladesh, as noted by [5], resonate with the Chilean context, where economic stresses, particularly due to the COVID-19 pandemic, may exacerbate dietary limitations, affecting health outcomes.

The results also show a centralization of healthy eating in Chile, highlighting regional disparities in the consumption of healthy foods in the vulnerable population. In the Zona Central, there is a higher frequency of fruit and vegetable consumption, with a monthly average of 19.8 ± 10.1 days and 23.8 ± 8.8 days, respectively. In contrast, the extreme regions, such as the Norte Grande and the Zona Austral, face significantly different realities. The Norte Grande, with a monthly average consumption of fats and sugar of 9.8 ± 10.7 days and 10.5 ± 11.1 days, respectively, shows an unhealthy consumption profile. The Zona Austral, on the other hand, has the lowest consumption of fruits (15.9 ± 9.4 days), vegetables (18.1 ± 8.9 days), and dairy (15.9 ± 11 days). These disparities are partly due to the geographical and climatic conditions of the different macro-zones [24]. The Zona Central, being the main area for fruit and vegetable production [25], facilitates access to fresh produce. In contrast, the Norte Grande, an arid region, and the Zona Austral, with conditions that do not favor mass production of fruits and vegetables [24,25], face significant challenges in accessing a balanced diet. This situation underscores the need to improve food governance and ensure equitable physical access to healthy foods across the country.

In addition, there is a potential of the geospatial warning system proposed in pinpointing areas of food insecurity, representing a good tool for the FSPFS to know where the most critical areas are to better localize the resources needed. From this perspective, the literature widely recognizes the potential of these systems. For example, Ref. [13] validated its precision in identifying vulnerable districts, aiding in resource allocation and planning towards Sustainable Development Goals. Ref. [16] emphasized its role in revealing spatial distribution and trends in Rajasthan, directing targeted interventions. Ref. [14] highlighted mapping's capacity to elucidate spatial patterns, although they caution that its success hinges on data quality and stakeholders' interpretative skills. Similarly, Ref. [15] demonstrated how mapping informs unmet needs, optimizing efforts to combat food insecurity in New Hampshire. However, some important limitations in this study are necessary to acknowledge. First, the use of a single-time data collection point during the diagnostic survey phase presents a "picture", limiting the ability to observe changes over time or to continuously integrate new data. This is compounded by the reliance on the HDDS, which, although useful, cannot encapsulate the nuances of nutritional status or food consumption patterns over time. Additionally, the program's focus on new families each year complicates the ability to track longitudinal progress, with the only measure of continuity being the communal, regional, or macro-zone data trends.

While the spatial analysis focuses on individual food groups, which provide valuable information, it would be beneficial to understand how these food groups interact within vulnerable contexts. Specifically, analyzing "meals" rather than just ingredients could offer a more comprehensive view of dietary practices. This approach would allow for a better understanding of the nutritional balance and cultural relevance of food consumption patterns in these populations. Considering meals as holistic units rather than isolated components could reveal insights into dietary habits, food security, and nutritional outcomes that are otherwise obscured by looking at ingredients alone. By shifting the focus to meals, interventions could be more effectively tailored to meet the actual dietary needs and preferences of vulnerable groups.

5. Conclusions

This study highlights that food insecurity remains a critical issue in Chile, particularly affecting vulnerable households as these exhibit limited dietary diversity, with insufficient intake of essential food groups like fruits, vegetables, and dairy, while consuming excessive fats and sugars. The analysis of intake frequency and the HDDS revealed that sociodemographic factors, food access issues, and water availability significantly influence dietary patterns. A notable sociodemographic finding is the gender disparity, with 86.6% of households led by women, indicating a need for gender-sensitive policies related to food. The study also observed that average age differences between male and female household heads suggest potential age-related vulnerabilities. Additionally, small households in extreme regions highlight specific resource needs, while employment patterns reveal that housework, pensions, and family farming are the predominant work activities, providing insight into livelihood sources.

The practical recommendations based on the results and analysis of this study are as follows: (1) When selecting households that could participate in the program, it is essential to analyze their demographic characteristics to ensure that the inclusion of these households is based on identifying social conditions that make them more vulnerable to having lower food diversity. (2) Understanding the distribution of consumption of critical food groups across Chilean territory can also aid in the prior planning of the logistics required to improve access to these foods in the participating households.

While this study provides a comprehensive view of dietary diversity in vulnerable Chilean households, it is important to acknowledge its limitations. The single-time data collection limits the ability to observe changes over time. Furthermore, reliance on the HDDS, though useful, does not fully capture the complexities of nutritional status and food consumption patterns. The prevalence of concerning consumption patterns, such as the under-consumption of fruits, vegetables, and dairy, and the over-consumption of fats and sugars, has direct implications for the nutritional health of vulnerable populations.

Recommendations for future studies include longitudinal tracking of households to assess changes in dietary diversity and nutritional status, as well as analyzing the interactions between different food groups within vulnerable contexts. Additionally, further investigation into how specific sociodemographic characteristics, such as the gender of the household head and family composition, influence food security and dietary diversity is suggested. Understanding these regional variations is vital for tailoring targeted interventions to address the specific dietary needs of each macro-zone.

Supplementary Materials: The following supporting information can be downloaded at: https://www.mdpi.com/article/10.3390/nu16172937/s1, Figures S1–S5: Communes with more than 50% of households below/above recommended for each food group across the different Chilean Macro-zone; Table S1. Intake of different food groups in Chilean vulnerable households.

Author Contributions: Conceptualization, M.d.V.M., K.S. and S.B.; methodology, M.d.V.M., K.S. and S.B.; software, M.d.V.M.; validation, K.S. and S.B.; formal analysis, M.d.V.M., K.S. and S.B.; investigation, M.d.V.M.; data curation, M.d.V.M.; writing—original draft preparation, M.d.V.M.; writing—review and editing, M.d.V.M., K.S. and S.B.; visualization, M.d.V.M.; supervision, K.S. and S.B.; funding acquisition, M.d.V.M. All authors have read and agreed to the published version of the manuscript.

Funding: This research was made possible thanks to ANID (previous CONICYT) from the Chilean Ministry of Education under the Becas Chile scholarship program, ref: 72210103.

Institutional Review Board Statement: The current research received ethical approval from the Human Ethical Review Committee (HERC) of the Royal (Dick) School of Veterinary Studies at the University of Edinburgh, with approval number HERC_2022_148 on 31 October 2022.

Informed Consent Statement: Not applicable.

Data Availability Statement: The datasets used in this study were authorized for analysis under a privacy agreement with the Ministry of Social Development and Family of Chile.

Acknowledgments: The authors gratefully acknowledge the assistance of Alexa Bellows, Cynthia Naydani, and Pablo Aguirre in the data analysis and visualization for this study. Special thanks are also extended to Shadia Sufan and Cristian Campos for their support in facilitating access to the data from Chile, and to the Subsecretary of Social Services for their cooperation.

Conflicts of Interest: The authors declare no conflicts of interest.

References

1. Muthini, D.; Nzuma, J.; Nyikal, R. Farm production diversity and its association with dietary diversity in Kenya. *Food Secur.* **2020**, *12*, 1107–1120. [CrossRef]
2. Larson, J.B.; Castellanos, P.; Jensen, L. Gender, household food security, and dietary diversity in western Honduras. *Glob. Food Secur.* **2019**, *20*, 170–179. [CrossRef]
3. Kennedy, G.; Ballard, T.; Dop, M. *Guidelines for Measuring Household and Individual Dietary Diversity*; Food and Agriculture Organization of the United Nations: Rome, Italy, 2011.
4. Ruel, M.T.; Deitchler, M.; Arimond, M. Developing Simple Measures of Women's Diet Quality in Developing Countries: Overview1, 2. *J. Nutr.* **2010**, *140*, 2048S–2050S. [CrossRef] [PubMed]
5. Kundu, S.; Al Banna, M.H.; Sayeed, A.; Sultana, M.S.; Brazendale, K.; Harris, J.; Khan, M.S.I. Determinants of household food security and dietary diversity during the COVID-19 pandemic in Bangladesh. *Public Health Nutr.* **2021**, *24*, 1079–1087. [CrossRef]
6. Kerr, R.B.; Kangmennaang, J.; Dakishoni, L.; Nyantakyi-Frimpong, H.; Lupafya, E.; Shumba, L.; Luginaah, I. Participatory agroecological research on climate change adaptation improves smallholder farmer household food security and dietary diversity in Malawi. *Agric. Ecosyst. Environ.* **2019**, *279*, 109–121. [CrossRef]

7. Pritchard, B.; Rammohan, A.; Vicol, M. The importance of non-farm livelihoods for household food security and dietary diversity in rural Myanmar. *J. Rural. Stud.* **2019**, *67*, 89–100. [CrossRef]
8. Arimond, M.; Wiesmann, D.; Becquey, E.; Carriquiry, A.; Daniels, M.C.; Deitchler, M.; Torheim, L.E. Simple food group diversity indicators predict micronutrient adequacy of women's diets in 5 diverse, resource-poor settings. *J. Nutr.* **2010**, *140*, 2059S–2069S. [CrossRef]
9. Martin-Prevel, Y.; Becquey, E.; Arimond, M. Food group diversity indicators derived from qualitative list-based questionnaire misreported some foods compared to same indicators derived from quantitative 24-hour recall in urban Burkina Faso. *J. Nutr.* **2010**, *140*, 2086S–2093S. [CrossRef]
10. Moursi, M.M.; Arimond, M.; Dewey, K.G.; Treche, S.; Ruel, M.T.; Delpeuch, F. Dietary diversity is a good predictor of the micronutrient density of the diet of 6-to 23-month-old children in Madagascar3. *J. Nutr.* **2008**, *138*, 2448–2453. [CrossRef]
11. Verger, E.O.; Ballard, T.J.; Dop, M.C.; Martin-Prevel, Y. Systematic review of use and interpretation of dietary diversity indicators in nutrition-sensitive agriculture literature. *Glob. Food Secur.* **2019**, *20*, 156–169. [CrossRef]
12. Becquey, E.; Martin-Prevel, Y. Micronutrient adequacy of women's diet in urban Burkina Faso is low. *J. Nutr.* **2010**, *140*, 2079S–2085S. [CrossRef] [PubMed]
13. Hossain, M.J.; Das, S.; Chandra, H.; Islam, M.A. Disaggregate level estimates and spatial mapping of food insecurity in Bangladesh by linking survey and census data. *PLoS ONE* **2010**, *15*, e0230906. [CrossRef]
14. Leroy, J.L.; Ruel, M.; Frongillo, E.A.; Harris, J.; Ballard, T.J. Measuring the food access dimension of food security: A critical review and mapping of indicators. *Food Nutr. Bull.* **2015**, *36*, 167–195. [CrossRef] [PubMed]
15. Wauchope, B.; Ward, S. *Mapping Food Insecurity and Food Sources in New Hampshire Cities and Towns*; Carsey Institute, University of New Hampshire: Durham, UK, 2012.
16. Swati, R.; Kavita, A. Measuring and mapping the state of food insecurity in Rajasthan, India. *Geogr. Environ. Sustain.* **2021**, *14*, 33–40. [CrossRef]
17. Hwang, M.; Smith, M. Integrating publicly available web mapping tools for cartographic visualization of community food insecurity: A prototype. *GeoJournal* **2012**, *77*, 47–62. [CrossRef]
18. Davis, J.; Magadzire, N.; Hemerijckx, L.M.; Maes, T.; Durno, D.; Kenyana, N.; May, J. Precision approaches to food insecurity: A spatial analysis of urban hunger and its contextual correlates in an African city. *World Dev.* **2022**, *149*, 105694. [CrossRef]
19. Mathenge, M.; Sonneveld, B.G.; Broerse, J.E. Mapping the spatial dimension of food insecurity using GIS-based indicators: A case of Western Kenya. *Food Secur.* **2023**, *15*, 243–260. [CrossRef]
20. Nica-Avram, G.; Harvey, J.; Goulding, J.; Lucas, B.; Smith, A.; Smith, G.; Perrat, B. Fims: Identifying, predicting and visualising food insecurity. In Proceedings of the Companion Proceedings of the Web Conference, New York, NY, USA, 20–24 April 2020; pp. 190–193.
21. Leisher, C. A comparison of tablet-based and paper-based survey data collection in conservation projects. *Soc. Sci.* **2014**, *3*, 264–271. [CrossRef]
22. EVS (Elige Vivir Sano). Estudio: Radiografía de la Alimentación en Chile. Resumen de Primeros Resultados. Available online: https://aam.cl/wp-content/uploads/2021/02/20210112-Radiografi%CC%81a-de-la-Alimentacio%CC%81n-EVS.pdf (accessed on 3 May 2021).
23. National Socioeconomic Characterization Survey. Ministry of Social Development and Family, Government of Chile. Food Insecurity Outcomes. Available online: https://datasocial.ministeriodesarrollosocial.gob.cl/fichaIndicador/814/1 (accessed on 3 May 2024).
24. Sarricolea, P.; Herrera-Ossandon, M.; Meseguer-Ruiz, Ó. Climatic regionalisation of continental Chile. *J. Maps* **2017**, *13*, 66–73. [CrossRef]
25. Meza, F.; Gil, P.; Melo, O. Agricultural uses. *Water Resour. Chile* **2021**, *8*, 243–258.
26. World Food Programme. *Manual for Food Security Assessment in Emergencies*, 2nd ed.; [Spanish version]; Food and Agriculture Organization of the United Nations: Rome, Italy, 2009.
27. Megbowon, E.T.; Mushunje, A. Assessment of food security among households in Eastern Cape Province, South Africa: Evidence from general household survey, 2014. *Int. J. Soc. Econ.* **2018**, *45*, 2–17. [CrossRef]

Disclaimer/Publisher's Note: The statements, opinions and data contained in all publications are solely those of the individual author(s) and contributor(s) and not of MDPI and/or the editor(s). MDPI and/or the editor(s) disclaim responsibility for any injury to people or property resulting from any ideas, methods, instructions or products referred to in the content.

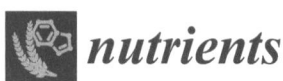 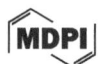

Article

Food Neophobia in Children: A Case Study in Federal District/Brazil

Priscila Claudino De Almeida [1,*], Eduardo Yoshio Nakano [2], Ivana Aragão Lira Vasconcelos [3], Renata Puppin Zandonadi [3], António Raposo [4,*], Ariana Saraiva [5], Hmidan A. Alturki [6] and Raquel Braz Assunção Botelho [3,*]

[1] Graduate Program in Human Nutrition, University of Brasília, Brasília 70910-900, Brazil
[2] Department of Statistics, University of Brasília, Brasília 70910-900, Brazil; eynakano@gmail.com
[3] Department of Nutrition, University of Brasília, Brasília 70910-900, Brazil; ivanaunb@gmail.com (I.A.L.V.); renatapz@unb.br (R.P.Z.)
[4] CBIOS (Research Center for Biosciences and Health Technologies), Universidade Lusófona de Humanidades e Tecnologias, Campo Grande 376, 1749-024 Lisboa, Portugal
[5] Department of Animal Pathology and Production, Bromatology and Food Technology, Faculty of Veterinary, Universidad de Las Palmas de Gran Canaria, Trasmontaña s/n, 35413 Arucas, Spain; ariana_23@outlook.pt
[6] King Abdulaziz City for Science & Technology, Wellness and Preventive Medicine Institute—Health Sector, Riyadh 11442, Saudi Arabia; halturki@kacst.edu.sa
* Correspondence: nprialmeida@gmail.com (P.C.D.A.); antonio.raposo@ulusofona.pt (A.R.); raquelbotelho@unb.br (R.B.A.B.); Tel.: +55-61-98220-2078 (P.C.D.A.); +55-61-98137-8620 (R.B.A.B.)

Abstract: A reluctance to eat and/or avoidance of novel foods is characterized as food neophobia (FN). FN restricts the diet to familiar foods when, in fact, it should be much more varied. FN can be a barrier to healthy foods, affecting the quality of diet, and impairing children's growth and development. Therefore, according to their caregivers' perceptions, this study aimed to evaluate FN in children from Federal District/Brazil. The Brazilian Children's Food Neophobia Questionnaire (BCFNeo), a specific instrument developed and validated in Brazil, was answered by caregivers of children aged 4 to 11 y/o. Sampling occurred through snowball recruitment, being convenient and non-probabilistic. The Health Sciences Ethics Committee approved the study. The analysis evaluated FN in total (BCFNeoTot) and in the following domains: general (FNgen), for fruits (FNfru), and for vegetables (FNveg). FN scores were compared between sex and child's age and categorized according to three ordinal levels. FN levels were compared using the Mann–Whitney U test. The Friedman test, followed by the Wilcoxon test with Bonferroni correction, was performed to analyze differences in FN according to the environment. Of the caregivers' answers for their children, 595 answers were included, because 19 were out of age. The prevalence of high FN was 42.9%. The domain with the highest prevalence of high FN was vegetables (48.6%). Children aged 8 to 11 y/o had a higher mean FN in two domains (FNgen $p = 0.047$ and FNveg $p = 0.038$) when compared to children aged 4 to 7 y/o. Boys were more neophobic in all domains (FNgen $p = 0.017$; FNfru $p = 0.010$; FNveg $p = 0.013$; BCFNeoTot $p = 0.008$), and FN tends not to decrease with age. The results showed that the children of the FD are more neophobic than Brazilian children in general, highlighting the importance of additional studies in FN determinants in this population and nutritional education interventions to reduce FN among FD children.

Keywords: child; food neophobia; prevalence

1. Introduction

A reluctance to eat and/or avoidance of novel foods is characterized as food neophobia (FN) [1]. This condition can restrict the diet to familiar foods when, in fact, it should be much more varied, especially for omnivores like humans. Therefore, FN describes a psychological trait whose intensity varies among individuals, raising questions of causality, correlation, and measurement [2].

Despite FN being a relevant topic in health promotion, it began gaining prominence in the late 20th century, particularly during the 1980s and 1990s. The first instrument to evaluate FN was created in 1992 by Pliner and Hobden [1]. In 1994, Pliner created an instrument focused on children [3]. It is relevant to choose the specific instrument, target group, and ways to measure this behavior [4].

FN intensely affects the consumption of healthy food, and it is a major barrier to consuming fruits and vegetables [5], affecting the diet quality and promoting deficiencies of certain essential nutrients, especially minerals and vitamins [6,7]. Children with FN may not acquire some of the skills associated with eating [6]. Deficiency or excess of some nutrients and malnutrition are critical and can lead to irreversible health consequences [6]. Children with neophobic behavior, who consume fewer and less-varied fruits and vegetables, are at a higher risk of becoming overweight [8]. Once FN is observed and quantified, strategies can be developed to overcome it, and valuable changes can occur in childhood and have significant impacts on adult life, such as obesity prevention [9].

Compared to other children from several countries, neophobic children were less likely to eat raw or cooked vegetables and legumes [10], berries [11], grapes [12], eggs [10], chicken [12], fish [11], cheese [12], and proteins [13]. They tend to eat more sweets [10], snacks [10], and fast food [14]. The energy consumption of neophobic children can be lower [12] or higher [10] or does not have significant differences among food neophobia levels, with a high intake of carbohydrates [10], lower intake of cholesterol [13], vitamin C [10], potassium [13], thiamin [10], phosphorus [13], folate [10], magnesium [13], iron [13], zinc [13], and selenium [13].

Some authors state that the distribution of the percentage of carbohydrates (50%) and fats (33%) does not significantly differ among the different levels of neophobia. However, the percentage of protein consumed by children is lower with increasing levels of neophobia (low: 16%; medium: 15%; high: 14%), possibly associated with higher sensory sensitivity towards protein-rich foods [13]. In addition, a higher degree of food neophobia also was not associated with lower consumption of functional foods (which included foods rich in bioactive compounds such as antioxidants, dietary fiber, omega-3 fatty acids, plant sterols, prebiotics, and probiotics) nor with a higher perceived risk associated with these foods [15]. Food neophobia is complex [4] and has many associated factors [16], such as gene traits [5] and prenatal experiences [17], flavor exposure in utero [5], flavor exposure during breastfeeding [5], parental influence on children's eating habits [16], heredity [5,18], sensory preferences [17], cognitive schemata [5], children's innate preference for sweet and savory flavors, the influence of the sensory aspect of the food, parents' pressure for the child to eat, parents' lack of encouragement and/or affection at mealtime, childhood anxiety, and feelings and emotions [16].

FN is common in childhood worldwide, especially at moderate and high levels [16]. This behavior is related to severe dietary restrictions and impacts on health [16], and it is expected between 2 and 3 years old [17] and between 2 and 5 years old [16]. After this period, FN tends to decrease until stabilization in adulthood [16,17]. In Brazil, previous studies showed that FN did not decrease with age among children from 4 to 11 years old [19], and the dietary intake of Brazilian children (0 to 10 y/o) had a high prevalence of inadequate micronutrient intake and poor diet quality [20]. According to the Brazilian Institute of Geography and Statistics (IBGE) [21], children consume fruits, vegetables, pork, roots, and tubers less frequently and consume more cookies, chips, soft drinks, ham, and sausages [21]. These worrying situations highlight the need for more research in the country.

Despite the studies performed in Brazil [19,22], no specific studies about FN in children in the Federal District (FD)/Brazil were observed [19,22]. The FD is located in a rich savanna with lots of biodiversity, being part of the second largest biome in South America, named "cerrado" [23]. Of the total residents of the FD, 55.5% were born locally, and nearly half in other Brazilian states [23]. Biodiversity and cultural diversity, represented by people from other Brazilian states, can be seen in the variety of local foods, which increases the chances for children to be exposed to different foods.

Thus, our study hypothesizes a high prevalence of food neophobia, which decreases with age, in both girls and boys living in the Federal District. Therefore, according to their caregivers' perceptions, the study aimed to assess food neophobia in children residing in the Federal District of Brazil. Considering the consequences and risks inherent to FN, those involved in multiprofessional follow-up and all caregivers involved with children need to be aware of it [16], and specific knowledge about this FN may allow more effective interventions [22].

2. Materials and Methods

It is a descriptive cross-sectional study. It was conducted with children (4 to 11 years old) from the FD. Following the Declaration of Helsinki guidelines, the study was analyzed and approved by the Health Sciences Ethics Committee, University of Brasilia, No. 5.438.498.

2.1. Participants

Sampling occurred through snowball recruitment, being convenient and non-probabilistic. The study included caregivers of Brazilian children (4 to 11 y/o) who live in the FD/Brazil. They needed to agree to participate and know about the child's eating behavior. The consent form had the conditions for participation in the research. Researchers excluded incomplete questionnaires.

Since there are no specific data on the FD population from 4 to 11 y/o, the minimum sample size was calculated considering 10 individuals per instrument item [24], resulting in 250 participants. Considering a significance level of 5% and power of 80%, this sample size guarantees that an effect size of 0.2 (small/medium) for the difference between the two groups will be statistically significant.

2.2. Instruments and Application

The Brazilian Children's Food Neophobia Questionnaire (BCFNeo) was chosen as it is still the only validated instrument in Portuguese to be used with caregivers of Brazilian children aged 4 to 11 years [8,9]. The instrument was composed of sociodemographic data, and BCFNeo [9] was available through the online platform Google forms®. We used social networks (such as Instagram®, Facebook®, and Twitter®), messaging apps, and email to reach participants. The data collection process occurred from November 2020 to November 2022.

To begin, the caregivers were questioned about their sociodemographic aspects (sex, age, degree of kinship, marital status, and educational level) and then about their children's (sex, nationality, diagnoses, age, and family income). Caregivers answered the instrument on their own. The instruction that only one caregiver should answer the instrument was given, and the caregiver could answer more than once if there was more than one child in the age group. The financial values, when presented, considered the conversion rate of USD 1.00 to BRL 4.93, the conversion value in January 2024. Considering the same conversion rate, the minimum wage (MW) for the analysis was BRL 1412.00, about USD 285.

The categorization of FN score followed a protocol previously validated [6]. The items were divided into three domains: neophobia in general, for fruits, and for vegetables. The domains had a similar number of items. Therefore, a better analysis of the score of the entire instrument (25 items) and each domain was performed. Each domain separately or the complete instrument allowed the assessment of the neophobic traits [6].

Data obtained from each item assumed values from 0 to 4. The general domain score comprises 9 items and presents punctuation from 0 to 36. The fruit FN score comprises 8 items with punctuation varying from 0 to 32. The FN vegetable domain score consists of 8 items and ranges from 0 to 32. Considering all domains, the FN total score comprises 25 items, and the total punctuation varies from 0 to 100 (9). The categorization of FN was defined according to scores: (i) up to 40 points: low neophobia, (ii) from 41 to 65 points: moderate neophobia, and (iii) 66 points or more: high neophobia. Therefore, for each domain, a low FN is up to 13 points, a moderate FN is between 14 and 21 points, and a high FN is from 22 points [6].

For some analyses, specific items of the instrument were used. These items refer to three environments children are exposed to: school, home, and a friend's home, influencing FN.

2.3. Statistical Analysis

The analysis used two age groups (4–7 and 8–11) and sex (female and male). The neophobia scores were compared between the sex and ages of the children (Student's *t*-test). These scores were also categorized according to three ordinal levels, and the Mann–Whitney U test was used to compare neophobia levels between sex and child's age. The Friedman test, followed by Wilcoxon test with Bonferroni correction, was performed to analyze differences in FN according to the environment by sex and child's age. The normality of the observations was tested using the Kolmogorov–Smirnov test with Lilliefors correction. All tests considered bicaudal hypotheses and a significance level of 5%. After extraction from the Google Forms® platform, analysis was performed using the SPSS® 20.0 software and Excel® 16.67. Descriptive statistics were presented as mean and standard deviation or frequencies and percentages.

3. Results

The sample comprised 595 participants after excluding 19 responses outside the age range (96.9% of individuals who accessed and completed the study were included). Caregivers were primarily female (n = 558; 93.8%); married or in a stable relationship (n = 489; 82.2%); living in urban areas (n = 586; 98.5%), aged between 19 and 66 y/o (mean age 39.41 ± 7.03 y/o). Most caregivers (Supplementary Table S1) were mothers (n = 534; 89.7%) with postgraduation (n = 255; 42.9%). The mean number of people living in the same house was 3.86 ± 0.97. Most (n = 328; 55.13%) had a monthly family income of more than ten minimum wages.

Regarding sex and age (Table 1), the sample is well balanced. Most children were boys (n = 336; 56.5%); the mean age was 6.93 ± 2.29 y/o. Most children (n = 367; 61.68%) had no medically diagnosed conditions; 228 (38.31%) presented one or more medical diagnoses.

The prevalence of low and high FN was 24.5% and 42.9%, respectively (Table 2). The domain of neophobia for fruits was the one with the lowest prevalence of high neophobia (37.0%), and the domain for vegetables had a higher neophobia prevalence (48.6%).

Table 3 shows that the mean score for FN was higher for children aged 8 to 11 y/o in the general domain ($p = 0.0047$) and in the vegetable domain ($p = 0.038$). High neophobia was most prevalent for boys in the general domain ($p = 0.011$), in the fruit domain ($p = 0.005$), in the vegetable domain ($p = 0.001$), and in total ($p = 0.023$).

To analyze if the environment (school, home, or a friend's house) could influence FN, we used specific items from the instrument that assessed FN for fruits and vegetables and based on the friend's influence, for these three environments. Each item has a score from 0 to 4 points.

Table 4 shows that children, in general, had lower FN towards fruits at school ($p = 0.000$), higher FN towards vegetables at a friend's house ($p = 0.000$), and, when under the influence of a friend, there was no difference ($p = 0.248$) between environments (home, school, and a friend's house). Younger children (4–7 y) had lower FN towards fruits ($p = 0.000$), vegetables ($p = 0.000$), and with friend´s influence (0.005) at school. Children ≥8 y/o had lower FN with friend´s influence at home ($p = 0.031$). Girls and boys had lower FN towards fruits at school ($p = 0.008$; $p = 0.005$), and boys had higher FN towards vegetables at friend´s houses ($p = 0.001$).

Table 1. Children's profiles (n = 595) and their sociodemographic data. Federal District/Brazil, 2020–2022.

		Sample	
	Categories	n	%
Sex	Male	336	56.5%
	Female	259	43.5%
Age	4 years old	120	20.2%
	5 years old	93	15.6%
	6 years old	71	11.9%
	7 years old	53	8.9%
	8 years old	90	15.1%
	9 years old	60	10.1%
	10 years old	68	11.4%
	11 years old	40	6.7%
Diagnoses [a]	No disease	367	61.68%
	Food allergies	31	5.21%
	Food intolerance	36	6.05%
	Autism spectrum disorder	114	19.15%
	Down's syndrome	29	4.87%
	Eating disorders [b]	3	0.50%
	Attention deficit hyperactivity Disorder/Anxiety	10	1.68%
	Others diagnoses [c]	45	7.56%

[a] Children may have one or more diagnoses. [b] Anorexia/bulimia/pediatric eating disorder, [c] such as other syndromes, respiratory diseases, and others.

Table 2. Neophobia classification (n = 595) and distribution. Federal District/Brazil, 2020–2022.

	Food Neophobia		
	Low (n; %)	Moderate (n; %)	High (n; %)
Domain of food neophobia in general * (FNgen)	126 (21.2%)	185 (31.1%)	284 (47.7%)
Domain of food neophobia for fruits * (FNfru)	188 (31.6%)	187 (31.4%)	220 (37.0%)
Domain of food neophobia for vegetables * (FNveg)	144 (24.2%)	162 (27.2%)	289 (48.6%)
TOTAL INSTRUMENT SCORE ** (BCFNeoTot)	146 (24.5%)	194 (32.6%)	255 (42.9%)

* Domain score: low (up to 13 points); moderate (14 to 21 points); high (22 points or more). ** Total score cutoff points: low—up to 40 points; moderate—from 41 to 65 points; high—66 points or more.

Table 3. Food neophobia score and classification distribution by sex and age group (n = 595). Federal District/Brazil, 2020–2022.

	Sex			Age		
	Girls (n = 259)	Boys (n = 336)	p	4–7 y (n = 337)	8–11 y (n = 258)	p
General neophobia (FNgen) Score						
Mean (SD)	19.58 (8.50)	21.25 (8.39)	0.017 *	19.92 (8.63)	21.31 (8.20)	0.047 *
Distribution						
Low (≤13)	58 (22.4%)	68 (20.2%)		82 (24.3%)	44 (17.1%)	
Moderate (14 to 21)	96 (37.1%)	89 (26.5%)	0.011 **	102 (30.3%)	83 (32.2%)	0.068 **
High (≥22)	105 (40.5%)	179 (53.3%)		153 (45.4%)	131 (50.8%)	
Fruit neophobia (FNfru) Score						
Mean (SD)	16.47 (8.32)	18.26 (8.39)	0.010 *	17.10 (8.66)	17.98 (8.03)	0.208 *
Distribution						
Low (≤13)	93 (35.9%)	95 (28.3%)		116 (34.4%)	72 (27.9%)	
Moderate (14 to 21)	87 (33.6%)	100 (29.8%)	0.005 **	99 (29.4%)	88 (34.1%)	0.237 **
High (≥22)	79 (30.5%)	141 (42.0%)		122 (36.2%)	98 (38.0%)	

Table 3. Cont.

	Sex			Age		
	Girls (n = 259)	Boys (n = 336)	p	4–7 y (n = 337)	8–11 y (n = 258)	p
Vegetable Neophobia (FNveg) Score						
Mean (SD)	18.91 (8.30)	20.62 (8.34)	0.013 *	19.25 (8.66)	20.69 (7.89)	0.038 *
Distribution						
Low ($\leq$13)	79 (30.5%)	65 (19.3%)		89 (26.4%)	55 (21.3%)	
Moderate (14 to 21)	71 (27.4%)	91 (27.1%)	0.001 *	96 (28.5%)	66 (25.6%)	0.049 **
High ($\geq$22)	109 (42.1%)	180 (53.6%)		152 (45.1%)	137 (53.1%)	
TOTAL (BCFNeoTot) Score						
Mean (SD)	54.96 (23.90)	60.13 (23.40)	0.008 *	56.27 (24.70)	59.98 (22.29)	0.056 *
Distribution						
Low (up to 40)	71 (27.4%)	75 (22.3%)		98 (29.1%)	48 (18.6%)	
Moderate (41 to 65)	91 (35.1%)	103 (30.7%)	0.023 **	98 (29.1%)	96 (37.2%)	0.082 **
High (66 or more)	97 (37.5%)	158 (47.0%)		141 (41.8%)	114 (44.2%)	

* Independent *t*-test; ** Mann–Whitney test.

Table 4. Score and distribution of food neophobia according to the environment by age group and sex (n = 595). Federal District/Brazil, 2020–2022.

		School Mean (SD)	Home Mean (SD)	Friend's House Mean (SD)	p *
Environment in Fruit Neophobia [1]	Total (n = 595)	1.96 (1.20) [A]	2.05 (1.23) [B]	2.07 (1.17) [B]	0.000
	Girls (n = 259)	1.80 (1.23) [A]	1.93 (1.22) [B]	1.90 (1.21) [AB]	0.008
	Boys (n = 336)	2.08 (1.16) [A]	2.14 (1.23) [AB]	2.20 (1.12) [B]	0.005
	4–7 y (n = 337)	1.82 (1.22) [A]	2.02 (1.25) [B]	2.01 (1.18) [A]	0.000
	8–11 y (n = 258)	2.14 (1.15) [A]	2.08 (1.19) [A]	2.15 (1.15) [A]	0.829
Environment in Vegetable Neophobia [2]	Total (n = 595)	2.30 (1.16) [A]	2.31 (1.23) [A]	2.42 (1.13) [B]	0.000
	Girls (n = 259)	2.16 (1.20) [A]	2.17 (1.21) [A]	2.29 (1.15) [A]	0.084
	Boys (n = 336)	2.40 (1.13) [A]	2.41 (1.24) [B]	2.53 (1.10) [B]	0.001
	4–7 y (n = 337)	2.13 (1.20) [A]	2.24 (1.25) [B]	2.30 (1.15) [B]	0.000
	8–11 y (n = 258)	2.51 (1.08) [A]	2.39 (1.20) [A]	2.58 (1.08) [A]	0.117
Neophobia with friends' influence [3]	Total (n = 595)	2.16 (1.07) [A]	2.17 (1.07) [A]	2.20 (1.06) [A]	0.248
	Girls (n = 259)	2.01 (1.12) [A]	2.05 (1.05) [A]	2.07 (1.07) [A]	0.380
	Boys (n = 336)	2.28 (1.01) [A]	2.27 (1.08) [A]	2.30 (1.05) [A]	0.576
	4–7 y (n = 337)	2.03 (1.08) [A]	2.13 (1.08) [B]	2.12 (1.06) [B]	0.005
	8–11 y (n = 258)	2.34 (1.02) [A]	2.23 (1.07) [B]	2.31 (1.06) [AB]	0.031

[1] At school, at home, or friend´s house: the taste of a new fruit; [2] at school, at home or friend´s house: the taste of a new vegetable; [3] at school, at home or friend´s house: a friend's acceptance would lead the child to taste the food. * Friedman test followed by Wilcoxon test with Bonferroni correction. Groups with different letters differ significantly.

Evaluating year-by-year and sex differences (Supplementary Table S2), total FN scores ranged from 52.42 to 65.14. Except for five and eight y/o, male children presented higher total FN. This was also observed in the FN of fruits and vegetables.

4. Discussion

This study evaluated FN in children from the Federal District/Brazil, following the perception of their caregivers. The prevalence of high FN was higher (42.9%) than in Brazil (33.4%) [19]. The analysis by age groups showed that older children (8–11 y/o) were more neophobic than younger (4–7 y/o). The difference was significant ($p < 0.05$) in vegetables and general neophobia. These results have not been confirmed in other local Brazilian studies [25,26]. In the first Brazilian study, evaluating children from 3 to 13 years in Uberaba/Minas Gerais, the youngest children tended to have the lowest interest in food, such as slow ingestion and satiety response. However, the authors found no significant difference in FN in the age group [25]. The second Brazilian study, performed with children aged 3 to 6 years in Natal/Rio Grande do Norte, found a greater tendency to FN in children aged 3–4 years compared to those aged 5–6 years ($p < 0.000$) [26]. A national study in Brazil found no significant difference in FN with age [19].

On the other hand, research in other countries has shown a reduction in FN as age advances. A study evaluated 5 national surveys conducted in Ireland on 3246 people aged 1 to 87 years and found that FN increased with age from 1 to 6 years, then decreased until early adulthood, where it remained stable until increasing with age in older adults (>54 years) [27]. An integrative review with a systematic approach showed a lack of patterns regarding sex or age with higher degrees of FN in children [8]. In our study, boys are more neophobic than girls, with a higher mean in general neophobia ($p = 0.017$), fruit neophobia ($p = 0.010$), vegetable neophobia ($p = 0.013$), and total FN ($p = 0.008$).

In Poland, 325 children from 2.5 to 7 years old [10], and in the United States, 85 children aged 3 to 12 years [28] were assessed, and no sex-related differences were found for FN. Unlike this study, two population studies conducted in Brazil and another in Ireland showed that FN was more prevalent among boys than girls [19,27]. Brazilian local studies varied in this regard. One of them did not find significant differences for FN concerning sex [25], and the other mentioned that girls aged 3–6 years were more neophobic than boys ($p = 0.0063$) [26].

The results on neophobic behavior and sex differences are difficult to explain. The studies that showed sex differences diversified on the justification [19,25,26]. When boys were more neophobic, the explanation was related to food preferences, suggesting that boys prefer less healthy foods, such as more meat and fatty foods, and girls prefer more fruits and vegetables. Furthermore, the sex variable can be determined by environmental effects such as personality [19].

When the girls were more neophobic, the explanation was related to the protective effect of neophobia and the role of women historically in choosing, organizing, and preparing the food offered to the families. Therefore, being more predisposed to avoid the new, they are more cautious, and this is a selective incentive that stimulates the most neophobic response [26]. A study suggested that FN was attributable to genetic factors, explaining approximately two-thirds of the variation in females [29].

Studies evaluated dietary intake in neophobic individuals and showed that energy intake among the levels of neophobia can be higher [10], lower [12], or equal [7]; that the percentage of carbohydrates can be higher (8) or equal [7]; and that dietary fat (including essential fatty acids) can be equal [7], but protein intake may be lower in more severe cases of neophobia [7]. Additionally, the low intake of fruits and vegetables may lead to a reduced intake of micronutrients such as vitamin C [10], potassium [13], thiamin [10], phosphorus [13], folate [10], magnesium [13], iron [13], zinc [13], and selenium [13]. However, neophobic individuals tend to eat more sweets [10], snacks [10], and fast food [14]. Some studies evaluated neophobia levels and did not find an association with lower consumption of functional foods [8], but the adherence to the Mediterranean diet—characterized by "high consumption of fresh or dried fruits and vegetables, legumes, and whole grains; moderate consumption of fish, dairy, and meat; low-to-moderate intake of red wine during meals; and the use of olive oil as the primary source of fat"—was inversely associated with food neophobia, suggesting that this personality trait may affect dietary pattern [13].

In Brazil, the federal units are different in geography, climate, food production, culture, and habits due to Brazilian territorial extension. The development of agriculture in the FD enhanced food production, and food became more accessible in terms of price and proximity to purchasing fresher food [30,31]. Greater access to a large variety of food does not necessarily mean the diet will be healthier. Most of the children in this study are from high-income families. The analysis of Brazilian food consumption [21] in children over ten y/o showed that the frequency of food consumption is more prominent in the higher-income strata. However, a higher per capita consumption of negative markers of diet quality (i.e., consumption of sweets, pizzas, fried and baked snacks, sandwiches) was observed in people with higher incomes, and a lower frequency of consumption of foods such as rice, corn, corn-based preparations, beans, pasta, and poultry [21].

In Brazil, four y/o children must be enrolled in early education and, at six, in elementary school [32,33]. There are studies [17,34] that considered social and environmental factors. These might also significantly influence and modulate children's food avoidances because the child may or may not feel safe in surroundings with unfamiliar food. Furthermore, there is growth in the potential of performing a specific behavior that a peer performs, or the teacher or parents may encourage to perform. For this reason, our study analyzed the influence of the different living surroundings (school, home, and friends' house) on FN of fruits and vegetables and friends' consumption of new foods. Our results showed that school may be the best place to stimulate the consumption of new fruits and vegetables for younger children and new fruits for girls and boys [17,34].

This result differed from the study by Damsbo-Svendsen et al. [34], which indicated that most children responded indifferently to unfamiliar foods at school (39.6%) or the youth center (30%). On the contrary, most children answered that they would surely try these foods at home (47.2%), at a relative's house (46.4%), and a friend's house (44.7%) [34]. Our study was carried out according to the caregivers' perception, and the above-mentioned study was carried out directly with the children.

In our study, the low FN prevalence of 24.5% was less than observed in Brazilian children (39.9%) [19]. The prevalence of high FN in FD was higher (42.9%) than in Brazil (33.4%) [19], indicating that children from FD could be more neophobic, and future research is necessary to evaluate the causes, allowing to change this scenario with one-off strategies and policies. Higher levels of FN, when persistent, should be included in the clinical domain as a subtype of eating disorders, leading to disruptions to personal and social life [5].

This study presents limitations to the Snowball Sampling (SS) method used to spread the research. SS is a cheap and popular sampling method in social research [35] that can be quickly disseminated. However, a strength of this method is that a minimum sample was defined before data collection to be representative. The sample may have reflected the SS method with most postgraduate caregivers and a high family income. However, these results can be explained since the FD was the federal unit with the highest human development index (0.814) and the country's highest monthly per capita income in 2022, about USD 680 (BRL 3357.00) [36].

Despite the limitation of convenience sampling [37] in this local study, in one city, we included children with food allergies and intolerances (representing 11.26% of the sample) and other conditions, as well as prevalence data for other studies in the FD. Other studies on FN usually do not bring data relating FN and food allergies or intolerances [11,19].

Another potential study limitation relates to the scale used to measure food neophobia. It is an indirect approach in which the questions pertain to what the caregiver thinks the child's behavior would be in a given scenario, rather than presenting the situation and directly assessing the child's reaction [2]. Caregivers' perceptions depend on memory, but it is believed that these caregivers, primarily mothers, often have extensive and usually quite comprehensive exposure to the eating habits, likes, and dislikes of the individuals under their care. Another possible research method for the study's subject would be similar to the one used in the prospective study by Nicklaus et al., 2005 [38], which involved behavioral measures through observing French children's lunches. However, this type of study also has limitations and is difficult to operationalize, which would significantly limit the studied sample size [2,38]. Additionally, Alley (2018) [2] highlights that the scores of scales used to assess food neophobia seem to possess strong psychometric properties, including predictive validity [2].

Food neophobia (FN) is a significant issue for children who suffer from conditions that require a special diet [36], and more studies are needed to assess this group in Brazil. Additionally, children with other behavioral disorders, such as Autism Spectrum Disorder (ASD), are also prone to FN, with a high prevalence of food neophobia reported in Brazil (73.9%) [37]. In our study, ASD children represent about 20% of the sample, and we included these children as part of a representative sample from the Federal District, given that all aspects related to food refusal can be exacerbated in ASD. This is due to their rigidity, difficulties in social environments, repetitive behaviors, and reluctance to accept new foods or changes in routine [39–41]. Furthermore, food refusal in these individuals may be influenced by food group type, smell, texture, color, temperature, and preferences for specific brands and packaging [41].

Mothers were the caregivers who mainly participated, probably because females are more interested in health and childcare [42]. Similar response rates were found in another study in Brazil [19]. This could lead to a sex bias, but it is minimized once the reproducibility of the instrument was assessed between different caregivers (two caregivers responded to the BCFNeo for the same children), and the result was good (ICC > 0.6) [19].

The pandemic may have influenced the results. A meta-analysis showed that one in five children <18y/o are globally experiencing anxiety symptoms, and one in four are globally experiencing depression symptoms at higher levels. These pooled estimates, which increased over time, double the prepandemic estimates [43]. This behavior and other factors caused by the pandemic could reflect changes in food consumption [28]. A systematic review conducted to summarize an overview of changes in eating habits due to the COVID-19 pandemic demonstrated that eating changed qualitatively [44]. The study included 157.900 children and adolescents from 39 full-text articles. The studies were conducted on five continents, and controversial results about eating habits were reported. Despite the results, the authors concluded that consuming fruits and vegetables increased during the COVID-19 pandemic [44]. However, our results showed high FN for fruits, not following the study that showed an increase in fruit intake during the pandemic.

As we had hypothesized, FN does not decrease with age, and there is a difference in FN according to gender. Older children were more neophobic than younger children. Boys are more neophobic than girls. More studies are needed to make local comparisons on FN in Brazilian children. Only two local studies outside the FD were found [25,26]; however, they did not use validated instruments specific to the target audience. It is necessary to compare FN among Brazilian states and to assess the peak of FN in this population since the national study [19] did not see differences in the expression of neophobia concerning age, and ours showed that older children could be more neophobic to some group foods.

Multilevel strategies enable the child to accept new foods and provide food familiarization, social learning, and associative learning [5]. It is necessary to have a holistic view of FN since this behavior is often underestimated and is considered a transitory condition [5]. Understanding the factors involved in FN is vital to making any progress to face it [9]. Effective prevention and treatment strategies depend on the knowledge of researchers and clinicians based on antecedent courses and interactions of FN [5]. Children with FN should be treated by a gastroenterologist, feeding therapist, clinical dietitian, sensory integration therapist, neurologist, psychologist, and other professionals [6]. One of the strengths of this study is that it used a validated instrument for the country, language, and target population, and an appropriate methodology that measures the level of FN through a score. Our result can improve public policies on healthy eating, government actions, and local and national movements and aimed at society. Furthermore, the instrument is divided into domains with their respective scores and questions about the context and environment in which FN occurs. This possibility allows, at the individual and clinical level, to assess which points are most urgent to be addressed and, thus, to evaluate periodically the best strategy to overcome FN, whether it is focused on food groups such as fruits, vegetables, school meals, or environments such as friends' houses, school, or one's own home.

5. Conclusions

The results allowed us to realize that the children of the FD are more neophobic than Brazilian children from another more extensive study, and between sex, boys are more neophobic. FN does not decrease with age. On the contrary, it can increase, suggesting that the FN needs further study in Brazil and more specific groups. Therefore, it is not easy to know whether increasing age, in this study, was a determinant of the increase in FN. It would be necessary to carry out a longitudinal study to verify this relationship.

Assessing FN with a validated instrument for the target audience enables differentiating the levels of this behavior. Future studies should adopt similar methodologies to ensure the comparability of results and analyze the differences among regions or countries. Our study not only evaluates the degree of FN but also identifies whether there is neophobia toward fruits, vegetables, or food in general. Other research could enhance this diagnosis through observational studies that track children's behavior during meals. Longitudinal studies may also be useful for examining changes in neophobia over time.

Based on the study data, schools seem to be a promising environment for addressing food neophobia in children. Therefore, it is crucial to implement public policies that encourage both public and private schools to engage in year-round nutrition-focused initiatives, such as cooking workshops, school gardens, and food tastings. These activities can increase children's exposure to new and regional foods, potentially reducing food neophobia over time.

Supplementary Materials: The following supporting information can be downloaded at: https://www.mdpi.com/article/10.3390/nu16172962/s1, Table S1: Characterization of caregivers and their children (n = 595). Brasília, Brazil, 2020–2022; Table S2: Average score according to age and sex of the children (n = 595). Brasília, Brazil, 2020–2022.

Author Contributions: Conceptualization, P.C.D.A., R.B.A.B. and I.A.L.V.; methodology, P.C.D.A., R.B.A.B., R.P.Z. and I.A.L.V.; validation, P.C.D.A., R.B.A.B. and E.Y.N.; formal analysis, E.Y.N.; investigation, P.C.D.A., A.R., A.S. and H.A.A.; writing—original draft preparation, P.C.D.A., R.B.A.B., R.P.Z. and I.A.L.V.; writing—review and editing, P.C.D.A., R.B.A.B., R.P.Z., E.Y.N., A.R., A.S., H.A.A. and I.A.L.V.; project administration, A.R. and R.B.A.B. All authors have read and agreed to the published version of the manuscript.

Funding: This work was funded by the Fundação para a Ciência e a Tecnologia (FCT) through the CBIOS projects https://doi.org/10.54499/UIDB/04567/2020, accessed on 24 August 2024 and https://doi.org/10.54499/UIDP/04567/2020, accessed on 24 August 2024.

Institutional Review Board Statement: The study was approved by the Health Sciences Ethics Committee, University of Brasilia, No. 5.438.498, on 30 May 2022, and followed the guidelines established by the Declaration of Helsinki.

Informed Consent Statement: Informed consent was obtained from all subjects involved in the study.

Data Availability Statement: The original contributions presented in the study are included in the article and Supplementary Materials, further inquiries can be directed to the corresponding authors.

Acknowledgments: The authors acknowledge the National Coordination of High Education Personnel Formation Programs (CAPES) and the Brazilian National Council for Scientific and Technologic Development (CNPq) for the scientific support.

Conflicts of Interest: The authors declare no conflicts of interest.

References

1. Pliner, P.; Hobden, K. Development of a scale to measure the trait of food neophobia in humans. *Appetite* **1992**, *19*, 105–120. [CrossRef]

2. Alley, T.R. Conceptualization and measurement of human food neophobia. In *Food Neophobia*; Elsevier: Amsterdam, The Netherlands, 2018; pp. 169–192.
3. Pliner, P. Development of Measures of Food Neophobia in Children. *Appetite* **1994**, *23*, 147–163. [CrossRef] [PubMed]
4. Damsbo-Svendsen, M.; Frøst, M.B.; Olsen, A. A review of instruments developed to measure food neophobia. *Appetite* **2017**, *113*, 358–367. [CrossRef]
5. Finistrella, V.; Gianni, N.; Fintini, D.; Menghini, D.; Amendola, S.; Donini, L.M.; Manco, M. Neophobia, sensory experience and child's schemata contribute to food choices. *Eat. Weight Disord.-Stud. Anorex. Bulim. Obes.* **2024**, *29*, 25. [CrossRef] [PubMed]
6. Bialek-Dratwa, A.; Szczepanska, E.; Szymanska, D.; Grajek, M.; Krupa-Kotara, K.; Kowalski, O. Neophobia-A Natural Developmental Stage or Feeding Difficulties for Children? *Nutrients* **2022**, *14*, 1521. [CrossRef]
7. Guzek, D.; Głąbska, D.; Lange, E.; Jezewska-Zychowicz, M. A Polish Study on the Influence of Food Neophobia in Children (10–12 Years Old) on the Intake of Vegetables and Fruits. *Nutrients* **2017**, *9*, 563. [CrossRef]
8. Firme, J.N.; De Almeida, P.C.; Batistela, E.; Zandonadi, R.P.; Raposo, A.; Botelho, R.B.A. Instruments to Evaluate Food Neophobia in Children: An Integrative Review with a Systematic Approach. *Nutrients* **2023**, *15*, 4769. [CrossRef]
9. Subramaniam, A.; Muthusamy, G. Food neophobia: Explored and unexplored terrains. *Int. J. Econ. Manag. Account.* **2024**, *1*, 129–147.
10. Kozioł-Kozakowska, A.; Piórecka, B.; Schlegel-Zawadzka, M. Prevalence of food neophobia in pre-school children from southern Poland and its association with eating habits, dietary intake and anthropometric parameters: A cross-sectional study. *Public Health Nutr.* **2018**, *21*, 1106–1114. [CrossRef]
11. Helland, S.H.; Bere, E.; Bjørnarå, H.B.; Øverby, N.C. Food neophobia and its association with intake of fish and other selected foods in a Norwegian sample of toddlers: A cross-sectional study. *Appetite* **2017**, *114*, 110–117. [CrossRef]
12. Cooke, L.; Carnell, S.; Wardle, J. Food neophobia and mealtime food consumption in 4-5 year old children. *Int. J. Behav. Nutr. Phys. Act.* **2006**, *3*, 1–6. [CrossRef]
13. Kutbi, H.A.; Asiri, R.M.; Alghamdi, M.A.; Albassami, M.Z.; Mosli, R.H.; Mumena, W.A. Food neophobia and its association with nutrient intake among Saudi children. *Food Qual. Prefer.* **2022**, *96*, 104372. [CrossRef]
14. Di Nucci, A.; Pilloni, S.; Scognamiglio, U.; Rossi, L. Adherence to Mediterranean Diet and Food Neophobia Occurrence in Children: A Study Carried out in Italy. *Nutrients* **2023**, *15*, 5078. [CrossRef]
15. Stratton, L.M.; Vella, M.N.; Sheeshka, J.; Duncan, A.M. Food neophobia is related to factors associated with functional food consumption in older adults. *Food Qual. Prefer.* **2015**, *41*, 133–140. [CrossRef]
16. Torres, T.d.O.; Gomes, D.R.; Mattos, M.P. Factors associated with food neophobia in children: Systematic review. *Rev. Paul. Pediatr.* **2021**, *39*, e2020089. [CrossRef]
17. Lafraire, J.; Rioux, C.; Giboreau, A.; Picard, D. Food rejections in children: Cognitive and social/environmental factors involved in food neophobia and picky/fussy eating behavior. *Appetite* **2016**, *96*, 347–357. [CrossRef]
18. Cooke, L.J.; Haworth, C.M.A.; Wardle, J. Genetic and environmental influences on children's food neophobia. *Am. J. Clin. Nutr.* **2007**, *86*, 428–433. [CrossRef]
19. de Almeida, P.C.; Vasconcelos, I.A.L.; Zandonadi, R.P.; Nakano, E.Y.; Raposo, A.; Han, H.; Araya-Castillo, L.; Ariza-Montes, A.; Botelho, R.B.A. Food Neophobia among Brazilian Children: Prevalence and Questionnaire Score Development. *Sustainability* **2022**, *14*, 975. [CrossRef]
20. De Carvalho, C.A.; Fonsêca, P.C.D.A.; Priore, S.E.; Franceschini, S.D.C.C.; De Novaes, J.F. Food consumption and nutritional adequacy in Brazilian children: A systematic review. *Rev. Paul. Pediatr.* **2015**, *33*, 211–221. [CrossRef]
21. Instituto Brasileiro de Geografia e Estatística—IBGE. *Pesquisa de Orçamentos Familiares 2017–2018: Análise do Consumo Alimentar Pessoal No Brasil*; Instituto Brasileiro de Geografia e Estatística—IBGE: Rio de Janeiro, Brazil, 2020.
22. de Almeida, P.C.; Rosane, B.P.; Nakano, E.Y.; Vasconcelos, I.A.L.; Zandonadi, R.P.; Botelho, R.B.A. Instrument to Identify Food Neophobia in Brazilian Children by Their Caregivers. *Nutrients* **2020**, *12*, 1943. [CrossRef]
23. Codeplan. *Companhia de Planejamento do Distrito Federal Pesquisa Distrital por Amostra de Domicílios—PDAD 2021: Distrito Federal*; Instituto Brasileiro de Geografia e Estatística—IBGE: Brasília, Brazil, 2022.
24. Cappelleri, J.C.; Jason Lundy, J.; Hays, R.D. Overview of Classical Test Theory and Item Response Theory for the Quantitative Assessment of Items in Developing Patient-Reported Outcomes Measures. *Clin. Ther.* **2014**, *36*, 648–662. [CrossRef]
25. Silva, T.A.; Jordani, M.T.; da Cunha Guimaraes, I.G.; Alves, L.; Moreno Braga, C.B.; Luz, S.d.A.B. Assessment of eating behavior and food neophobia in children and adolescents from uberaba-mg. *Rev. Paul. Pediatr.* **2020**, *39*, e2019368. [CrossRef]
26. De Medeiros, R.T.P. Caracterização da Neofobia Alimentar em Crianças de Três a Seis Anos. Master's Thesis, Federal University of Rio Grande do Norte, Rio Grande do Norte, Brazil, 2008.
27. Hazley, D.; Stack, M.; Walton, J.; McNulty, B.A.; Kearney, J.M. Food neophobia across the life course: Pooling data from five national cross-sectional surveys in Ireland. *Appetite* **2022**, *171*, 105941. [CrossRef]
28. Tan, C.C.; Holub, S.C. Maternal feeding practices associated with food neophobia. *Appetite* **2012**, *59*, 483–487. [CrossRef]
29. Knaapila, A.; Tuorila, H.; Silventoinen, K.; Keskitalo, K.; Kallela, M.; Wessman, M.; Peltonen, L.; Cherkas, L.F.; Spector, T.; Perola, M. Food neophobia shows heritable variation in humans. *Physiol. Behav.* **2007**, *91*, 573–578. [CrossRef]
30. da Silva Oliveira, M.N.; Wehrmann, M.E.S.d.F.; Sauer, S. Agricultura Familiar no Distrito Federal: A busca por uma produção sustentável. *Sustentabilidade em Debate* **2015**, *6*, 53–69. [CrossRef]

31. Companhia de planejamento do Distrito Federal—CODEPLAN; Secretaria de Estado do Planejamento, do Orçamento e Gestão. *Agricultura Familiar No Distrito Federal: Dimensões e Desafios*; Companhia de planejamento do Distrito Federal—CODEPLAN: Brasília, Brazil, 2015.
32. Ministério Da Educação. *Conselho Nacional de Educação Parecer CNE/CEB no 7/2019, Aprovado em 4 de Julho de 2019*; Ministério Da Educação: Brasília, Brazil, 2019.
33. Brazilian Law. *Lei No 12.796, de 4 de Abril de 2013*; Brazilian Law: Brasília, Brazil, 2013.
34. Damsbo-Svendsen, M.; Frøst, M.B.; Olsen, A. Development of novel tools to measure food neophobia in children. *Appetite* **2017**, *113*, 255–263. [CrossRef]
35. Pasikowski, S. Snowball Sampling and Its Non-Trivial Nature. *Przegląd Badań Eduk. Educ. Stud. Rev.* **2024**, *2*, 105–120. [CrossRef]
36. IBGE—Instituto Brasileiro De Geografia E Estatística. Estatísticas IBGE l Cidades@ l Distrito Federal l Panorama. Available online: https://cidades.ibge.gov.br/brasil/df/panorama (accessed on 1 March 2022).
37. Emerson, R.W. Convenience Sampling Revisited: Embracing Its Limitations Through Thoughtful Study Design. *J. Vis. Impair. Blind.* **2021**, *115*, 76–77. [CrossRef]
38. Nicklaus, S.; Boggio, V.; Chabanet, C.; Issanchou, S. A prospective study of food variety seeking in childhood, adolescence and early adult life. *Appetite* **2005**, *44*, 289–297. [CrossRef]
39. Lázaro, C.; Pondé, M.P. Narratives of mothers of autism spectrum disorders subjects: Focus on eating behaviour. *Matern. Child Nutr.* **2018**, *14*, e12587. [CrossRef]
40. Monteiro, M.A.; dos Santos, A.A.A.; Gomes, L.M.M.; Rito, R.V.V.F. Autism Spectrum Disorder: A Systematic Review About Nutritional Interventions. *Rev. Paul. Pediatr.* **2020**, *38*, e2018262. [CrossRef]
41. Marshall, J.; Hill, R.J.; Ziviani, J.; Dodrill, P. Features of feeding difficulty in children with Autism Spectrum Disorder. *Int. J. Speech-Lang. Pathol.* **2014**, *16*, 151–158. [CrossRef] [PubMed]
42. Davidson, D.J.; Freudenburg, W.R. Gender and environmental risk concerns: A review and analysis of available research. *Environ. Behav.* **1996**, *28*, 302–339. [CrossRef]
43. Racine, N.; McArthur, B.A.; Cooke, J.E.; Eirich, R.; Zhu, J.; Madigan, S. Global Prevalence of Depressive and Anxiety Symptoms in Children and Adolescents During COVID-19: A Meta-analysis. *JAMA Pediatr.* **2021**, *175*, 1142–1150. [CrossRef]
44. Pourghazi, F.; Eslami, M.; Ehsani, A.; Ejtahed, H.S.; Qorbani, M. Eating habits of children and adolescents during the COVID-19 era: A systematic review. *Front. Nutr.* **2022**, *9*, 1004953. [CrossRef] [PubMed]

Disclaimer/Publisher's Note: The statements, opinions and data contained in all publications are solely those of the individual author(s) and contributor(s) and not of MDPI and/or the editor(s). MDPI and/or the editor(s) disclaim responsibility for any injury to people or property resulting from any ideas, methods, instructions or products referred to in the content.

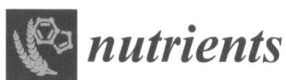 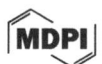

Article

Barriers and Enablers for Equitable Healthy Food Access in Baltimore Carryout Restaurants: A Qualitative Study in Healthy Food Priority Areas

Shuxian Hua [1], Vicky Vong [2], Audrey E. Thomas [3], Yeeli Mui [1] and Lisa Poirier [1,*]

[1] Department of International Health, Johns Hopkins Bloomberg School of Public Health, Baltimore, MD 21205, USA; shua8@jhmi.edu (S.H.)
[2] Department of Health Policy and Management, Johns Hopkins Bloomberg School of Public Health, Baltimore, MD 21205, USA; vvong1@jhmi.edu
[3] Department of Health, Behavior, and Society, Johns Hopkins Bloomberg School of Public Health, Baltimore, MD 21205, USA
* Correspondence: lpoirie4@jhmi.edu

Abstract: Black neighborhoods in the U.S., historically subjected to redlining, face inequitable access to resources necessary for health, including healthy food options. This study aims to identify the enablers and barriers to promoting equitable healthy food access in small, independently owned carryout restaurants in under-resourced neighborhoods to address health disparities. Thirteen in-depth interviews were conducted with restaurant owners in purposively sampled neighborhoods within Healthy Food Priority Areas (HFPAs) from March to August 2023. The qualitative data were analyzed using inductive coding and thematic analysis with Taguette software (Version 1.4.1). Four key thematic domains emerged: interpersonal, sociocultural, business, and policy drivers. Owners expressed mixed perspectives on customers' preferences for healthy food, with some perceiving a community desire for healthier options, while others did not. Owners' care for the community and their multicultural backgrounds were identified as potential enablers for tailoring culturally diverse menus to meet the dietary needs and preferences of their clientele. Conversely, profit motives and cost-related considerations were identified as barriers to purchasing and promoting healthy food. Additionally, owners voiced concerns about taxation, policy and regulation, information access challenges, and investment disparities affecting small business operations in HFPAs. Small restaurant businesses in under-resourced neighborhoods face both opportunities and challenges in enhancing community health and well-being. Interventions and policies should be culturally sensitive, provide funding, and offer clearer guidance to help these businesses overcome barriers and access resources needed for an equitable, healthy food environment.

Keywords: independently owned restaurants; healthy food access; food desert; food policy; nutrition program

Citation: Hua, S.; Vong, V.; Thomas, A.E.; Mui, Y.; Poirier, L. Barriers and Enablers for Equitable Healthy Food Access in Baltimore Carryout Restaurants: A Qualitative Study in Healthy Food Priority Areas. *Nutrients* **2024**, *16*, 3028. https://doi.org/10.3390/nu16173028

Academic Editors: Ariana Saraiva and António Raposo

Received: 23 August 2024
Revised: 5 September 2024
Accepted: 6 September 2024
Published: 8 September 2024

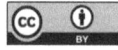

Copyright: © 2024 by the authors. Licensee MDPI, Basel, Switzerland. This article is an open access article distributed under the terms and conditions of the Creative Commons Attribution (CC BY) license (https://creativecommons.org/licenses/by/4.0/).

1. Introduction

Over the past 50 years, Americans have significantly increased their consumption of food prepared outside the home, constituting 34% of the total household calories consumed [1]. In 2022, spending on food away from home in the U.S. was 16% higher than the previous year [2], contributing more than 570 additional calories per day to the American diet, on average [3]. While these figures encompass all meals prepared outside the home, particular attention has been directed towards those prepared by fast-food services such as carryouts (i.e., small, independently owned restaurants with primarily pickup services and limited seating), which provide mostly energy-dense, nutrient-poor options [4].

Despite overall improvements in the nutritional quality of fast-food meals in the U.S. from 2003 to 2016, studies have shown that they still do not match the dietary quality of full-service restaurants [5]. Moreover, disparities in access to healthy prepared foods are evident at the neighborhood level, with a disproportionate concentration of fast-food restaurants located in predominantly low-income, African American census tracts, while non-Hispanic White neighborhoods have a higher prevalence of non-fast-food restaurants overall [6]. These inequities in healthy food access are manifestations of 'structural racism', defined as macro-level conditions (e.g., laws, institutional policies, and entrenched norms) that restrict the opportunities, resources, power, and well-being of individuals and populations based on race/ethnicity [7]. Consequently, experts in nutrition, food security, and food systems are increasingly exploring the role of structural drivers in shaping disparities in access to healthfully prepared food [8].

Efforts to address these disparities have included a variety of intervention strategies ranging from expanding menus with healthy options, using financial incentives and educational campaigns to promote healthy choices, reducing portion sizes, and offering healthier substitutes [9–11]. A systematic comparison of 27 interventions conducted in both rural and urban areas throughout the U.S. revealed that the only interventions demonstrating sufficient evidence of effectiveness involved point-of-purchase information combined with increased availability of healthy menu items, underscoring the significance of healthier food procurement in restaurants for increasing healthy food access [12]. A scoping review that examined the motivations and obstacles for procuring healthy foods faced by corporate-owned establishments compared to independently owned restaurants found that the latter demonstrated a stronger commitment to the well-being of their customers and local communities but had constraints related to available financial resources [13].

Despite the extensive body of research on restaurant interventions, there is limited knowledge regarding the structural factors influencing healthy food access in carryout restaurants. Previous studies have shown that business decisions and interpersonal dynamics shape menu offerings. Carryout restaurant owners have reported receiving negative feedback from customers when offering healthy choices and expressed concerns that such offerings might have a detrimental impact on their business [14]. Other research has highlighted concerns around low customer demand for healthy foods, potential revenue loss, and non-financial challenges related to sourcing healthy ingredients [15]. A closer examination of these concerns which decode policies shaping the neighborhood food environment, offers a promising path forward for establishing a healthier and more equitable carryout food system. To identify key areas for implementing interventions or policies designed to improve access to healthy food in carryout restaurants, this paper seeks to answer the following questions: What are the barriers and enablers for promoting equitable access to healthy food in Baltimore's carryout food system at the interpersonal, sociocultural, and business levels? Additionally, what are the policy drivers influencing small business operations and their provision of healthy foods?

2. Materials and Methods

2.1. Study Context

In Baltimore, Maryland, equitable access to healthcare resources and healthy food is intricately linked to historical and social factors, particularly structural racism and redlining [16]. The urban food environment has been significantly influenced by racial and economic segregation, which began to take shape in the early 20th century with the implementation of a racial housing covenant in 1910, restricting African Americans and other racial minorities from buying or occupying homes in neighborhoods designated as "white only" [17]. Such covenants, alongside other forms of structural racism in housing, have led to substantial disparities in access to resources, including but not limited to quality education, employment, food and healthcare [7]. As of 2018, Baltimore City had a population of approximately 600,000, with 31% of black residents living in an HFPA, compared to only 9% of White residents live in Priority Areas [18]. To be considered as a HFPA, an area must have the lowest-tier Healthy Food Availability Index (HFAI), a score based on the presence of basic food staples and healthy food options ranging from 0 to 28.5. Additionally, the median household income must be at or below 185% of the federal poverty level, over 30% of households must not have a vehicle, and the distance to the supermarket must be greater than a quarter of a mile [18].

Meanwhile, the immigrant population in Baltimore City has been rapidly growing, with an 11.5% increase from 2010 to 2021 [19]. Today, immigrants constitute only 8% of the total population, yet they own 21% of the city's businesses, notably investing in neighborhood enterprises such as corner stores and carryout restaurants [20–22]. However, challenges such as language barriers and undocumented status often lead to their underrepresentation in research studies, leaving their needs and concerns underserved [23].

2.2. Sampling and Participant Recruitment

We used purposive and random sampling for recruitment. Zip codes were purposively selected based on fulfilling the criteria of an HFPA (as defined in Section 2.1) by the city government. These criteria were chosen to focus on carryout restaurants most likely experiencing inequitable access to healthy food. Demographic data were obtained from the 2020 Census. To ensure geographic diversity, zip codes were purposively selected to balance representation, aiming for roughly equal representation from east and west Baltimore. In total, 10 zip codes were selected.

Carryout restaurants were eligible if they met the following criteria: (1) the owner was 18 years or older and (2) the carryout restaurant was located in Baltimore City. A list of carryout restaurants in each selected zip code was obtained from November 2022 data provided by the Maryland Department of Health. These restaurants were randomized using a random number generator to create the order in which research assistants would attempt recruitment. The goal was to recruit at least one restaurant per zip code. Additionally, specific restaurants were also recommended by the project's Community Advisory Board (CAB) comprised of a carryout restaurant owner and food access planners from the Baltimore City Department of Planning. The intention was for the recruitment phase to continue until at least one restaurant from each zip code was successfully recruited into the study or until data saturation was reached, as determined collectively by the research team. Data saturation was determined when no new themes or information emerged from the subsequent interviews [24]. Ultimately, the team was able to recruit at least one restaurant from eight of the ten zip codes. The research team approached 190 restaurants and successfully interviewed 13 restaurant owners or managers. Roughly 33% (66) of the restaurants approached were permanently closed, the owner was not available at 22% (42), 13% (26) did not meet inclusion criteria, 12% (22) were closed repeatedly or were unable to be located, 11% (21) did not want to participate, and 1.5% (3) were interested, but were lost to follow-up when trying to schedule an interview.

2.3. Data Collection

From March to August 2023, thirteen interviews were conducted with carryout restaurant owners by four trained research assistants. These interviews were semi-structured and based on an in-depth interview (IDI) guide developed by the research team, which included the following 5 sections of questions: general information, carryout operations, food shopping and sourcing, relationships with the community, and food policy (Supplementary Materials). Interviews lasted between 30 and 60 min and were conducted in-person, over the phone, or via Zoom and recorded using the voice memos application, with prior consent obtained from all participants. Participants received a USD 25 gift card as compensation.

2.4. Data Management and Analysis

Audio files of interviews were transcribed using Scribie's cloud-based transcription service as of 8 April 2016 [25]. Cleaned transcripts were uploaded into Taguette software (Version 1.4.1) for qualitative data analysis [26]. A codebook was developed inductively through group discussion. Three research assistants independently coded half of the transcripts, then met with the research team to discuss the codebook's applicability to the transcripts overall. Following several rounds of discussion, the revised codebook was used to code the remaining transcripts. Thematic analysis was used to analyze qualitative data. Codes were organized into themes encompassing interpersonal, sociocultural, business, and policy drivers with sub-themes identified. All themes were reviewed in collaboration with CAB members on 21 August 2023.

3. Results

Thirteen carryouts from eight zip codes participated in the study. Table 1 presented their descriptive characteristics. Of these, six carryouts were inherited from previous generations, while seven were established by new entrepreneurs. Regarding their offerings, twenty-three percent of the carryouts offer Italian cuisine such as pasta and pizza, with an equal percentage serving seafood. Fifteen percent offer general American items like breakfast sandwiches and hot dogs, and another fifteen percent are stores specializing in fried chicken. Ethnic cuisines, such as Soul food (which originated in the American South and has significance to African American culture), Caribbean, and Asian food each make up eight percent. Thirty-eight percent are in neighborhoods with the lowest (<USD 750,000) small business investment.

Table 1. Characteristics of thirteen carryout restaurants in HFPAs in Baltimore City, Maryland.

	Characteristics	n (%)
Carryout Level	Type of Cuisine	
	Italian	3 (23)
	Seafood	3 (23)
	General/Mixed/American	2 (15)
	Chicken Meals	2 (15)
	Soul Food	1 (8)
	Caribbean	1 (8)
	Asian	1 (8)
Neighborhood or Zip Code Level [1]	Average HFAI	
	>9.5	5 (38)
	≤9.5	8 (62)
	Median Household Income (in dollars)	
	>40,000	9 (69)
	≤40,000	4 (31)
	Household without Vehicles Available (%)	
	>30%	13 (100)
	≤30%	0
	Total Amount Invested in Small Businesses per 50 Businesses (in dollars)	
	>1,000,000	4 (31)
	750,000–1,000,000	4 (31)
	<750,000	5 (38)

[1] Data on median household income and the percentage of households without vehicles are sourced from the U.S. Census Bureau and reported at the zip code level. The average HFAI and total amount invested in small businesses per 50 businesses are sourced from the Baltimore Neighborhood Indicators Alliance and reported at the community statistical area/neighborhood level.

3.1. Interpersonal Drivers

3.1.1. Perceptions of Consumer Preferences

Owners expressed mixed perceptions about customers' preferences for healthier food. Some owners observed that customers in the city, who have less access to high-quality food establishments compared to those in the surrounding county, demonstrate a preference for healthy options. One owner positioned this reality against the common perception that city customers merely dislike healthy food and emphasized that they should be offered healthy choices like those in more affluent areas (Table 2, quote 1). Aligned with this perception of healthy food preferences, owners also observed the growing demand for vegetables and vegetarian options and are accommodating these requests (Table 2, quote 2).

Table 2. Supporting quotes for interpersonal drivers.

Themes	Sub-Themes		Supporting Examples
Interpersonal Drivers	Perceptions of consumer preferences	1.	"'Cause majority the perception where the assumption is basically, Oh, city people don't like healthy stuff. But that's, that's not just true. Because they love. You have to give them the same quality that you would give them in the county or somewhere that is-let's say people are more fortunate or have a little bit more money."
		2.	"And this is just something that's just started happening. They'll ask, if we have any vegetarian options and I'm like, 'Well, right now, the best that I can do-We do serve some vegetables, but as far as a particular vegetarian dish. We haven't really looked into that as of yet. Maybe in the future.'"
		3.	"I have no idea how to make that healthy. Just the vegan, I guess."
		4.	"Cheap, hot, fast. I mean, it's not the healthiest thing in the world, but people are on a certain budget. Sometimes they don't want to spend $18 for a plate over here or somewhere."
		5.	"A lot of people say they like their grits and the breakfast sandwiches. So I think if we tried to change them up, it could go either good or bad. I'm not really sure, but I think that people like them the way it is now."
		6.	"I think the most challenging part is the language barrier, kind of. My mom is pretty... She's not fluent at all in English. And so it's sometimes pretty hard for her to understand the customers, kind of have the customers understand her."
	Care for consumer well-being	7.	"The old menu, it seemed to me it's like a less quality type of cuisine, cheaper brands. So, what I'm doing is I'm trying to get better quality stuff and drop the prices. So right now, this area, if you only have $4, you can only get pretty much a cheeseburger, a hamburger and it's all greasy stuff. So now what I'm trying to offer is a side salad with tuna salad on the side. Offer more vegetables, offer more things they haven't tasted as far as spices and stuff like that."
		8.	"Some people want clubs. We didn't have them before when we first opened. They want cold cuts, turkey, not red meat. And you have people that do not eat pork bacon. We have turkey bacon because of religion or they just don't want it."
		9.	"Well, we have a lot of customers, like people with disabilities, they come sometimes and we say, 'We don't need anything.' And some days, we prepare them food and we give it to them."
		10.	"And I tell you, in my store nobody goes hungry. My cashiers and everybody know that it doesn't matter how they look, if they look poor or they look rich. If they come to you, they're hungry. You give them, they eat something. So that's something they've been telling me that goes a long way."
		11.	"Somebody found a [bay] leaf in the rice and the person thought this was something really nasty and he was really angry with my employee on the phone. I knew exactly what it was, I said, 'can you bring him back and I'll replace it for you?' So when he came back and I opened my spices that I put in the rice and I pulled it out and I said, 'this is what it is'. I said, this is all-natural stuff that I put in rice. That's what I make my rice taste better. I just don't give you boil rice or I don't just slap the rice there and give it to you."
	Maximizing transactions	12.	"And that all stemmed from basically making so much, such a great profit off this place. It was extremely lucrative. However, I do not know what pushed him into the realm of just going strictly towards selling seafood. But that's not all he did. Like I said, he owned businesses like buildings where he rented out the businesses. So he kind of did like real estate."
		13.	"I mean, naturally Baltimore has a bad rap period, so I don't go anywhere else in Baltimore. I go from here and home."
		14.	"So, it kind of goes down to the manager we had over in the old market. She was a vegan and she would always ask me, and I'm like, 'I cannot purchase these things in this market 'cause there's no demand for it over there.' But over here there is."
		15.	"I did business the wrong way. I was treating customers... I was almost racist."

Conversely, some owners believed that city consumers refrain from making healthy food choices due to personal preferences, as well as other factors such as budgetary constraints and communication challenges. This perception contributed to owners' reluctance to introduce healthier menu items due to anticipated low sales. A hot dog vendor in a food market, who admitted to "having no idea how to make that healthy" (Table 2, quote 3), speculated that Baltimore customers prioritize budget considerations when making their food choices, leading them to opt for cheaper fast-food options (Table 2, quote 4). Another breakfast carryout owner perceived that customers in less-resourced areas prefer the food they are accustomed to, suggesting it would be challenging to acclimate them to different options, including healthy ones (Table 2, quote 5). The belief that customers have unchangeable dietary habits was common among owners with limited English proficiency who spoke with native-speaking customers, as communication challenges contributed to misunderstandings of consumers' preferences (Table 2, quote 6).

3.1.2. Care for Consumer Well-Being

Owners showcased different ways of demonstrating care for their customers and the community. Some owners upgraded the healthfulness and affordability of the menus to make healthy food more accessible to those who previously had limited access to such options (Table 2, quote 7). They also catered to customers with dietary restrictions. Recognizing that consuming certain meats is taboo for people practicing specific diets or religions, owners introduced alternative protein options, such as poultry (Table 2, quote 8). Moreover, some owners demonstrated care for the community by expressing a commitment to serving food to anyone who comes to them in need, regardless of their ability to pay or physical disabilities, thus challenging social stigmas associated with marginalization (Table 2, quote 9). For owners, the motivation to foster a positive relationship with the community, treating every customer equally regardless of their socioeconomic status, is seen as advantageous for sustaining the business in the long run (Table 2, quote 10).

3.1.3. Maximizing Transactions

A smaller number of owners discussed the transactional nature of running a food business, expressing a desire to maximize profits from their customers without offering much in return. One seafood carryout owner explained how the carryout was initially established by the original owner, who viewed it as a property investment for profit (Table 2, quote 12). Another owner, despite operating their establishment downtown with significant daily customer traffic from tourists and local workers, opted to live outside of Baltimore City due to its "bad reputation" (Table 2, quote 13). This profit-oriented mindset influenced their decisions on the types of food to offer, diverging from a focus on customer and community well-being to prioritizing the market viability of the food. As mentioned by the same owner who chose to live outside the city, the decision to introduce vegan options came after relocating to an area that attracted a different customer demographic (Table 2, quote 14).

3.2. Sociocultural Drivers

Multicultural Ownership Shapes Food Offerings

The cultural aspect of food offerings emerged as a recurring theme. Alongside commonly found fast-food-style items like fried chicken, sandwiches, pizza, and subs, many owners incorporated menu items reflecting their own cultural backgrounds (Table 3, quotes 1–2). For instance, a Black-owned carryout shared their motivation for offering "Soul food," a term they used to denote African American cuisine, to provide novel options in a predominantly African American community already saturated with other types of carryouts (Table 3, quote 3). A few owners, originating from countries with food cultures distinct from those of the U.S., sought to blend home flavors and traditional dishes into their Americanized menus. This gradual introduction aims to acquaint customers with "something solid" (Table 3, quote 4) beyond the familiar "finger food", as described by a Caribbean-origin owner (Table 3, quote 5). Similarly, an Afghan owner of a fried chicken carryout described introducing a grilled meat and rice dish to improve the healthfulness of the otherwise calorie-dense menu. The dish, containing multiple food groups (grains, vegetables, and dairy), not only enhances the nutritional content of the carryout's menu but also provides the owner with an opportunity to share his cultural roots with his customers (Table 3, quote 6). This integration of different food cultures potentially enriches the diversity of the local food environment and may open up opportunities to provide customers with healthier food options.

Table 3. Supporting quotes for sociocultural drivers.

Themes	Sub-Themes	Supporting Examples
Sociocultural Drivers	Multicultural Ownership Shapes Food Offerings	1. "It's gonna be fast food, Chinese food, we have three, and also the Latin food." 2. "We have homemade spaghetti, homemade meatballs." 3. "And just being within that neighborhood, it's just your typical carryout, the Chinese food, subs, sandwiches. So he just wanted to bring something different. So he decided to do a soul food type, something home-cooked." 4. "It's exciting to them too. Because, I mean, they were customers getting pizza, pizza, pizza. Now they come and they're getting food, they're getting rice, they're getting something solid." 5. "I don't want to do a drastic change, because they are accustomed to the finger food, so we want to take it gradually. So, I'll be slowly starting to introduce the jerk chicken, the peas and rice, the curry chicken, and they love that. So, I want to- as I build the clientele with that, I'll kind of expand the menu to oxtail and... all of the different Caribbean foods." 6. "I started about six, seven years with the healthy stuff that they cannot get in the city. They have to go far away to get the healthy stuff like chicken oil rice. I do many things like steak oil rice and fish oil rice, those are grilled items. I do not use a lot of spice. I use all natural ingredients, yogurt is my base. And then I put just a little salt, black pepper and garlic. I marinate my meat and it goes on the grill, and I don't fry them. Even the rice I cook, I put a very little bit of oil. I make sure it is done because I eat... Rice is very big in Asia. I know how to cook it. So I cook them really healthy way and then I put lettuce, a salad like the Romanie lettuce with tomatoes, and then put the rice on the side, and put the meat on the rice."

3.3. Business Drivers

Cost of Business Impacts Carryouts' Ability to Offer Healthy Options

Cost was a consistent theme occurring throughout the interviews, including both food costs and operational costs to keep the business running, such as rent, utility fees, taxes, and employee salaries. When discussing food costs, owners shared that they based their food purchasing decisions on price differences among suppliers. For small businesses like carryouts, adopting this cost-effective strategy is crucial for survival in a challenging macroeconomic climate (Table 4, quote 1). One owner highlighted the challenge of food price inflation over time, explaining that escalating food prices complicate the procurement of a diverse range of ingredients to meet customers' varying preferences and dietary needs (Table 4, quotes 2–3). Beyond the challenges of sourcing cost-effective ingredients from suppliers, owners were also concerned about the additional costs associated with expanding their menu offerings. One owner of a pizza and sub carryout had plans to introduce a chicken dish would require "not too much oil" and would be "easy for older people to eat." However, he mentioned that the specific equipment needed to cook this dish is expensive, causing him to delay the introduction of the new item to build up the necessary cooking capacity across months (Table 4, quotes 4–5). Ultimately, the increase in these costs will be reflected in the food prices charged to customers (Table 4, quote 6).

Table 4. Supporting quotes for business drivers.

Themes	Sub-Themes	Supporting Examples
Business Drivers	Cost of business impacts carryouts' ability to offer healthy options	1. "So whatever is cheaper, they give us, so we survive. Because our small business- the rent, taxes, and employees, so if it's too high, we cannot survive. First day before ordering, we call and check the price. How much is the price for French fries? He said $33 for a box. Other said $32, so we get $32. Because it's a penny, a penny we make it. We have homemade spaghetti, homemade meatballs." 2. "It can kind of be challenging sometimes because the prices go up all the time." 3. "So, I might go out and say, 'Okay, I want to do this special today, this special, this special,' and then when I go to the Restaurant Depot, I'll get the stuff. And then some people, 'Oh, well, I don't like this, I don't like that'. So we try to incorporate it and have as many substitutions as possible, because everyone does not have the same favor. That's really one of the big challenges is—making sure that we have a substitution for something." 4. "This is the same food. But taste is different. And the equipment is new coming, so change. No too much oil. So people like it…Taste is a yummy taste, old people easily eat." 5. "Because this type of equipment is like cookers. If you boil in a cooker and you boil in another pot, there's a difference. If you cook in a machine, it tastes, and you can easily eat. We—maybe two months after, because the equipment is very expensive. 14,000 for one. I need three equipment, so adds up to 42,000. So, one by one… I already bought one. And after two, three months, I will buy one more. Then we start the new menu." 6. "My gas, electric. The same gas and electric I used as I did last year, at least $400 more a month. So I have to raise my prices to cover that $400."

3.4. Policy Drivers

3.4.1. Taxation

Many carryout owners voiced concerns over the increasing Maryland sales and business taxes, fearing that their business cannot "survive" due to rising costs and inflation (Table 5, quote 1). While specific taxation such as business tax and sales tax were a common complaint for the carryout owners, some noted that the taxation also negatively affected the consumers. Taxation dynamics can directly influence profitability, and if not properly communicated or understood, customers might mistakenly believe that the business is overcharging (Table 5, quote 2). A carryout owner was blamed by their customers, facing multiple complaints regarding Maryland's sales tax affecting the cost of food items on the menu.

Table 5. Supporting quotes for policy drivers.

Themes	Sub-Themes	Supporting Examples
Policy Drivers	Taxation	1. "Because our small business- the rent, taxes, and employees, so if it's too high, we cannot survive." 2. "So they [Customers] gotta understand that it's not us doing it, but it's the Maryland sales tax. Then a lot of people complain, a lot of people complain about it… But if you go anywhere, no matter where you go, you have to pay Maryland's sales tax."

Table 5. *Cont.*

Themes	Sub-Themes		Supporting Examples
Policy Drivers	Government regulations and policy	3.	"Each carryout is not the same. Say if we wanted to do fountain drinks, you have to have a certain permit for fountain drinks. You gotta have a certain permit if you wanna do alcohol...you gotta have a certain permit if you wanna, actually have a sit-down spot."
		4.	"We make sure we keep everything up to date. 'Cause they [Health Department] definitely do get on you if you don't have your right licenses and whatnot. And, the city does come in periodically and, they do checks and if stuff is not right, they will shut you down because we do know of a few places that have been, shut down because stuff wasn't in order."
		5.	"Instead of paying $0.03 for a [styrofoam] box, you're paying a $1.03 for this eco-friendly platter box. So yeah, over the past couple of years, they've [Maryland] really hit carryouts and restaurants hard with all these regulations and bag bans... there's no point."
		6.	"We wait a whole year just to open because waiting on this bench inspection, waiting on the city [Health Department] to come, it was a challenge."
		7.	"It's gonna be the fire department inspection, then... a city inspection, the building inspection."
		8.	"We had to call and make an appointment, and then they call and cancel. And then we have to make the appointment again."
		9.	"If we went to add something [on the menu], we had to pay extra and we had to call the city and let them know, and they had to come and check everything we're gonna do, so then they gonna say, 'Yes, you can put it or not.'"
		10.	"It's [Carryouts] not like chains, where there's a lot of funding. There's a lot of room for mistakes, room for leeway. So, I think in terms of that, we do need a little bit more attention so that we can actually keep afloat and manage."
	Information Challenges	11.	"So it's stuff [grants] out there, but you really have to do your groundwork really, and it's not as easy as people think it is to get some of these grants for minorities or whatnot."
		12.	"I'm not so sure because I'm in the process of the whole thing, [SNAP] application, new application and everything, but I think you have to have a certain amount of items in the store and carry... You must carry certain items in the store."
		13.	"We had to wait five months just to get an IRS [EIN] number, it's like the social security number for the place... a USA or American citizen, they gonna get [it] in the next day...it was a different process because we got something called ITIN number, it's like an identification number. And they say, 'Oh, if you come with a social security number, it's gonna be different.'"
		14.	"We had to get the manager food licenses, and we had to go to Virginia because there is no classes here [Baltimore] on my language."
	Uneven investment across neighborhoods	15.	"Once they [policymakers] get their juice, that's all they care about. And I really think that they should stop and think about people sometimes."
		16.	"[There have been] a myriad of businesses that've been in and out of this whole block here... I think it'd be upsetting if this place ever closed because of the city not helping us out more... I think the mayor needs to help support mom and pop establishments."
		17.	"Downtown Baltimore does need a little bit more support and help from the government. 'Cause obviously it's very impoverished very... The literacy rates are low. It's very... It's just getting by, you know?... I think whether it be homes, just communities and the businesses that are in this area, I think it'd be nice to get a little bit more support from the government in that kind of aspect."
		18.	"I think almost on a daily basis there is a lot of people on drugs, a lot of homeless people that come in, which kind of disrupts the environment for a lot of our other customers as well. And it's just overall kind of hard to deal with stuff like that."
		19.	"The ones [Carryouts] that really don't care about the business or their neighborhood, they'll let drug dealing in their store, they're going to let anything happen in their store."

3.4.2. Government Regulations and Policy

Maryland's state-level policies often necessitate swift and sometimes costly changes to business practices, challenging carryout owners to adapt while maintaining service quality. Several carryout owners shared that the Health Department and other enforcers of general policy regulations have hindered or prevented business operations due to their inadequate and untimely delivery of information. These miscommunications range from information about permits, health inspections, and supply ordinances (Table 5, quotes 3–8).

Carryout owners described the city's various inspections as a "challenge" since they had to cease operation waiting for repeated inspections from different government entities such as the Fire Department, and permit approval without a concrete timeline (Table 5, quotes 6–7). Furthermore, some carryout owners cited difficulty in scheduling these appointments (Table 5, quotes 8). This oversight is even present when carryout owners want to change or add menu items (Table 5, quote 9). Additionally, one carryout owner was concerned over increasing supply costs due to following the 2019 Baltimore City Foam Ban [27], an ordinance to support environmental sustainability efforts by banning foam to-go boxes in favor of compostable options (Table 5, quote 5).

When carryout owners were asked how to improve policies that would benefit their business operations, most carryout owners advocated for additional funding due to the variety of daily challenges that their small businesses face compared to corporate chains (Table 5, quote 10).

3.4.3. Information Challenges

Some carryout owners reported difficulties in accessing beneficial information and resources regarding grant applications, business loans, and participating in the Supplemental Nutrition Assistance Program (SNAP) or Restaurant Meals Program (RMP), which may benefit their business and communities. SNAP is a federal program that provides low- or no-income individuals and families with food purchasing benefits to supplement the cost of groceries to ensure adequate health and nutrition [28]. Meanwhile, RMP is a sub-program of SNAP, operating as a state-optional program that allows certain SNAP beneficiaries, who are unable to prepare or store food for themselves, to buy prepared meals at restaurants with their SNAP benefits [29]. In recent years, the Maryland Department of Human Services has tried to support small businesses by providing grants, loans, and federal benefits opportunities, but carryout owners expressed that they were unaware that such programs existed. Those that did know explained that the application process and information was "not easy" and requires one to "really have to do your own groundwork" to seek information, especially for grants made specifically for minority small business owners (Table 5, quote 11). One carryout owner explained his SNAP application process, but was perplexed by the SNAP program's initiative and navigation regarding the menu item requirements (Table 5, quote 12).

Factoring in foreign-born carryout owners, accessing resources to apply for and obtain licenses presents a bigger challenge due to language barriers or undocumented status. One carryout owner shared that they felt treated differently during the business ownership process compared to American owners due to their immigration status, having to wait 5 months for their tax and business identification information (Table 5, quote 13). Another owner expressed the need to travel to another state to attend classes for permits in their language (Table 5, quote 14).

3.4.4. Uneven Investment across Neighborhoods

Investment disparities persist in Baltimore, with specific zip codes and neighborhoods with low incomes receiving minimal attention from policymakers. This presents an ongoing challenge that many carryout owners face. Existing establishments are less likely to be improved and supported by the local government as owners believe that the city's politics and leaders influence the investments or disinvestments and allocation of funds (Table 5, quotes 15–17). One carryout owner blames and mistrusts their policymakers, "Once they get their juice, that's all they care about". Other carryout owners echoed this strained relationship with city officials, believing there is a lack of support for their businesses resulting in high turnover rates and inconsistent investments (Table 5, quote 16).

In addition, many carryout owners described how these conditions resonate throughout the community and culminate in crime, worse living conditions, inequitable food access, and declining business longevity (Table 5, quotes 17–18). One carryout owner criticized other carryouts, stating that they allow crime to occur in their vicinities to increase foot traffic (Table 5, quote 19). Although these were the issues highlighted, many carryout owners carried the sentiment that there needs to have more financial support for small business owners. One carryout owner indicated that there were specific areas within the city that need more funding from the government (Table 5, quote 17).

4. Discussion

In this study, we identified barriers, enablers, and policy influences associated with providing equitable healthy food access in Baltimore, MD, carryout restaurants. We found that the menu offerings in carryout restaurants are determined by individual-level factors, such as restaurant owners' perceptions of what customers like and owners' cultural identities; interpersonal-level factors, such as the relationship between carryouts and customers; and institutional-level factors, such as food costs. At the policy level, difficulties in accessing funding information and constant regulation of carryout restaurants strongly affected the owners' bottom lines. All these factors are intertwined.

Owners' opinions in this study were divided on whether customers are interested in healthy menu offerings, reflecting a broader issue observed in the literature. Customer demand was identified as both an enabler and a constraint in a scoping review of restaurant interventions [13]. The mixed perspective on customer preferences can be attributed to several factors. Firstly, economic constraints are a significant determinant of food choices in low-income neighborhoods, such as those in HFPAs in Baltimore. Many restaurant owners, both in this study and others, have voiced that customers often prioritize affordability in their food decisions, leading them to opt for cheaper, energy-dense foods rather than healthier options, which are perceived as more expensive [14,15]. Beyond food cost, people's food preferences are also influenced by their social networks, nutrition knowledge, media influence, work demands, and lifestyle choices [30]. Overall, interventions using pricing strategies suggest that lowering prices could increase purchases of healthy foods [13,31]. This indicates that if restaurants could source healthier ingredients at lower costs, use alternative cooking methods (e.g., grilling versus frying), or receive subsidies for offering healthier prepared food at cheaper prices, it might increase the promotion of healthier menu options. Secondly, cultural preferences and habitual eating patterns also play a critical role in food choices. In communities with long-standing dietary traditions, there may be resistance to changing established eating habits, such as consuming large portions and meat-heavy meals, even in the face of diet-related diseases [32]. Some owners may interpret this resistance as a lack of interest in healthy foods, when in fact, it could be a reluctance to deviate from tradition and cultural values. This can create a cycle where the perceived lack of demand discourages owners from offering healthier options, which in turn limits customer exposure to such options.

Owners' motivation to maximize profits has been identified as a barrier. Although several owners in this study, as well as in other research, have claimed to be committed to serving their communities [13], the need to "survive" often leads carryout owners to prioritize expenses over the potential revenue that new healthy menu items might generate. Other studies have found that many restaurant owners, both in fast-food and casual dining, prioritize maximizing their sales and profits over the healthy food offerings. Profit is the primary consideration when making changes to their menu [15].

We discovered that macro forces such as regulations, policies, and taxation affect independent carryout restaurants by influencing their economic viability, potentially creating barriers to offer healthy food. As components of a broader economic ecosystem, small businesses often find themselves disproportionately affected by policies that may either overlook their circumstances or impose undue burdens due to their limited financial resources. For example, the foam ban implemented by Baltimore City in 2019 inadvertently burdened carryout owners with increased costs for alternative food package materials [27], which owners indicated had significant financial repercussions. In contrast, it is plausible to anticipate that such policies may have a lesser impact on chain or upscale restaurants, with research suggesting that these larger establishments may even reap financial benefits from "green" initiatives like the foam ban in the long term [33]. Moreover, small restaurant owners highlighted the challenge of operating within narrow net profit margins, particularly when revenue is consistently allocated to taxes and operating fees. This suggests that government support, such as creating grants for small businesses to support sustainability initiatives and offset operational costs, could mitigate this issue [34]. Despite these findings, we observe that much of the existing research on the intersection of policy and healthy food availability in restaurants focuses on nutritional guidelines [35,36], rather than the larger systems impacting small businesses' ability to operate and procure healthy foods. Thus, there is a pressing need for a comprehensive exploration of policy impacts on small, independent restaurants within a systemic framework.

Carryout owners also revealed financial inequities, especially in uneven neighborhood investments. These disparities stem from structural racism policies like redlining, which restricted resources for communities of color, including food access [37]. Many of the carryouts we interviewed served fried chicken, reflecting the prevalence of "chicken box stores" in Baltimore. These unhealthy food outlets are driven by a perceived supply and demand for unhealthy foods within the community [38]. Since all our participants were recruited from neighborhoods within HFPAs, it is not surprising that discussions frequently touched on the unhealthy food supply and demand and the impact of neighborhood underinvestment. Issues such as higher crime rates, vacant houses, and poor cleanliness deter patronage and negatively affect the community food system [39]. One possible solution includes mechanisms like universal basic income (UBI). A scoping review of the effects of basic income-like interventions in high-income countries found that such interventions led to improved nutrition, reduced property crime, and reduced financial strain [40]. Implementing UBI could provide financial stability for residents, enabling them to make healthier food choices and contribute to a more equitable food system.

When asked about food policy, food assistance programs like the SNAP and RMP, which benefit community members, were discussed during interviews and CAB meetings. Restaurant owners expressed confusion or lack of awareness regarding these programs, often using the terms interchangeably and being uncertain about the application process. Despite the RMP being established in Maryland four years ago, this indicates inadequate communication from program implementers. Research suggests this issue is widespread among small businesses in the U.S. due to minimal marketing efforts [41], despite these programs' potential to improve nutritional outcomes [42,43]. To enhance healthy food choices and support local businesses, marketing efforts for the RMP in Maryland should focus on independent restaurants. This could increase access to healthier food options and stimulate the circulation of SNAP dollars throughout the local economy [44].

Administrative burdens underlie the challenges of being a carryout owner, constraining their ability to provide community benefits through social programs, grants, or basic operational certificates. These challenges are further exacerbated for immigrant carryout owners, who have increasingly become the business owners in Baltimore [21]. These burdens include language barriers, complex documentation, and fees, which can hinder access to basic public services [45]. Immigrant carryout owners expressed frustration over possible mistreatment from bureaucracies due to their status. One owner with limited English proficiency, who self-identified as undocumented, faced difficulties obtaining food handler licenses, necessitating travel to another state for translated documents. Limited English proficiency also leads to miscommunication [46], overlooking customers' healthfulness requirements in purchasing food. Furthermore, immigrant owners also voiced that they struggled more with obtaining necessary business ownership documentation, such as Individual Taxpayer Identification Number (ITIN), Tax ID, and Employer Identification Number (EIN) compared to their U.S. citizen counterparts.

4.1. Implications for Policy

The findings from this study highlight several critical implications for policy aimed at improving healthy food access in urban, under-resourced neighborhoods. First, the use of subsidies to incentivize the provision of healthier prepared foods at lower prices could address financial disparities and promote equitable resource allocation across different communities. Second, implementing UBI may ensure that resources and investments are equitably distributed among individuals, households, neighborhoods, and communities, thereby providing residents with the financial stability needed to make healthier food choices. Third, food assistance programs such as the SNAP and RMP should increase their marketing efforts and encourage the participation of independent restaurants. This would allow small businesses to benefit from government funding, while also expanding access to healthier food options for low-income populations. By addressing these areas, policymakers can support small, independent carryout restaurants in their efforts to offer healthier menu options and create a more equitable food system.

4.2. Limitations and Strengths

To our knowledge, this study is the first to examine structural policy drivers and their relation to barriers and enablers for providing healthy food options in the context of carryouts in urban areas with limited healthy food access and high poverty rates. Our study successfully interviewed a variety of restaurant owners, including those newer to business and those inheriting family businesses. Though we have a small sample size due to recruitment challenges (owners with busy schedules, not present, or not wanting to participate), our interviews reached data saturation. We captured both the operational and personal experiences of running a carryout restaurant business, exploring the narrative intersections of sociocultural, business, and policy factors that shape the carryout food system. Additionally, we obtained geographic variety within the city (east vs. west), enabling discussions on investments and disinvestments surrounding small-business-like carryouts and their communities.

Our findings are robust due to data saturation. Many concerns voiced by carryout owners related to food offerings are interconnected. While studies show customers want healthier foods, many owners do not believe this [47]. At the same time, owners enter the business to make a profit, but as inflation, taxes, and general operating costs increase, they need to raise the prices of their offerings, ultimately impacting customers with budget constraints. This results in less revenue for owners to afford healthier, usually more expensive foods, creating a cycle that hampers restaurant operations. This is especially dire in this study since the establishments are already located in areas with minimal healthy food access. However, if restaurant owners lack access to evidence, current practices will prevail. This highlights the need for clearer, more accessible research, programs, and policies to help owners improve offerings and understand customer demand.

However, several important limitations arose. First, the small sample size may not provide a fully comprehensive view, and future studies with larger samples are necessary to generalize these findings more broadly. Second, we were only able to interview carryouts from eight out of the intended thirteen zip codes, with some participating carryouts in the same zip code. In the five zip codes that we were unable to recruit carryouts, we noticed several limiting factors that prevented us from engaging with carryout owners. These zip codes have historically higher poverty rates and marginalization, potentially causing distrust of researchers from perceived "privileged" institutions. Furthermore, some carryouts mentioned time constraints, and we could only interview owners fluent in English.

This study aimed to capture potential barriers and enablers for ensuring equitable access to nutritious food in Baltimore's carryout food system from the perspectives of carryout restaurant owners. We did not obtain perspectives from customers nor ask about the carryout owner's race and identity, which warrant improved study design and further studies.

5. Conclusions

This qualitative paper discusses the structural factors affecting healthy food access in small, independently owned carryout restaurants located in urban, under-resourced neighborhoods from the stakeholders' perspectives. These factors are multi-leveled and multifaceted, spanning intrapersonal, interpersonal, sociocultural, community, and policy domains. Future programs and interventions should address the identified barriers and leverage existing community strengths. Nutrition assistance programs, such as the RMP and SNAP, should increase outreach to business operators and provide application guidance within low-income communities to eventually reach eligible participants. The study also reveals a communication gap between policymakers and small business operators regarding support for sustaining small businesses in these areas. Researchers and public health professionals should work to ensure that messages from this underrepresented population effectively reach policymakers.

Supplementary Materials: The following supporting information can be downloaded at: https://www.mdpi.com/article/10.3390/nu16173028/s1, Document S1: IDI guide.

Author Contributions: S.H. and V.V. have both contributed equally to the manuscript preparation. Y.M. and L.P. contributed to designing and supervising the study. S.H., V.V. and A.E.T. carried out data collection and analysis. All authors validated the coding framework. All authors were involved in writing the initial manuscript draft. All authors were involved in reviewing and editing the manuscript, and all authors approved the final manuscript. All authors have read and agreed to the published version of the manuscript.

Funding: This work was supported by the 2022 Bloomberg American Health Initiative Spark Award.

Institutional Review Board Statement: The study was approved by the Johns Hopkins Bloomberg School of Public Health Institutional Review Board (IRB 00022949) on 17 November 2022. Verbal consent was obtained from all subjects involved in the study. Verbal consent was witnessed and formally recorded.

Informed Consent Statement: Oral informed consent was obtained from all subjects involved in the study.

Data Availability Statement: All data generated or analyzed during this study are included in this published article. The raw data supporting the conclusions of this article will be made available by the authors on request due to privacy reasons.

Acknowledgments: The authors wish to express their gratitude to the restaurant staff and members of the CAB who contributed their time and shared their valuable insights on shaping this initiative. We also want to thank the research assistants, Veronica Velez-Burgess and Christina LiPuma, for their involvement in data collection.

Conflicts of Interest: The authors declare no conflicts of interest.

References

1. Saksena, M.J.; Okrent, A.M.; Anekwe, T.D.; Cho, C.; Dicken, C.; Effland, A.; Elitzak, H.; Guthrie, J.; Hamrick, K.S.; Hyman, J.; et al. *America's Eating Habits: Food Away From Home*; EIB-196; U.S. Department of Agriculture: Washington, DC, USA, 2018. Available online: https://www.ers.usda.gov/webdocs/publications/90228/eib-196.pdf?v=7152 (accessed on 17 March 2024).
2. U.S. Department of Agriculture. Food Prices and Spending. 2024. Available online: https://www.ers.usda.gov/data-products/ag-and-food-statistics-charting-the-essentials/food-prices-and-spending/ (accessed on 8 April 2024).
3. Duffey, K.J.; Popkin, B.M. Energy Density, Portion Size, and Eating Occasions: Contributions to Increased Energy Intake in the United States, 1977–2006. *PLoS Med.* **2011**, *8*, e1001050. [CrossRef] [PubMed]

4. Kirkpatrick, S.I.; Reedy, J.; Kahle, L.L.; Harris, J.L.; Ohri-Vachaspati, P.; Krebs-Smith, S.M. Fast-Food Menu Offerings Vary in Dietary Quality, but Are Consistently Poor. *Public Health Nutr.* **2014**, *17*, 924–931. [CrossRef] [PubMed]
5. Liu, J.; Rehm, C.D.; Micha, R.; Mozaffarian, D. Quality of Meals Consumed by US Adults at Full-Service and Fast-Food Restaurants, 2003–2016: Persistent Low Quality and Widening Disparities. *J. Nutr.* **2020**, *150*, 873–883. [CrossRef] [PubMed]
6. Powell, L.M.; Chaloupka, F.J.; Bao, Y. The Availability of Fast-Food and Full-Service Restaurants in the United States. *Am. J. Prev. Med.* **2007**, *33*, S240–S245. [CrossRef]
7. Braveman, P.A.; Arkin, E.; Proctor, D.; Kauh, T.; Holm, N. Systemic And Structural Racism: Definitions, Examples, Health Damages, And Approaches To Dismantling: Study Examines Definitions, Examples, Health Damages, and Dismantling Systemic and Structural Racism. *Health Aff.* **2022**, *41*, 171–178. [CrossRef]
8. Hines, A.L.; Brody, R.; Zhou, Z.; Collins, S.V.; Omenyi, C.; Miller, E.R.; Cooper, L.A.; Crews, D.C. Contributions of Structural Racism to the Food Environment: A Photovoice Study of Black Residents With Hypertension in Baltimore, MD. *Circ Cardiovasc. Qual. Outcomes* **2022**, *15*, e009301. [CrossRef]
9. Lee-Kwan, S.H.; Bleich, S.N.; Kim, H.; Colantuoni, E.; Gittelsohn, J. Environmental Intervention in Carryout Restaurants Increases Sales of Healthy Menu Items in a Low-Income Urban Setting. *Am. J. Health Promot.* **2015**, *29*, 357–364. [CrossRef]
10. Ayala, G.X.; Castro, I.A.; Pickrel, J.L.; Williams, C.B.; Lin, S.-F.; Madanat, H.; Jun, H.-J.; Zive, M. A Restaurant-Based Intervention to Promote Sales of Healthy Children's Menu Items: The Kids' Choice Restaurant Program Cluster Randomized Trial. *BMC Public Health* **2016**, *16*, 250. [CrossRef]
11. Perepezko, K.; Tingey, L.; Sato, P.; Rastatter, S.; Ruggiero, C.; Gittelsohn, J. Partnering with Carryouts: Implementation of a Food Environment Intervention Targeting Youth Obesity. *Health Educ. Res.* **2018**, *33*, 4–13. [CrossRef]
12. Valdivia Espino, J.N.; Guerrero, N.; Rhoads, N.; Simon, N.-J.; Escaron, A.L.; Meinen, A.; Nieto, F.J.; Martinez-Donate, A.P. Community-Based Restaurant Interventions to Promote Healthy Eating: A Systematic Review. *Prev. Chronic Dis.* **2015**, *12*, 140455. [CrossRef]
13. Fuster, M.; Handley, M.A.; Alam, T.; Fullington, L.A.; Elbel, B.; Ray, K.; Huang, T.T.-K. Facilitating Healthier Eating at Restaurants: A Multidisciplinary Scoping Review Comparing Strategies, Barriers, Motivators, and Outcomes by Restaurant Type and Initiator. *Int. J. Environ. Res. Public Health* **2021**, *18*, 1479. [CrossRef]
14. Noormohamed, A.; Lee, S.H.; Batorsky, B.; Jackson, A.; Newman, S.; Gittelsohn, J. Factors Influencing Ordering Practices at Baltimore City Carryouts: Qualitative Research to Inform an Obesity Prevention Intervention. *Ecol. Food Nutr.* **2012**, *51*, 481–491. [CrossRef]
15. Glanz, K.; Resnicow, K.; Seymour, J.; Hoy, K.; Stewart, H.; Lyons, M.; Goldberg, J. How Major Restaurant Chains Plan Their Menus. *Am. J. Prev. Med.* **2007**, *32*, 383–388. [CrossRef]
16. Ogungbe, O.; Yeh, H.-C.; Cooper, L.A. Living Within the Redlines: How Structural Racism and Redlining Shape Diabetes Disparities. *Diabetes Care* **2024**, *47*, 927–929. [CrossRef]
17. Power, G. Apartheid Baltimore Style: The Residential Segregation Ordinances of 1910–1913. *Md. Law Rev.* **1983**, *42*, 309. Available online: https://digitalcommons.law.umaryland.edu/cgi/viewcontent.cgi?article=2498&context=mlr (accessed on 20 June 2024).
18. Misiaszek, C.; Buzogany, S.; Freishtat, H. *Baltimore City's Food Environment: 2018 Report*; Johns Hopkins Center for a Livable Future: Baltimore, MD, USA, 2018; p. 53. Available online: https://clf.jhsph.edu/sites/default/files/2019-01/baltimore-city-food-environment-2018-report.pdf (accessed on 20 June 2024).
19. Cullum Clark, J.H. *Immigrants and Opportunity in America's Cities (Blueprint for Opportunity Series No. 3)*; The George W. Bush Institute: Dallas, TX, USA, 2022. Available online: https://gwbushcenter.imgix.net/wp-content/uploads/Immigrants-and-Opp-3.pdf (accessed on 20 June 2024).
20. Department of Planning Policy & Data Analysis Division. Baltimore City Foreign Born Demographics Dashboard. Available online: https://baltplanning.maps.arcgis.com/apps/dashboards/e8ee9a972a16408a810418955f173f6b (accessed on 20 June 2024).
21. Kallick, D.D. *Immigrant Small Business Owners: A Significant and Growing Part of the Economy*; FISCAL POLICY INSTITUTE: Washington, DC, USA, 2012. Available online: https://fiscalpolicy.org/wp-content/uploads/2012/06/immigrant-small-business-owners-FPI-20120614.pdf (accessed on 20 June 2024).
22. Song, H.-J.; Gittelsohn, J.; Kim, M.; Suratkar, S.; Sharma, S.; Anliker, J. A Corner Store Intervention in a Low-Income Urban Community Is Associated with Increased Availability and Sales of Some Healthy Foods. *Public Health Nutr.* **2009**, *12*, 2060–2067. [CrossRef]
23. Chang, C.; Minkler, M.; Salvatore, A.L.; Lee, P.T.; Gaydos, M.; Liu, S.S. Studying and Addressing Urban Immigrant Restaurant Worker Health and Safety in San Francisco's Chinatown District: A CBPR Case Study. *J. Urban Health* **2013**, *90*, 1026–1040. [CrossRef] [PubMed]
24. Sandelowski, M. Sample Size in Qualitative Research. *Res. Nurs. Health* **1995**, *18*, 179–183. [CrossRef] [PubMed]
25. Scribie. 2024. Available online: https://www.scribie.com/ (accessed on 20 June 2024).
26. Rampin, R.; Rampin, V. Taguette: Open-Source Qualitative Data Analysis. *J. Open Source Softw.* **2021**, *6*, 3522. [CrossRef]
27. Baltimore Office of Sustainability. Baltimore City Foam Ban. 2018. Available online: https://www.baltimoresustainability.org/baltimore-city-foam-ban/ (accessed on 20 June 2024).
28. U.S. Department of Agriculture. Supplemental Nutrition Assistance Program (SNAP). 2024. Available online: https://www.fns.usda.gov/snap/supplemental-nutrition-assistance-program (accessed on 13 April 2024).

29. U.S. Department of Agriculture. Restaurant Meals Program. 2024. Available online: https://www.fns.usda.gov/snap/retailer/restaurant-meals-program (accessed on 13 April 2024).
30. Ravikumar, D.; Spyreli, E.; Woodside, J.; McKinley, M.; Kelly, C. Parental Perceptions of the Food Environment and Their Influence on Food Decisions among Low-Income Families: A Rapid Review of Qualitative Evidence. *BMC Public Health* **2022**, *22*, 9. [CrossRef]
31. Gittelsohn, J.; Trude, A.; Poirier, L.; Ross, A.; Ruggiero, C.; Schwendler, T.; Anderson Steeves, E. The Impact of a Multi-Level Multi-Component Childhood Obesity Prevention Intervention on Healthy Food Availability, Sales, and Purchasing in a Low-Income Urban Area. *Int. J. Environ. Res. Public Health* **2017**, *14*, 1371. [CrossRef] [PubMed]
32. Sumlin, L.L.; Brown, S.A. Culture and Food Practices of African American Women With Type 2 Diabetes. *Diabetes Educ.* **2017**, *43*, 565–575. [CrossRef] [PubMed]
33. Namkung, Y.; Jang, S. Are Consumers Willing to Pay More for Green Practices at Restaurants? *J. Hosp. Tour. Res.* **2017**, *41*, 329–356. [CrossRef]
34. U.S. Small Business Administration. COVID-19 Relief Options. Available online: https://www.sba.gov/funding-programs/loans/covid-19-relief-options (accessed on 25 May 2024).
35. Madanaguli, A.; Dhir, A.; Kaur, P.; Srivastava, S.; Singh, G. Environmental Sustainability in Restaurants. A Systematic Review and Future Research Agenda on Restaurant Adoption of Green Practices. *Scand. J. Hosp. Tour.* **2022**, *22*, 303–330. [CrossRef]
36. Piekara, A. Sugar Tax or What? The Perspective and Preferences of Consumers. *Int. J. Environ. Res. Public Health* **2022**, *19*, 12536. [CrossRef]
37. Huang, S.J.; Sehgal, N.J. Association of Historic Redlining and Present-Day Health in Baltimore. *PLoS ONE* **2022**, *17*, e0261028. [CrossRef]
38. Mui, Y.; Ballard, E.; Lopatin, E.; Thornton, R.L.J.; Pollack Porter, K.M.; Gittelsohn, J. A Community-Based System Dynamics Approach Suggests Solutions for Improving Healthy Food Access in a Low-Income Urban Environment. *PLoS ONE* **2019**, *14*, e0216985. [CrossRef]
39. Mui, Y.; Gittelsohn, J.; Jones-Smith, J.C. Longitudinal Associations between Change in Neighborhood Social Disorder and Change in Food Swamps in an Urban Setting. *J. Urban Health* **2017**, *94*, 75–86. [CrossRef]
40. Gibson, M.; Hearty, W.; Craig, P. The Public Health Effects of Interventions Similar to Basic Income: A Scoping Review. *Lancet Public Health* **2020**, *5*, e165–e176. [CrossRef]
41. Robertson, B. *Food Equity through Restaurant Meals: An Evaluation of Los Angeles County's Restaurant Meals Program*; Occidental College, Urban and Environmental Policy: Los Angeles, CA, USA, 2020. Available online: https://www.oxy.edu/sites/default/files/assets/UEP/Comps/2020/barbara_robertson_food_equity_through_restaurant_meals.pdf (accessed on 4 July 2024).
42. Ettinger De Cuba, S.; Chilton, M.; Bovell-Ammon, A.; Knowles, M.; Coleman, S.M.; Black, M.M.; Cook, J.T.; Cutts, D.B.; Casey, P.H.; Heeren, T.C.; et al. Loss of SNAP Is Associated with Food Insecurity and Poor Health in Working Families with Young Children. *Health Aff.* **2019**, *38*, 765–773. [CrossRef]
43. Miller, D.P.; Morrissey, T.W. SNAP Participation and the Health and Health Care Utilisation of Low-Income Adults and Children. *Public Health Nutr.* **2021**, *24*, 6543–6554. [CrossRef] [PubMed]
44. Canning, P.; Stacy, B. The Supplemental Nutrition Assistance Program (SNAP) and the Economy: New Estimates of the SNAP Multiplier. 2019. Available online: https://ageconsearch.umn.edu/record/291963/?v=pdf (accessed on 25 May 2024). [CrossRef]
45. Moynihan, D.; Herd, P.; Harvey, H. Administrative Burden: Learning, Psychological, and Compliance Costs in Citizen-State Interactions. *J. Public Adm. Res. Theory* **2015**, *25*, 43–69. [CrossRef]
46. Banaji, M.R.; Fiske, S.T.; Massey, D.S. Systemic Racism: Individuals and Interactions, Institutions and Society. *Cogn. Res.* **2021**, *6*, 82. [CrossRef] [PubMed]
47. Huse, O.; Schultz, S.; Boelsen-Robinson, T.; Ananthapavan, J.; Peeters, A.; Sacks, G.; Blake, M.R. The Implementation and Effectiveness of Outlet-level Healthy Food and Beverage Accreditation Schemes: A Systematic Review. *Obes. Rev.* **2023**, *24*, e13556. [CrossRef]

Disclaimer/Publisher's Note: The statements, opinions and data contained in all publications are solely those of the individual author(s) and contributor(s) and not of MDPI and/or the editor(s). MDPI and/or the editor(s) disclaim responsibility for any injury to people or property resulting from any ideas, methods, instructions or products referred to in the content.

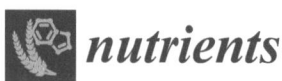 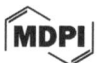

Article

The Role of Nutrition in Maintaining the Health and Physical Condition of Sports Volunteers

Mateusz Rozmiarek

Department of Sports Tourism, Faculty of Physical Culture Sciences, Poznan University of Physical Education, 61-871 Poznan, Poland; rozmiarek@awf.poznan.pl

Abstract: Nutrition plays a key role in maintaining health and physical condition, particularly for active individuals, including athletes. It can therefore be assumed that individuals performing physically demanding tasks during the organization of sporting events, such as volunteers, should also pay attention to their nutrition. While the importance of diet for athletes has been widely studied, the impact of nutrition on sports volunteers remains under-researched. Volunteers often have to cope with varying degrees of physical and mental exertion, which may affect their nutritional needs. A qualitative study was conducted using in-depth individual interviews (IDIs) with 17 sports volunteers who had experience in organizing various sporting events. Participants were purposefully selected based on specific inclusion criteria, which included active involvement in sports volunteering (with a minimum of two years of experience in volunteer activities) as well as volunteering experience at sports events of various scales. The interviews aimed to understand the eating habits, dietary awareness, and impact of nutrition on health and physical fitness. The data were transcribed and subjected to thematic analysis, focusing on coding responses and identifying recurring themes. Most participants did not place much importance on their diet, making random food choices due to a busy lifestyle and lack of time. Only a few volunteers consciously adjusted their diet when they had knowledge of the physically demanding tasks they were expected to perform during their volunteer work. The majority of volunteers relied on less reliable sources of nutritional information, such as blogs or social media, rather than credible sources of knowledge. This study revealed that many individuals involved in sports volunteering are unaware of the impact of diet on their fitness and health. There is a need for nutritional education for this group to improve their awareness of the importance of a balanced diet in the context of increased physical activity. It is also advisable to provide better nutritional conditions during sporting events and to promote the use of professional sources of information about healthy eating.

Keywords: volunteering; sport; nutrition; volunteer management; dietary habits; health; physical conditions; energy intake; diet; nutritional education

Citation: Rozmiarek, M. The Role of Nutrition in Maintaining the Health and Physical Condition of Sports Volunteers. *Nutrients* 2024, *16*, 3336. https://doi.org/10.3390/nu16193336

Academic Editors: Ariana Saraiva and António Raposo

Received: 20 August 2024
Revised: 25 September 2024
Accepted: 26 September 2024
Published: 1 October 2024

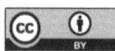

Copyright: © 2024 by the author. Licensee MDPI, Basel, Switzerland. This article is an open access article distributed under the terms and conditions of the Creative Commons Attribution (CC BY) license (https://creativecommons.org/licenses/by/4.0/).

1. Introduction

Nutrition plays a key role in maintaining health as well as optimal physical and mental condition, especially among physically active individuals [1]. Athletes, in particular, pay close attention to dietary aspects, adjusting their nutrition to meet their training and competition needs to maximize performance and improve results [2]. However, the importance of proper nutrition is not limited to those directly involved in sports. Individuals supporting the organization of sporting events, such as organizers, technical staff, or sports volunteers, may also face significant physical and mental demands due to their responsibilities [3].

Volunteers involved in organizing sporting events form a specific group that not only plays essential roles in the management of sports events but also engages in various physical activities related to their duties [4]. These may include tasks requiring appropriate levels of strength, endurance, agility, or fitness, such as setting up courses, assisting with the arrangement of sports equipment, or performing other organizational duties that may be challenging for the average person. Therefore, a balanced diet may also be crucial for sports volunteers to maintain high energy levels, focus, and the ability to perform tasks effectively, which ultimately contributes to the quality and efficiency of sports event organization. Proper nutrition in this group can support not only their health but also contribute to the success and smooth execution of events.

Most of the existing research on the impact of diet on physical condition or performance focuses on professional athletes [5,6], which limits the perspective on other, equally important social groups. While professional athletes represent a group with specific dietary needs, sports volunteers, who are required to maintain an adequate level of physical fitness, remain largely overlooked in scientific studies. To date, there is a lack of systematic analyses of their eating habits and dietary needs, even though their lifestyle may require distinct dietary recommendations.

Sports volunteers working in conditions that demand significant physical activity will have increased energy and nutrient requirements in terms of their diet. Work during sports events such as marathons, triathlons, or track and field competitions often involves long hours of intense activity, presenting them with unique nutritional challenges. Proper dietary adjustments are crucial to maintain both physical health and fitness during their volunteer duties. Similar to athletes, their increased caloric needs resulting from physical activity should be met with a diet rich in macronutrients such as carbohydrates, proteins, and fats to meet the body's energy and recovery needs [7]. It is also important to emphasize that adequate hydration and supplementation with certain micronutrients, such as iron or vitamins, can play a key role in optimizing physical performance [8].

However, not all volunteers are expected to maintain high levels of physical fitness, as some of them fill roles that require more organizational or administrative skills. Examples of such roles include managing participant registrations, overseeing race offices, distributing starter kits, supporting VIP guests, or working in media and communication tasks. In these cases, the ability to work in a team and precision and information management skills are essential, rather than physical fitness. For these volunteers, adhering to general healthy eating principles is fundamental, as confirmed by studies on the differing nutritional needs depending on the level of physical activity [9].

The nutritional needs of sports volunteers, like those of athletes, can vary depending on individual metabolic factors such as basal metabolic rate, body composition, or tolerance to specific food components. Personalizing their diet could therefore be a crucial factor and a significant challenge for this group [10], although for many sports event organizers, this may seem unrealistic, as volunteers are often viewed as auxiliary staff. However, according to scientific research, the eating habits of individuals performing physically demanding tasks can change depending on the intensity of their activity and the roles they assume [11]. Volunteers who dedicate more time to organizing and participating in sports events may be more aware of their dietary needs and strive to better adjust their eating habits to meet their energy demands, even during the preparation stages of their duties. On the other hand, those less involved in sports volunteering may not always realize the importance of optimizing their diet.

Additionally, stress and fatigue resulting from long hours of volunteering can negatively affect food choices, further complicating the maintenance of proper fitness and health levels [12,13]. Another important issue is what volunteers eat, or if they eat at all, during sports events. Proper nutrition directly impacts their well-being, especially given the physical demands of their roles. However, appropriate food options are not always available to them during such events. Volunteers may have limited access to balanced meals, leading them to opt for quick, highly processed foods with low nutritional value, which negatively affects their health and performance [14]. For this reason, ensuring appropriate nutritional conditions during such events should be a priority to support both the health and efficiency of volunteers, regardless of other factors [15].

This study aimed to analyze the daily dietary choices of participants, their understanding of the significance of diet for health and physical fitness—an aspect that is crucial for many volunteer roles—and to identify the sources of nutritional knowledge influencing their dietary approach. The following research hypotheses were formulated:

Hypothesis 1. *Most sports volunteers do not attach significant importance to their daily diet, resulting in random food choices that are not aligned with their energy needs, given the intense nature of their volunteer activities.*

Hypothesis 2. *Sports volunteers who do not pay attention to their diet and rely on random meals exhibit lower physical fitness during sports events compared to those who consciously plan their meals according to their energy requirements.*

Hypothesis 3. *Sports volunteers use various sources of nutritional information, with professional sources being less frequently utilized compared to less reliable sources, such as blogs or social media.*

The results of this study will provide a better understanding of how dietary habits affect the health and physical fitness of sports volunteers and how the level of dietary awareness and sources of information impact their well-being. The final conclusions could form the basis for developing recommendations to improve the diet and health of individuals involved in organizing sports events.

2. Materials and Methods

This study was qualitative in nature and employed in-depth individual interviews (IDIs) as the primary research method [16]. Fontana and Frey [17] described in-depth individual interviews as one of the best ways to understand people and explore topics in depth. The individual approach to respondents, compared to, for example, moderated or unmoderated focus groups, leads to results containing more details, as well as greater engagement in discussing sensitive topics or those related to private life [18].

The choice of this research method was driven by the specific nature of this study, which generated a need for obtaining in-depth, complex information about eating habits, dietary awareness, and the perception of the impact of nutrition on physical condition by sports volunteers. The qualitative approach allowed for flexibility in the investigation and the adaptation of questions to the individual experiences of the participants [19], enabling a deeper understanding of their motivations, challenges, and barriers related to nutrition.

2.1. Sample Selection

Seventeen sports volunteers with experience in various types of sports events held over the past two years were invited to participate in this study. All study participants were involved in the 2023 European Games and were recruited from the pool of volunteers from this event. In our study, we applied specific criteria to standardize the attributes of the volunteers. Participants were intentionally selected based on precise inclusion criteria, which included active involvement in sports volunteering, requiring a minimum of two years of experience and participation in sports events of various scales. Additionally, we considered factors related to having a similar number of male and female participants (9 women and 8 men) as well as diversity in terms of education and occupation (for those who were not students or pupils). This approach aimed to ensure group homogeneity and minimize potential bias, resulting in reliable findings. The participants engaged in assisting various sports disciplines and performed different volunteer roles, which allowed for a better understanding of the specific nutritional requirements arising from diverse tasks. Table 1 presents an anonymized list of the study participants.

Table 1. Table of participants.

Alias	Gender	Age	Education Level	Occupation
V1	Male	25	Master's	Teacher
V2	Male	19	Secondary	Student
V3	Female	20	Secondary	Student
V4	Female	18	Primary	Pupil
V5	Male	22	Bachelor's	Tour guide
V6	Male	20	Secondary	Student
V7	Female	18	Primary	Pupil
V8	Male	24	Vocational secondary	Electrician
V9	Male	21	Bachelor's	Paramedic
V10	Female	23	Master's	Sociologist
V11	Male	28	Master's	Insurance agent
V12	Female	19	Secondary	Student
V13	Female	25	Master's	Psychologist
V14	Female	18	Primary	Pupil
V15	Male	23	Master's	Corporate employee
V16	Female	19	Secondary	Student
V17	Female	20	Secondary	Casual worker

2.2. Justification for Sample Size

The sample size (n = 17) was determined according to the principles of qualitative research, where the number of participants is often guided by the point of data saturation. Data saturation means that no new, significant themes or information emerge from further interviews that could impact the understanding of the research topic. In this study, saturation was reached after conducting 17 interviews, confirming that this sample was sufficient to obtain comprehensive data. This sample size is also supported by numerous scientific publications dedicated to qualitative research methodology [20,21].

2.3. Procedure

This study was conducted using semi-structured interviews, which allowed for open-ended questions and provided respondents with the freedom to express themselves. This approach facilitated the collection of more nuanced responses and the discovery of themes that may not have been initially anticipated in the research protocol. The interviews focused on three main areas: the volunteers' daily eating habits, their nutritional awareness regarding meal planning, and their sources of nutritional information. This method provided a comprehensive view of the group's dietary behaviors and diverse approaches to healthy eating and its significance while performing volunteer roles at sports events.

To avoid research bias or variation in the questions asked, all interviews were conducted by one person—the author of this study. Interviews with volunteers were conducted from 1 July to 15 August 2023. Each interview lasted approximately one and a half hours, although the topics discussed were part of a broader exploration of dietary issues in the context of sports volunteering. Interviews were recorded with the participants' consent.

The interviews were carried out in accordance with research ethics standards. Before the interviews began, participants were informed about the purpose of the study, its nature, and the voluntary nature of their participation. Each participant gave informed consent to participate in the study and to the recording of the interview. They were also assured of the anonymity and confidentiality of the collected data. The results of this study were presented in a manner that does not allow for the identification of individual participants.

2.4. Data Analysis

The interview data were subjected to thematic analysis in four stages: (1) transcription of data and preliminary reading of the materials; (2) coding of participants' responses and identification of recurring themes; (3) grouping of codes into larger thematic categories; (4) interpretation of results and drawing conclusions based on identified themes. Each stage of the analysis was conducted with adherence to the standards of qualitative research rigor, which enhanced the credibility and validity of the data interpretation.

In order to ensure greater transparency and rigor in the analysis, an iterative and multi-stage approach to thematic analysis was applied. After the initial transcription of the interviews, the transcripts were read multiple times to fully understand the participants' responses. The data was coded on two levels: (1) open coding, which identified potentially relevant themes, and (2) axial coding, which grouped thematic connections and enabled the identification of key motifs. This process was supported by analytical tools such as NVivo, ensuring systematic coding.

All codes were then compared and grouped to refine thematic categories. The results of the analysis were confronted with the limited available studies in related thematic areas, which allowed for embedding the findings in a broader context. The researcher applied a rigorous approach to coding and categorizing the data. To minimize subjectivity and enhance the objectivity of the results, the researcher repeatedly verified the identified themes and compared them with the initial codes to ensure consistency in interpretation.

3. Results

This study was conducted with a group of 17 sports volunteers involved in organizing various sports events, including distance runs, triathlons, and track and field competitions. These volunteers performed a range of roles, from logistical organization to direct support for participants, requiring varying levels of physical activity. This study involved interviews about their dietary habits, dietary changes based on their volunteer activities, and sources of nutritional information. Below are the main findings from these interviews, illustrated with quotes from the respondents.

3.1. Daily Dietary Habits of Sports Volunteers

In the studied group of volunteers, the vast majority (n = 14) did not pay much attention to their daily diet. Their dietary choices were mostly random. One participant noted "Honestly, I eat whatever is at hand—I work intensely, and when you're on the go all day, you don't pay attention to what you eat" (V8). Another volunteer added "Diet isn't something I think about daily. I live with my parents, so I eat whatever is available at home" (V4). Another participant admitted, "Even if I wanted to eat healthier, I often just don't have the time. I study, work, and meet friends in my free time, so eating takes a back seat" (V5).

However, a few individuals attempted to plan their meals, although they often settled for whatever was available at the moment. For example, one participant said "I try to plan my meals, but I don't always succeed. When I'm away from home, I sometimes end up at McDonald's, but it's better to eat something than nothing" (V6). Another added "I don't have time to regularly think about what I eat, but I try to eat healthily when I can" (V3). Another volunteer mentioned "Sometimes I end up eating in a rush, but when I can, I choose fruits or make sandwiches myself" (V10).

Only three volunteers (n = 3) demonstrated full dietary awareness and made an effort to tailor their nutrition to their body's needs. One of them stated "Regular consumption of vegetables is crucial for me. Since I started paying more attention to my diet, I feel much better" (V11). Another volunteer added, "I make sure to drink plenty of water and avoid processed foods. I've noticed that a healthy diet not only improves my physical fitness but also my concentration" (V13). Meanwhile, another volunteer remarked "I eat regularly because I know how important proper nutrition is for recovery after an intense day" (V1).

3.2. Nutritional Awareness and Meal Planning among Sports Volunteers

In this study, the majority of participants (n = 14) did not place significant importance on their diet, both in terms of the quality of their meals and their alignment with the intensity and type of sports events they were involved in. These volunteers often relied on the available meals provided by the event organizers, eating randomly without much planning, and did not consider the energy needs associated with more demanding roles. One participant noted, "I always eat whatever is served on site. Often it's sandwiches or some snacks, but I don't pay attention to whether it's good for me" (V2). Another respondent mentioned, "During long events, I'm often forced to eat whatever is available, even if it's not the healthiest. You just need to eat something to have the energy" (V12). Another participant said, "Most of the time we eat what is offered to us, if there's even something planned. Sometimes the organizer only gave me an apple for the whole day, and I had to make do with that, though it was very tough" (V14).

Most of these individuals did not perceive the connection between diet and physical condition during their volunteer work. Their eating habits were largely random, and healthy eating was not a priority. As one volunteer noted, "I don't really worry about what I eat. Most of the time, I'm busy, so I eat whatever is available without much thought" (V16). Another respondent added, "My diet is very random. If there's nothing to eat and there's a kebab or some fast-food restaurant nearby, that's what I eat. Healthy food isn't a priority for me, especially during intense volunteer days" (V15).

Only three respondents (n = 3) demonstrated a conscious approach to their diet, adjusting their eating habits to match the intensity of their volunteer work. These individuals paid attention to their energy needs, particularly for physically demanding roles. One volunteer observed, "When I'm involved from early morning setting up the running course and placing barriers, I know I need to eat something substantial before and after. I always choose oatmeal for breakfast and then an energy bar during the event" (V1). Another participant added, "During events like triathlons, I always carry bananas and electrolyte water with me. I need to stay well-hydrated and replenish energy because it's really long events" (V13). These volunteers highlighted that diet plays a crucial role in maintaining their physical condition and health during long volunteer days. One of them noted, "If I don't eat a proper meal before the event, I get tired quickly. I know that good nutrition is essential to survive the whole day on my feet, and the organizer doesn't always provide decent food" (V11). For these individuals, meal planning and including healthy snacks, such as nuts, fruits, or yogurt, was an important part of their preparation for engaging in sports volunteering.

3.3. Sources of Nutritional Knowledge among Sports Volunteers

Volunteers obtained their nutritional knowledge from various sources. A small portion of the volunteers (n = 3) used professional and reliable sources, such as scientific articles, specialized nutrition websites, athlete guidelines, or even consultations with dietitians. As one participant noted, "I read a lot about nutrition, especially in the context of sports, as I try to run recreationally three times a week. I've also consulted with a dietitian a few times in my life because I know that what I eat directly affects how I feel" (V1). Another participant added, "I regularly read blogs run by experts in healthy eating. I believe that well-balanced meals are important for maintaining high fitness levels" (V13). Notably, this trio was the oldest in the group, which might suggest that as people age, their awareness and interest in professional sources of nutritional information increase. Over time, life experiences and the need to maintain good health may lead to a greater inclination to use reliable sources of knowledge, contributing to their greater attention to a balanced diet.

Among the remaining volunteers (n = 14), most admitted they did not actively seek nutritional information and relied mainly on intuition and available options. One participant said, "I don't specifically look for information about food. I eat what I have, and I don't think about it" (V4). Another added, "I don't worry too much about what I eat. I usually eat whatever is at hand without checking if it's healthy" (V9). There were also volunteers who mentioned occasionally using more popular sources of nutritional information, such as blogs, social media, and advice from friends. They often referred to using tips available online through popular search engines. As one volunteer mentioned, "I look for information on Instagram or articles that pop up in Google. I try to choose reliable sources, but I admit that sometimes I go with what friends suggest" (V10). Another volunteer added, "I don't always pay attention to where the food information comes from. I often just browse what's easily available online" (V17). Another participant noted, "I've read blogs or general advice about healthy eating, but I'm not sure how reliable those sources were" (V7).

4. Discussion

The conducted research revealed significant relationships between the level of nutritional awareness among sports volunteers and their dietary habits and perception of the impact of diet on physical condition. The results indicate some concerning trends with important implications for both understanding the needs of volunteers and for potential interventions aimed at improving their health and effectiveness during sports events.

4.1. Awareness of Diet and Dietary Habits

The results of this study revealed significant gaps in nutritional awareness among sports volunteers, which may have serious consequences for their health and physical condition. Most respondents did not pay attention to the quality of their diet, consistent with previous research highlighting widespread issues with meal planning even among individuals engaged in intense physical activities [22]. The literature emphasizes that poor nutrition, such as frequent consumption of fast food, can lead to health problems, including increased risk of obesity and metabolic diseases [23,24].

The findings also show that volunteers often eat randomly, relying on available options during events, which may lead to deficiencies in key nutrients. In the context of sports, inadequate nutrition can affect performance, as confirmed by Manore and colleagues [25]. Deficiencies in protein, carbohydrates, and micronutrients can lead to muscle weakness, slowed recovery, and overall deterioration in physical performance [26]. Similar effects may therefore affect volunteers engaged in physically demanding roles during sports events, who are also at risk of potential nutritional deficiencies due to poorly balanced diets.

Interestingly, even those volunteers who attempt to plan their meals were not always able to adjust their diet to the dynamic conditions of sports events, suggesting a need for better nutritional organization in such situations. Optimal meal planning, especially before prolonged and intense activities, is crucial for maintaining adequate energy levels and effectiveness [27]. Research indicates that improving meal planning and increasing nutritional awareness can significantly impact health and overall well-being [2].

4.2. The Significance of Diet in the Context of Health and Physical Condition

The results of this study suggest that the vast majority of volunteers are not fully aware of the impact of diet on health and physical condition, and as such, they do not adjust their dietary habits to the specific physical demands of sports volunteering. These practices are inconsistent with the findings of Hawley et al. [27], who emphasized the importance of diet periodization, meaning adjusting calorie, macronutrient, and micronutrient intake to the specific energy needs of an activity. Our results revealed a lack of understanding of the role diet plays in maintaining physical condition and health, a point already established by Logue et al. [28] in the context of active athletes. Our participants often viewed food merely as a means to satisfy hunger, rather than a crucial element for their physical performance. These findings suggest a need for education and increased awareness within this group to enable better alignment of their diet with their body's needs.

On the other hand, individuals with a higher level of dietary awareness reported difficulties in maintaining consistent dietary habits. Similar issues were described in studies by Boyle et al. [29], who found that physically active individuals often encounter barriers such as lack of time, access to appropriate food, and logistical challenges, leading to irregular and often haphazard meal consumption. Participants from this group clearly indicated that their dietary choices were situation-dependent, which could lead to suboptimal health outcomes in the long term.

4.3. Lack of Knowledge and Intervention Opportunities

The results of this study reveal significant gaps in nutritional knowledge among sports volunteers. These findings align with Barbee's observations [30], who noted that many people rely on unverified sources, which can lead to the adoption of incorrect nutritional advice. Our research shows that the majority of volunteers use unreliable sources of nutritional information, such as social media or lifestyle articles. The increased availability of information on the internet, including blogs and social media, contributes to the spread of unverified nutritional information [31]. Consequently, this can negatively impact the quality of dietary decisions and the effectiveness of dietary strategies.

One of the key challenges is therefore to provide appropriate sources, resources, and tools for sports volunteers so that they can make more informed nutritional decisions. In this context, it is crucial to implement specific strategies and interventions. For example, sports event organizers could provide pre-event nutrition briefings that give volunteers information on optimal nutrition and how to adjust their diet to their level of activity. Additionally, it is important to ensure that healthy meal options are available at event locations. Such measures can support volunteers in maintaining an appropriate level of energy and physical condition, which in turn enhances the overall quality of event organization.

Moreover, research by Sánchez-Díaz et al. [32] indicates that a low level or complete lack of nutrition education often leads to suboptimal dietary decisions that can impair physical condition. Although these studies pertain to professional athletes, their findings can also be applied to sports volunteers.

Lack of nutritional knowledge and reliance on unverified sources among sports volunteers not only limits their ability to optimally support their health and physical condition but may also contribute to long-term health issues. As highlighted by Devlin and Belski [33], low levels of knowledge about basic nutrition principles affect the ability to properly adjust the diet to the intensity of physical tasks. As a result, meeting increased energy needs becomes extremely challenging, which can lead to chronic fatigue, nutrient deficiencies, and issues with recovery after exertion. Spronk et al. [34] note that a lack of access to professional nutritional advice among physically active individuals, which can also be related to volunteers, often results in decisions based on popular myths and trends that lack scientific support. Thus, implementing educational intervention programs is crucial to increasing awareness about healthy eating and its impact on physical performance. In the context of sports volunteering, such knowledge could translate into improvements in both the quality of volunteer work and their health, minimizing the risk of injuries and exhaustion.

4.4. Strengths and Limitations

A strong point of the conducted study was the use of individual interviews, which allowed for a deep exploration of participants' personal experiences and motivations, providing multidimensional and rich data. This approach made it possible to understand the dynamics between nutritional knowledge and dietary choices, as well as their impact on health and physical condition, which is crucial in research on dietary habits. Additionally, the analysis covered volunteers' dietary awareness, enabling the identification of differences in approach between various participant groups and the identification of barriers to practicing healthy eating. The specific context of this study—volunteers involved in sports events, characterized by a high level of physical activity—makes it unique and provides valuable data on the impact of diet on physical performance in this group, which has not been extensively studied from this perspective before.

However, this study has certain limitations that may affect the generalization of the results. First, this study was conducted in one country, Poland, which may limit the applicability of the findings to a broader population of sports volunteers. Further research with a larger and more diverse participant group is needed to better understand the influence of factors such as cultural differences, education level, and socioeconomic environment on dietary habits. Additionally, the use of interviews may lead to subjectivity in responses, especially regarding the self-assessment of dietary habits. In the future, it would be worthwhile considering supplementing this study with quantitative methods, such as dietary diaries or anthropometric measurements, which could provide more objective data. Quantitative methods allow for more precise and less participant-biased results, as well as enable the analysis of a larger amount of data, increasing the reliability of conclusions. This approach also facilitates the identification of trends and correlations that may be invisible in qualitative data. Their use can therefore significantly enhance the quality of research, leading to more accurate and universal conclusions, which are particularly important in the context of future studies on population health and dietary habits.

5. Conclusions

The results of this study show that the dietary habits of sports volunteers are varied, but in most cases, they are not given much attention. The majority of participants consumed random meals, often relying on available, highly processed products. Only a few respondents demonstrated full awareness of their diet and made an effort to adjust their nutrition to the physical demands of volunteering. These results suggest a need for greater education on healthy eating, especially in the context of increased physical exertion and the challenges associated with working during sports events. Further research should also take into account the differences in the nutritional needs of volunteers depending on the type of sports event and the cultural contexts in which these events occur, in order to better tailor dietary recommendations to variable conditions.

These conclusions also highlight the importance of providing appropriate meals during sports events. Volunteers who do not have access to a balanced diet may experience increased fatigue and decreased effectiveness, which can negatively impact the organization of events. Therefore, event organizers should ensure conditions that support healthy eating, which would not only benefit the volunteers' health but also enhance the quality of their work and contribute to the success of the events being organized.

Funding: This research received no external funding.

Institutional Review Board Statement: This study, conducted among sports volunteers, adhered to the principles of the Declaration of Helsinki, even though it did not require approval from an Ethics Committee. The research relied on in-depth interviews, which do not interfere with participants' health or introduce experimental procedures. All participants provided informed consent, ensuring full respect for their autonomy and privacy. Additionally, participants' personal data were protected according to current privacy standards, and the analysis of results was based on anonymous information, fully complying with the requirements for confidentiality and participant protection.

Informed Consent Statement: Informed consent was obtained from all subjects involved in this study.

Data Availability Statement: The original contributions presented in the study are included in the article, further inquiries can be directed to the corresponding author.

Conflicts of Interest: The author declares no conflicts of interest.

References

1. Shao, T.; Verma, H.K.; Pande, B.; Costanzo, V.; Ye, W.; Cai, Y.; Bhaskar, L.V.K.S. Physical Activity and Nutritional Influence on Immune Function: An Important Strategy to Improve Immunity and Health Status. *Front. Physiol.* **2021**, *12*, 751374. [CrossRef] [PubMed]
2. Thomas, D.T.; Erdman, K.A.; Burke, L.M. Nutrition and Athletic Performance. *Med. Sci. Sports Exerc.* **2016**, *48*, 543–568. [CrossRef] [PubMed]
3. Cuskelly, G.; Hoye, R.; Auld, C. *Working with Volunteers in Sport: Theory and Practice*; Routledge: London, UK, 2006.
4. Cuskelly, G. Volunteer Retention in Community Sport Organisations. *Eur. Sport Manag. Q.* **2004**, *4*, 59–76. [CrossRef]
5. Zajac, A.; Poprzecki, S.; Maszczyk, A.; Czuba, M.; Michalczyk, M.; Zydek, G. The Effects of a Ketogenic Diet on Exercise Metabolism and Physical Performance in Off-Road Cyclists. *Nutrients* **2014**, *6*, 2493–2508. [CrossRef] [PubMed]
6. De Bruin, A.P.K.; Oudejans, R.R.D.; Bakker, F.C. Dieting and Body Image in Aesthetic Sports: A Comparison of Dutch Female Gymnasts and Non-Aesthetic Sport Participants. *Psychol. Sport Exerc.* **2007**, *40*, 507–520. [CrossRef]

7. Burke, L.M.; Hawley, J.A.; Wong, S.H.S.; Jeukendrup, A.E. Carbohydrates for Training and Competition. *J. Sports Sci.* **2011**, *29* (Suppl. S1), S17–S27. [CrossRef]
8. Lukaski, H.C. Vitamin and Mineral Status: Effects on Physical Performance. *Nutrition* **2004**, *20*, 632–644. [CrossRef]
9. Wirnitzer, K.; Motevalli, M.; Tanous, D.; Gregori, M.; Wirnitzer, G.; Leitzmann, C.; Hill, L.; Rosemann, T.; Knechtle, B. Supplement Tntake in Half-Marathon, (Ultra-)Marathon and 10-km Runners—Results from the NURMI Study (Step 2). *J. Int. Soc. Sports Nutr.* **2021**, *18*, 64. [CrossRef]
10. Jeukendrup, A. A Step Towards Personalized Sports Nutrition: Carbohydrate Intake During Exercise. *Sports Med.* **2014**, *44* (Suppl. S1), 25–33. [CrossRef]
11. Cermak, N.M.; van Loon, L.J. The Use of Carbohydrates During Exercise as an Ergogenic Aid. *Sports Med.* **2013**, *43*, 1139–1155. [CrossRef]
12. Maughan, R.J.; Shirreffs, S.M. Nutrition for Sports Performance: Issues and Opportunities. *Proc. Nutr. Soc.* **2012**, *71*, 112–119. [CrossRef] [PubMed]
13. Birkenhead, K.L.; Slater, G. A Review of Factors Influencing Athletes' Food Choices. *Sports Med.* **2015**, *45*, 1511–1522. [CrossRef] [PubMed]
14. Monteiro, C.A.; Cannon, G.; Moubarac, J.C.; Levy, R.B.; Louzada, M.L.; Jaime, P.C. The UN Decade of Nutrition, the NOVA Food Classification and the Trouble with Ultra-Processing. *Public Health Nutr.* **2019**, *21*, 5–17. [CrossRef] [PubMed]
15. Seaman, A.N. Concessions, Traditions, and Staying Safe: Considering Sport, Food, and the Lasting Impact of the COVID-19 Pandemic. *Sport J.* **2021**, *41*, 1–9.
16. Milena, Z.R.; Dainora, G.; Alin, S. Qualitative Research Methods: A Comparison Between Focus-Group And In-Depth Interview. *Ann. Univ. Oradea Econ. Sci.* **2008**, *4*, 1279–1283.
17. Fontana, A.; Frey, J.H. The interview. From structured questions to negotiated text. In *Handbook of Qualitative Research*, 2nd ed.; Lincoln, Y.S., Denzin, N.K., Eds.; Sage: Thousand Oaks, CA, USA, 2000; pp. 645–672.
18. Kaplowitz, M.D. Statistical analysis of sensitive topics in group and individual interviews. *Qual. Quant.* **2000**, *34*, 419–431. [CrossRef]
19. Russell, C.; Gregory, D.; Ploeg, J.; DiCenso, A.; Guyatt, G. Qualitative Research. In *Evidence-Based Nursing: A Guide to Clinical Practice*; DiCenso, A., Guyatt, G., Ciliska, D., Eds.; Elsevier Mosby: St. Louis, MO, USA, 2005; pp. 120–136.
20. Hennink, M.; Kaiser, B.N. Sample Sizes for Saturation in Qualitative Research: A Systematic Review of Empirical Tests. *Soc. Sci. Med.* **2022**, *292*, 114523. [CrossRef]
21. Boddy, C.R. Sample Size for Qualitative Research. *Qual. Mark. Res.* **2016**, *19*, 426–432. [CrossRef]
22. Economos, C.D.; Bortz, S.S.; Nelson, M.E. Nutritional Practices of Elite Athletes: Practical Recommendations. *Sports Med.* **1993**, *16*, 381–399. [CrossRef]
23. Schröder, H.; Fito, M.; Covas, M.I. Association of Fast Food Consumption with Energy Intake, Diet Quality, Body Mass Index and the Risk of Obesity in a Representative Mediterranean Population. *Br. J. Nutr.* **2007**, *98*, 1274–1280. [CrossRef]
24. Jaworowska, A.; Blackham, T.; Davies, I.G.; Stevenson, L. Nutritional Challenges and Health Implications of Takeaway and Fast Food. *Nutr. Rev.* **2013**, *71*, 310–318. [CrossRef] [PubMed]
25. Manore, M.; Meyer, N.L.; Thompson, J. *Sport Nutrition for Health and Performance*; Human Kinetics: Champaign, IL, USA, 2009.
26. Amawi, A.; AlKasasbeh, W.; Jaradat, M.; Almasri, A.; Alobaidi, S.; Hammad, A.A.; Bishtawi, T.; Fataftah, B.; Turk, N.; Al Saoud, H.; et al. Athletes' Nutritional Demands: A Narrative Review of Nutritional Requirements. *Front. Nutr.* **2024**, *10*, 1331854. [CrossRef] [PubMed]
27. Hawley, J.A.; Burke, L.M. Effect of Meal Frequency and Timing on Physical Performance. *Br. J. Nutr.* **1997**, *77* (Suppl. 1), S91–S103. [CrossRef] [PubMed]
28. Logue, D.; Madigan, S.M.; Delahunt, E.; Heinen, M.; Mc Donnell, S.J.; Corish, C.A. Low Energy Availability in Athletes: A Review of Prevalence, Dietary Patterns, Physiological Health, and Sports Performance. *Sports Med.* **2018**, *48*, 73–96. [CrossRef] [PubMed]
29. Boyle, M.; Stone-Francisco, S.; Samuels, S.E. Environmental Strategies and Policies to Support Healthy Eating and Physical Activity in Low-Income Communities. *J. Hunger Environ. Nutr.* **2007**, *1*, 3–25. [CrossRef]
30. Barbee, M. *Politically Incorrect Nutrition: Finding Reality in the Mire of Food Industry Propaganda*; Vital Health Publishing: Hulbert, OK, USA, 2004.
31. Vasconcelos, C.; Costa, R.L.D.; Dias, Á.L.; Pereira, L.; Santos, J.P. Online Influencers: Healthy Food or Fake News. *Int. J. Internet Mark. Advert.* **2021**, *15*, 149–175. [CrossRef]
32. Sánchez-Díaz, S.; Yanci, J.; Castillo, D.; Scanlan, A.T.; Raya-González, J. Effects of Nutrition Education Interventions in Team Sport Players. A Systematic Review. *Nutrients* **2020**, *12*, 3664. [CrossRef]
33. Devlin, B.L.; Belski, R. Exploring General and Sports Nutrition and Food Knowledge in Elite Male Australian Athletes. *Int. J. Sport Nutr. Exerc. Metab.* **2015**, *25*, 225–232. [CrossRef]
34. Spronk, I.; Heaney, S.E.; Prvan, T.; O'Connor, H.T. Relationship Between General Nutrition Knowledge and Dietary Quality in Elite Athletes. *Int. J. Sport Nutr. Exerc. Metab.* **2015**, *25*, 243–251. [CrossRef]

Disclaimer/Publisher's Note: The statements, opinions and data contained in all publications are solely those of the individual author(s) and contributor(s) and not of MDPI and/or the editor(s). MDPI and/or the editor(s) disclaim responsibility for any injury to people or property resulting from any ideas, methods, instructions or products referred to in the content.

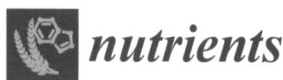 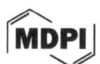

Article

Adaptation of the Food Literacy (FOODLIT) Tool for Turkish Adults: A Validity and Reliability Study

Yasemin Ertaş Öztürk [1,*], Sevtap Kabalı [1], Yasemin Açar [1], Duygu Ağagündüz [2] and Ferenc Budán [3,*]

[1] Department of Nutrition and Dietetics, Ondokuz Mayıs University, 55200 Samsun, Türkiye; sevtap.kkurtaran@omu.edu.tr (S.K.); dytyaseminacar@gmail.com (Y.A.)
[2] Department of Nutrition and Dietetics, Gazi University, 06490 Ankara, Türkiye; duyguturkozu@gazi.edu.tr
[3] Institute of Physiology, Medical School, University of Pécs, H-7624 Pécs, Hungary
* Correspondence: yasemnertas@gmail.com (Y.E.Ö.); budan.ferenc@pte.hu (F.B.)

Abstract: Background: Food literacy is associated with sustainable food systems and encourages individuals to adopt healthy eating habits. However, there is no validated method that can be used to measure food literacy related to sustainable food systems of Turkish adults. This research aimed to assess the validity and reliability of the Turkish adaptation of the "Food Literacy (FOODLIT) Tool" for Turkish adults. Methods: The study involved 328 people aged 19 to 58 years. The FOODLIT-Tool is a five-point Likert-type scale consisting of 24 items and five factors ("culinary competencies", "production and quality", "selection and planning", "environmentally safe" and "origin"). Results: The Cronbach's alpha coefficient was applied to assess internal consistency reliability, showing an excellent scale coefficient of 0.927. The model was evaluated with a confirmatory factor analysis (CFA). The findings of the CFA suggested that the fit indices were acceptable ($\chi^2/df = 1.257$, comparative fit index: 0.991, goodness-of-fit index: 0.977, normed fit index: 0.990 and root mean error of approximation: 0.028). Furthermore, there was a positive relationship between the FOODLIT-Tool score and the "Sustainable and Healthy Eating Behaviors Scale" (SHEB) score ($r = 0.518$, $p < 0.001$). Conclusion: Our study shows that the Turkish version of the FOODLIT-Tool integrated with sustainable food systems is a valid and reliable measurement tool for assessing the food literacy of Turkish adults.

Keywords: food literacy; sustainability; validity and reliability; nutrition; Turkish adults; measurement tool

Citation: Ertaş Öztürk, Y.; Kabalı, S.; Açar, Y.; Ağagündüz, D.; Budán, F. Adaptation of the Food Literacy (FOODLIT) Tool for Turkish Adults: A Validity and Reliability Study. *Nutrients* **2024**, *16*, 3416. https://doi.org/10.3390/nu16193416

Academic Editors: Ariana Saraiva and António Raposo

Received: 19 September 2024
Revised: 4 October 2024
Accepted: 7 October 2024
Published: 9 October 2024

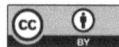

Copyright: © 2024 by the authors. Licensee MDPI, Basel, Switzerland. This article is an open access article distributed under the terms and conditions of the Creative Commons Attribution (CC BY) license (https://creativecommons.org/licenses/by/4.0/).

1. Introduction

Food literacy is a factor that has recently gained increasing importance and encourages healthy eating habits. According to Vidgen and Galleos (2014), food literacy is "the acquisition of the knowledge, skills and behaviors necessary to plan, manage, select, prepare and eat foods to determine nutrient needs and consumption. In other words, it is the structure that empowers individuals and communities to maintain diet quality" [1]. Food literacy has many determinants and influencing factors. These are essentially listed as food/health choices, skills and behaviors, culture, emotions, knowledge and food systems [2]. All the components mentioned above provide individuals and societies with the freedom to choose food and provide a critical perspective on food choice. On the other hand, inadequacy in food literacy may lead to a lack of information about the process of food from farm to fork [3,4]. Inadequate literacy, together with easy access to unhealthy foods in the food supply chain and the loss of culinary skills during food preparation, may lead to inappropriate consumer behaviors in the food system [4,5].

In recent years, there has been a global change in food systems due to individual and environmental factors [6]. More than half of the United Nations' 17 Sustainable Development Goals to be achieved by 2030 are related to health, environment and food systems [7]. Studies have shown that the production, processing, packaging, distribution and consumption steps of food are responsible for one-third of total greenhouse gas emissions [8]. In this context, a sustainable food system should meet the needs of individuals from a health and nutrition perspective and ensure access to healthy and safe food [9,10]. Similar to this trend, food literacy encompasses a wide range of issues, from individual and public health to the food system and its interaction with the environment. Recent studies on food literacy suggest that the term should include multifaceted decision-making concepts related to food and the food system. In this respect, the sustainable food system can be integrated into the conceptual framework of food literacy, and issues such as sustainability and food safety can be addressed in the process from food production to consumption [11–14].

Rosas et al. conducted the Food Literacy Project (FOODLIT-PRO) [15], which aimed to integrate the sustainable food system and food literacy into the conceptual framework and subsequently revealed the Food Literacy Wheel (FLW) [16]. With this project, the definition, determinants and influential factors of food literacy have been comprehensively presented. In line with sustainable food systems, the FLW includes health, nutrition, cultural, social, sustainability, industry, policy, learning and psychological contexts as influential factors. In addition, the wheel includes a series of stages such as food selection, purchasing, preservation, planning and culinary skills. In this context, in addition to the assessment of consumers' food literacy status, the need to evaluate the heterogeneous factors and determinants of food literacy has emerged [16,17]. The need to assess sustainable food systems that integrate all health, environmental, social and economic perspectives emphasizes both the food literacy of consumers and the importance of the food supply chain [18]. In recent years, instruments assessing consumers' food literacy have been developed [19,20]. However, there is no validated method that can be used to measure food literacy related to sustainable food systems of Turkish adults. In this study, we aimed to assess the validity and reliability of the "Food Literacy Tool (FOODLIT-Tool)" for Turkish adults.

The importance of the validity and reliability of the FOODLIT-Tool for Turkish adults can be listed as follows: (1) In addition to measuring consumers' food literacy, this tool takes into account different perspectives (environmentally safe, production and quality, selection and planning, culinary skills, origin). (2) This tool provides targets for understanding and intervention in the food supply chain. (3) This tool focuses not only on the level of knowledge about food but also on sustainability, meal planning, food safety and food preparation skills. We believe that this study will contribute to future studies on the assessment of food literacy related to sustainable food systems.

2. Materials and Methods

2.1. Adaptation to Turkish Language and Content Validity

The original instructions and items of the FOODLIT-Tool (Supplementary Material S1) underwent translation into Turkish and subsequent back translation into English in accordance with the suggested recommendations [21]. Two independent academicians with advanced English and a linguist translated the tool to Turkish. Afterward, the Turkish version of the tool was back translated into English by two independent nutrition experts who had never seen the original English version of the tool. After the translation of the tool was finalized, Turkish form was sent to ten nutrition experts and they gave their opinions on content. Experts rated the items and the item-based content validity ratio and content validity index (CVI) for each factor, and total was calculated. The CVI values were >0.800, and it was above the critical value [22].

A pilot study was conducted on a sample of 17 people to examine the acceptability and understanding of the items. Participants studied the tool and were invited to express their comments on each item. Minor suggestions (e.g., synonym alteration) for increasing the understanding were accepted and considered for two items. The final Turkish version of the tool is presented in Supplementary Material S2.

2.2. Participants and Data Collection

This study was conducted on 328 participants (73.5% women) from December 2023 to February 2024. Data were obtained through the Google Forms web platform. Any adults

(19–65 years) who speak Turkish language were included in the study. People with any psychiatric disorder, following a special dietary regimen, and pregnant or lactating women were not included. Adherence to the inclusion and exclusion criteria was achieved through initial inquiries regarding the relevant criteria. The presence of psychiatric illness was assessed based on whether it was diagnosed by a physician. The study questionnaire was administered to participants at a ratio above 1:20 (500 subjects), providing equal representation of both sexes; however, in the end, the data from all persons who volunteered to participate were analyzed. Mean age of the participants was 26.6 ± 8.36 years; 62.6% of them had undergraduate or higher educational degree, 71.6% were single, and 22.6% were low-income status.

The research received approval from the Ondokuz Mayıs University Clinical Research Ethics Committee (decision number: 2023/357-B.30.2.ODM.0.20.08/554, date: 8 November 2023), following the principles of the Helsinki Declaration.

2.3. Measures

2.3.1. Food Literacy Tool

The FOODLIT-Tool was created by Rosas et al. [18] through a qualitative investigation of the definition, determinants and influential aspects of food literacy [15]. The construction of a conceptual and empirical framework encompasses the fundamental knowledge, competencies and behaviors connected to food. It also considers the factors that facilitate or hinder these aspects, as well as the various areas of interaction that aim to address broader concerns related to global sustainability in food systems [16] as part of the FOODLIT-PRO [15]. The tool contains 24 items, five factors (F1: Culinary competencies, F2: Production and quality, F3: Selection and planning, F4: Environmentally safe, F5: Origin) and Likert-type scoring system (0—never/totally disagree, 1—sometimes/disagree, 2—frequently/agree, 3—always/totally agree). Each item is scored between 0 and 3 points. The total score and the scores of the sub-factors are obtained by totaling the relevant items. The original Cronbach's alpha value is 0.831.

2.3.2. Sustainable and Healthy Eating Behaviors Scale

"Sustainable and Healthy Eating Behaviors" (SHEB) Scale was originally developed by Żakowska-Biemans et al. [23] and adapted into Turkish by Köksal et al. [24]. The Turkish version of the scale consists of 32 items and seven factors that are SHEB_F1: "Quality labels (regional and organic)", SHEB_F2: "Seasonal food and avoiding food waste", SHEB_F3: "Animal welfare", SHEB_F4: "Meat reduction", SHEB_F5: "Healthy and balanced diet", SHEB_F6: "Local food" and SHEB_F7: "Low fat". Likert-type scale was used and scored 1 to 7. Respondents were asked to rate each item as 'never', 'very rarely', 'rarely', 'sometimes', 'often', 'very often' or 'always'. Higher scores obtained indicate that the individual had the characteristics evaluated by the relevant factors. The Cronbach's alpha value is 0.912.

2.4. Statistical Analysis

Internal consistency reliability was assessed using Cronbach's alpha coefficients, which uses a polychronic correlation matrix since it is more suitable than the Pearson correlation for ordinal data [25]. In order to test the constant validity of the FOODLIT-Tool, a confirmatory factor analysis (CFA) was conducted. Since the original tool was developed based on a framework and the items were parts of the conceptual and empirical framework with a mixed methodology [16], no exploratory factor analysis was conducted. The model was tested using the diagonally weighted least squares (DWLS) procedure. In order to determine whether the model had a good fit, the following fit indices were examined: chi-square/df, Comparative Fit Index (CFI), Good of Fit Index (GFI), Tucker–Lewis Fit Index (TLI), the Non-Normed Fit Index (NNFI), the Incremental Fit Index (IFI), the adjusted goodness of fit index (AGFI), the Standardized Root Mean Square Residual (SRMR) and the Root Mean Square Error of Approximation (RMSEA). We accepted chi-square/df < 2.0, CFI, GFI, TLI, NNFI, IFI values of ≥ 0.90, AGFI > 0.85 and RMSEA and SRMR ≤ 0.10 as cut-off values [26–29]. Also, we examined the concurrent validity of the tool by performing a correlation analysis between the FOODLIT-Tool and SHEB Scale total and sub-factors. Statistical findings were obtained using IBM SPSS 28 and R software (version 4.4.1), and the type-1 error level was set at α = 0.05.

3. Results

The model was evaluated with subjects who responded to every item on the scale (n = 328) with a participant-to-item ratio of >10:1. The skewness and kurtosis results showed that the item answers exhibited a normal univariate distribution, with acceptable ranges for skewness and kurtosis being −2 to +2 and −7 to +7, respectively. After removing ten outliers, the multivariate normality was established (Mahalanobis distance maximum value = 48.600, $p < 0.001$).

The answers to the items are shown in Figure 1. The majority of the participants (91%) totally agreed with i21, which is "I am aware of the time of year of each food". The item most disagreed (61%) with was i14, which is "I control the calories and/or other nutritional characteristics of the food I eat daily".

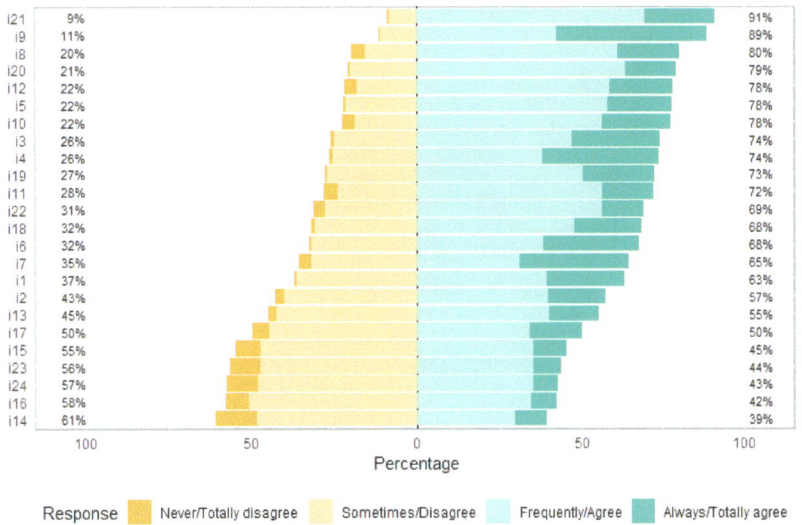

Figure 1. Responses to the FOODLIT-Tool items.

The Cronbach's alpha coefficients of total and factors are presented in Table 1. Accordingly, the total and sub-factor scores are reliable.

Table 1. Reliability of the factors and total tool.

Factors	Items	Item Number	Cronbach's Alpha
F1: Culinary competencies	i1, i2, i3, i4, i5, i6, i7, i8	8	0.871
F2: Production and quality	i10, i11, i12	3	0.883
F3: Selection and planning	i14, i17, i18, i19, i22, i23, i24	7	0.903
F4: Environmentally safe	i9, i13, i20, i21	4	0.763
F5: Origin	i15, i16	2	0.866
Total	all items	24	0.927

The goodness of fit index for the CFA analysis (five factors and 24 items) is presented in Table 2, and the coefficients for the full model are presented in Figure 2.

Table 2. The goodness of fit index.

	χ^2/df	CFI	GFI	TLI	NNFI	IFI	AGFI	SRMR	RMSEA
Model	1.257	0.991	0.977	0.990	0.990	0.991	0.971	0.061	0.028

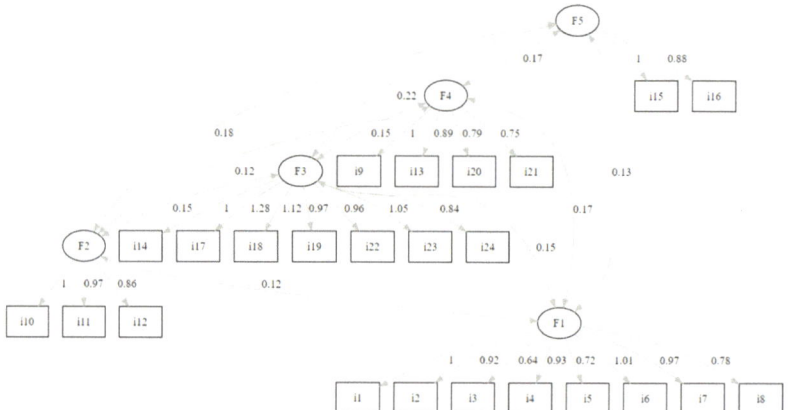

Figure 2. Confirmatory factor analysis for the coefficients of the model.

To assess concurrent validity, correlational analysis between the FOODLIT-Tool and the SHEB Scale was conducted and is reported in Figure 3. Positive correlations were observed between the FOODLIT-Tool factors and the SHEB Scale sub-factors ($p < 0.05$). The strongest associations were between the FOODLIT-Tool and the SHEB Scale (r = 0.518, $p < 0.001$) and the FOODLIT-Tool and the SHEB_F1 factor (r = 0.528, $p < 0.001$).

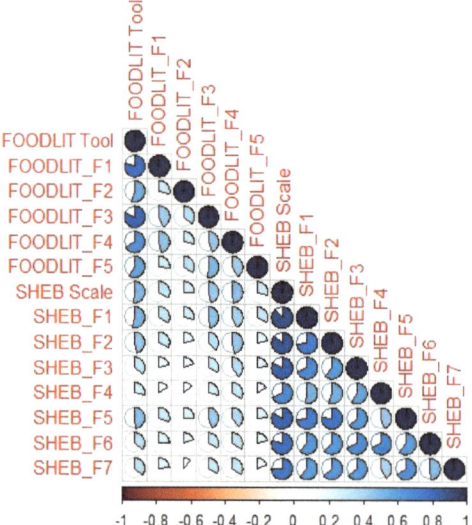

Figure 3. Correlations between the FOODLIT-Tool and the SHEB Scale. The ratio of the pies represents the correlation of the coefficient levels. All relationships were statistically significant ($p < 0.05$). FOODLIT: Food literacy; SHEB: Sustainable and Healthy Eating Behaviors; SHEB_F1: "Quality labels (regional and organic)"; SHEB_F2: "Seasonal food and avoiding food waste"; SHEB_F3: "Animal welfare"; SHEB_F4: "Meat reduction"; SHEB_F5: "Healthy and balanced diet"; SHEB_F6: "Local food"; SHEB_F7: "Low fat".

4. Discussion

Food literacy refers to an individual's capacity to understand, perceive and engage with the intricate food system over the course of their lifetime. Food literacy encompasses an individual's understanding, abilities, beliefs and behaviors related to eating [30]. Enhancing food literacy not only improves individualized nutrition, health and wellness but also enables individuals to understand the impact of their food choices on the environment and how their food selections affect others [30,31]. The macro perspective of food literacy separates it into three primary areas: food, nutrition and health; agriculture, environment and ecology; and social development and equity. Food literacy is viewed as a component of food, health, sustainable environments and social equality [32].

Recently, there has been an increasing interest in examining the connection between food literacy and its impact on health outcomes. Individuals with a deficiency in basic knowledge about food are at a higher risk of developing ailments such as obesity, chronic heart disease, diabetes and cancer [33,34]. People with low food literacy may be unaware of how many calories are in a serving of their meal, as well as how much salt or sugar it contains [35]. They may have a limited understanding of the potential advantages or disadvantages of the dietary components. They may lack knowledge about the appropriate dietary choices for their age or health condition, leading to uncertainty about which foods they should consume more or less frequently [34,36]. In this context, it is important to increase the food literacy awareness levels of individuals.

Sustainable diets are defined by the Food and Agriculture Organization as follows: "Sustainable Diets are those diets with low environmental impacts which contribute to food and nutrition security and to healthy life for present and future generations. Sustainable diets are protective and respectful of biodiversity and ecosystems, culturally acceptable, accessible, economically fair and affordable; nutritionally adequate, safe and healthy; while optimizing natural and human resources" [37]. These diets aim to improve food security, promote health for current and future generations, and mitigate environmental impact [38].

Food literacy is a key aspect of sustainability since it plays a role in promoting social, economic and environmental sustainability. Food literacy cultivates an understanding of the connection between food consumption and the environment. Possessing a high level of literacy can contribute to mitigating the impact of humans on the environment by making informed and sustainable dietary choices [39,40]. The outcomes of good food literacy prevent the loss of resources such as soil, water and energy at all stages of the food supply chain and reduce greenhouse gas emissions that cause climate change [4,41]. Cullen et al. [42] defined food literacy through the viewpoint of community food security as the acquisition of knowledge in three domains: (1) the impact of food on personal health and well-being; (2) the multifaceted nature of the food system encompassing societal, economic, cultural, environmental and political perspectives; and (3) the comprehensive food system, spanning from production to waste management. This notion underscores the necessity of cultivating knowledge, skills and habits pertaining to food to improve decision-making that benefits individuals and fosters a sustainable food system.

This study aimed to assess the validity and reliability of the Turkish adaption of the FOODLIT-Tool among the Turkish population. This study consisted of a total of 328 people. This scale is suitable for utilization among adult individuals. It is hypothesized that those working in various fields of healthcare, specifically nutrition and dietetics, could utilize this scale to enhance the advancement of nutritional knowledge, skills and behaviors. The number of scales in Türkiye available to assess adults' food literacy is limited. This study is expected to fill a gap in the literature and lead to further research on food literacy. Various food literacy scales are utilized globally, such as the Food and Nutrition Literacy Instrument [19], the Self-Perceived Food Literacy Scale [43,44], the International Food Literacy Questionnaire [45] and the Food Literacy Behavior Checklist [46]. Participants with higher levels of food literacy consumed considerably more fruits, vegetables and fish than those with lower levels of food literacy. Furthermore, it was underlined that assessing the literacy levels of persons during the initial patient encounter and prior to providing dietary guidance will enhance the enhancement of nutritional well-being [19,43–46].

Our results showed that the Turkish version of the FOODLIT-Tool is valid and reliable, with 24 items and five factors. The factors are culinary competencies, production and quality, selection and planning, environmentally safe and origin. These factors are measured by a total of eight, three, seven, four and two items, respectively. The overall FOODLIT-Tool questionnaire has reliable internal consistency (Cronbach's α = 0.927). The Cronbach's α coefficients for the five factors (culinary competencies, production and quality, selection and planning, environmentally safe and origin) were 0.871, 0.883, 0.903, 0.763 and 0.866, respectively, which are higher than the original scale (0.54 to 0.73). The five-factor model (Figure 2) showed confirmatory factor analysis and an acceptable goodness of fit index (χ^2/df = 1.257, CFI = 0.991, GFI = 0.977, TLI = 0.990, NNFI = 0.990, IFI = 0.991, AGFI = 0.971, SRMR = 0.061 and RMSEA = 0.028) (Table 2). In the original scale, Rosas et al. found fit indices as χ^2/df = 3.958, SRMR = 0.055, RMSEA = 0.055, CFI = 0.907, and GFI = 0.917 [18]. We accepted chi-square/df < 2.0, CFI, GFI, TLI, NNFI, IFI values of $\geq$0.90, AGFI > 0.85, and RMSEA and SRMR $\leq$ 0.10 as cut-off values [26–29]. It can be seen that the fit indices we found as a result of the analyses performed in this study are within the accepted range and have similar values to the original scale. These results show that the Turkish version of the FOODLIT-Tool is a valid and reliable scale in determining food literacy.

The answers to the items are shown in Figure 1. Participants did not care about controlling the calories and nutritional characteristics of the food they ate daily. Individuals with an obsession with healthy eating, such as orthorexia nervosa, may have conditions such as controlling the calories of the foods consumed and being anxious about healthy food consumption. These conditions develop with the desire for a healthy diet, and concerns about health, nutrition and food quality are at the forefront [47,48].

We used the SHEB Scale, which was adapted into Turkish by Köksal et al. [24], indicating that the factors of the SHEB Scale are similar to those of the FOODLIT-Tool. Both scales prioritize promoting the consumption of seasonal and regional foods while mitigating food waste within the framework of sustainability. The second factor of the SHEB Scale, titled "seasonal food and avoiding food waste", includes the following items related to food waste: "I don't waste food", "I reuse leftovers from food", "I buy regional food", "I eat seasonal fruits and vegetables", "In season, I shop at farmer's markets", "I avoid sugary drinks", "I limit my salt usage". In the FOODLIT-Tool, the items related to food waste are given as "I buy local/national trade products to support local/national business", "I eat food according to its seasonality", "I am aware of the time of year of each food". The two scales are similar in that they emphasize issues such as consuming seasonal foods, supporting local/national products/producers and not wasting food waste and recycling it. We found positive relationships between the FOODLIT-Tool factors and the SHEB Scale sub-factors. All relationships were statistically significant (p < 0.05). When the mean values of the SHEB Scale's sub-factors were compared, the quality labels factor (factor 1), which includes regional and organic items, had the highest value [24]. These findings show that quality is an important criterion for creating consumer awareness and food literacy in choosing local products that are healthier, unprocessed and contain fewer preservatives. A few studies have explored the associations between food literacy and sustainable and healthy eating behaviors; Kabasakal-Cetin et al. [49] examined the impact of food literacy and sustainable eating behaviors on the intake of ultra-processed foods. They found that lower food literacy (β = −0.140, p = 0.004) and sustainable and healthy eating behaviors (β = −0.104, p = 0.032) predicted increased intake of ultra-processed foods. In another study, Mortaş et al. investigated the relationship between food and nutrition literacy and sustainable, healthy eating behaviors among young adults. They found that there were significant relationships between the SHEB Scale and the Food and Nutrition Literacy Instrument [48]. Our findings are consistent with these studies, showing that food literacy is associated with sustainability and healthy eating skills. Increased food literacy was positively connected with sustainable eating behavior in adults [20,50–52].

This study has highlighted a number of issues that affect both individual and public health and well-being, such as encouraging consumers to make food choices related to sustainability and health, environmental safety, origin, food supply chain and food safety, meal planning and culinary skills. We believe that the FOODLIT-Tool integrated with sustainable food systems is a useful and valid tool that can be used to comprehensively assess the food literacy levels of consumers in Türkiye. Furthermore, the FOODLIT-Tool can be used in longitudinal studies to assess changes in consumers' food literacy over time. National policies can be developed to create educational programs for consumers based on the FOODLIT-Tool results and to eliminate deficiencies. In this context, in addition to providing information about the process from production to consumption of food, consumer education on sustainable food systems can be planned. The effectiveness of planned food-literacy education can be determined by using this tool to identify the aspects of the target groups that need to be improved. These food literacy components can be included in Good Manufacturing Practices to raise awareness of food producers at the national level. Thus, steps can be taken to encourage food producers and consumers to encourage the adoption of sustainable food production and consumption behaviors.

However, several limitations also need to be acknowledged. At first, we utilized self-reported health data and did not employ any screening tools to verify physiological abnormalities. The research predominantly focuses on women; subsequent studies should incorporate a greater representation of Turkish men, as their perspectives can differ.

5. Conclusions

The results of the study show that the Turkish adaptation of the FOODLIT-Tool is valid and reliable. We believe that this tool will serve as a reliable instrument for assessing the level of food literacy among individuals residing in Türkiye and subsequently uncover the influence of food literacy on culinary competencies, production and quality, selection and planning, environmental safety and origin of the food. Ultimately, it will provide assistance for future research endeavors aimed at determining the level of food literacy in comparable environments and age cohorts. Enhancing food literacy will provide individuals and communities with an understanding of sustainable food systems and will encourage maintaining healthy dietary patterns. We consider that it would be beneficial to evaluate food literacy for a healthier society, a clean environment and a sustainable agricultural supply. The education sector employees, food producers and policy makers can create this awareness through their co-operation.

Supplementary Materials: The following supporting information can be downloaded at: https://www.mdpi.com/article/10.3390/nu16193416/s1. File S1: The original items of FOODLIT-Tool; File S2: Food Literacy Tool Turkish Version.

Author Contributions: Conceptualization, Y.E.Ö.; methodology, Y.E.Ö., S.K. and Y.A.; validation, Y.E.Ö., S.K. and Y.A.; formal analysis, Y.E.Ö. and D.A.; data curation, Y.E.Ö., S.K. and Y.A.; writing—original draft preparation, Y.E.Ö., S.K. and Y.A.; writing—review and editing, Y.E.Ö., S.K., Y.A., D.A. and F.B.; visualization, Y.E.Ö.; supervision, Y.E.Ö., D.A. and F.B. All authors have read and agreed to the published version of the manuscript.

Funding: This research received no external funding.

Institutional Review Board Statement: The study was conducted in accordance with the Declaration of Helsinki, and was approved by the Ondokuz Mayıs University Clinical Research Ethics Committee (protocol code: 2023/357-B.30.2.ODM.0.20.08/554 and approval date: 8 November 2023).

Informed Consent Statement: Informed consent was obtained from all subjects involved in the study.

Data Availability Statement: Dataset available upon request from the authors due to privacy.

Acknowledgments: The authors would like to acknowledge the participants for taking their time and voluntarily completing surveys.

Conflicts of Interest: The authors declare no conflicts of interest.

References

1. Vidgen, H.A.; Gallegos, D. Defining food literacy and its components. *Appetite* **2014**, *76*, 50–59. [CrossRef] [PubMed]
2. Truman, E.; Lane, D.; Elliott, C. Defining food literacy: A scoping review. *Appetite* **2017**, *116*, 365–371. [CrossRef] [PubMed]
3. Conrad, Z.; Niles, M.T.; Neher, D.A.; Roy, E.D.; Tichenor, N.E.; Jahns, L. Relationship between food waste, diet quality, and environmental sustainability. *PLoS ONE* **2018**, *13*, e0195405. [CrossRef] [PubMed]
4. Lisciani, S.; Camilli, E.; Marconi, S. Enhancing food and nutrition literacy: A key strategy for reducing food waste and improving diet quality. *Sustainability* **2024**, *16*, 1726. [CrossRef]
5. Mengi Çelik, Ö.; Karacil Ermumcu, M.S.; Ozyildirim, C. Turkish version of the 'food and nutrition literacy questionnaire for Chinese school-age children for school-age adolescents: A validity and reliability study. *BMC Public. Health* **2023**, *23*, 1807. [CrossRef]
6. Barrett, C.B. Actions now can curb food systems fallout from COVID-19. *Nat. Food* **2020**, *1*, 319–320. [CrossRef]
7. United Nations. Sustainable Development Goals. Available online: https://sdgs.un.org/goals (accessed on 3 April 2024).
8. Crippa, M.; Solazzo, E.; Guizzardi, D.; Monforti-Ferrario, F.; Tubiello, F.N.; Leip, A. Food systems are responsible for a third of global anthropogenic GHG emissions. *Nat. Food* **2021**, *2*, 198–209. [CrossRef]
9. Spiker, M.; Reinhardt, S.; Bruening, M. Academy of nutrition and dietetics: Revised 2020 standards of professional performance for registered dietitian nutritionists (competent, proficient, and expert) in sustainable, resilient, and healthy food and water systems. *J. Acad. Nutr. Diet.* **2020**, *120*, 1568–1585.e28. [CrossRef]
10. Campbell, C.G.; Feldpausch, G. Teaching nutrition and sustainable food systems: Justification and an applied approach. *Front. Nutr.* **2023**, *10*, 1167180. [CrossRef]
11. Yuen, E.Y.; Thomson, M.; Gardiner, H. Measuring nutrition and food literacy in adults: A systematic review and appraisal of existing measurement tools. *Health Lit. Res. Pr.* **2018**, *2*, e134–e160. [CrossRef]
12. Widener, P.; Karides, M. Food system literacy: Empowering citizens and consumers beyond farm-to-fork pathways. *Food Cult. Soc.* **2014**, *17*, 665–687. [CrossRef]
13. Nguyen, H. Sustainable Food Systems: Concept and Framework. Food and Agriculture Organization of the United Nations. 2018. Available online: https://openknowledge.fao.org/items/8d2575e3-e701-4b1d-8e20-d9c83179c848 (accessed on 5 April 2024).
14. Park, D.; Choi, M.K.; Park, Y.K.; Park, C.Y.; Shin, M.J. Higher food literacy scores are associated with healthier diet quality in children and adolescents: The development and validation of a two-dimensional food literacy measurement tool for children and adolescents. *Nutr. Res. Pr.* **2022**, *16*, 272–283. [CrossRef]
15. Rosas, R.; Pimenta, F.; Leal, I.; Schwarzer, R. FOODLIT-PRO: Food literacy domains, influential factors and determinants—A qualitative study. *Nutrients* **2019**, *12*, 88. [CrossRef] [PubMed]
16. Rosas, R.; Pimenta, F.; Leal, I.; Schwarzer, R. FOODLIT-PRO: Conceptual and empirical development of the food literacy wheel. *Int. J. Food Sci. Nutr.* **2021**, *72*, 99–111. [CrossRef]
17. Amouzandeh, C.; Fingland, D.; Vidgen, H.A. A scoping review of the validity, reliability and conceptual alignment of food literacy measures for adults. *Nutrients* **2019**, *11*, 801. [CrossRef] [PubMed]
18. Rosas, R.; Pimenta, F.; Leal, I.; Schwarzer, R. FOODLIT-tool: Development and validation of the adaptable food literacy tool towards global sustainability within food systems. *Appetite* **2022**, *168*, 105658. [CrossRef]
19. Demir, G.; Özer, A. Development and validation of food and nutrition literacy instrument in young people, Turkey. *Prog. Nutr.* **2022**, *3*, 4. [CrossRef]
20. Kubilay, M.N.; Yüksel, A. Validity and reliability study of the Turkish adaptation of the Sustainable Food Literacy Scale. *Gümüşhane Üniversitesi Sağlık Bilim. Derg.* **2023**, *12*, 1562–1570. [CrossRef]
21. Brislin, R.W. Back-translation for cross-cultural research. *J. Cross-Cult. Psychol.* **1970**, *1*, 185–216. [CrossRef]
22. Ayre, C.; Scally, A.J. Critical values for Lawshe's content validity ratio: Revisiting the original methods of calculation. *Meas. Eval. Couns. Dev.* **2014**, *47*, 79–86. [CrossRef]
23. Żakowska-Biemans, S.; Pieniak, Z.; Kostryra, E.; Gutkowska, K. Searching for a measure integrating sustainable and healthy eating behaviors. *Nutrients* **2019**, *11*, 95. [CrossRef]
24. Köksal, E.; Bilici, S.; Çitar Dazıroğlu, M.E.; Erdoğan Gövez, N. Validity and reliability of the Turkish version of the Sustainable and Healthy Eating Behaviors Scale. *Br. J. Nutr.* **2023**, *129*, 1398–1404. [CrossRef] [PubMed]
25. Holgado-Tello, F.P.; Chacón-Moscoso, S.; Barbero-García, I.; Vila-Abad, E. Polychoric versus Pearson correlations in exploratory and confirmatory factor analysis of ordinal variables. *Qual. Quant.* **2010**, *44*, 153–166. [CrossRef]
26. Hu, L.T.; Bentler, P.M. Cutoff criteria for fit indexes in covariance structure analysis: Conventional criteria versus new alternatives. *Struct. Equ. Model.* **1999**, *6*, 1–55. [CrossRef]
27. Mulaik, S.A.; James, L.R.; Van Alstine, J.; Bennett, N.; Lind, S.; Stilwell, C.D. Evaluation of goodness-of-fit indices for structural equation models. *Psychol. Bull.* **1989**, *105*, 430. [CrossRef]
28. Hooper, D.; Coughlan, J.; Mullen, M.R. Evaluating model fit: A synthesis of the structural equation modelling literature. In Proceedings of the 7th European Conference on Research Methodology for Business and Management Studies, London, UK, 19–20 June 2008; pp. 195–200. [CrossRef]
29. Shi, D.; Lee, T.; Maydeu-Olivares, A. Understanding the model size effect on SEM fit indices. *Educ. Psychol. Meas.* **2019**, *79*, 310–334. [CrossRef]

30. Teng, C.C.; Chih, C. Sustainable food literacy: A measure to promote sustainable diet practices. *Sustain. Prod. Consum.* **2022**, *30*, 776–786. [CrossRef]
31. Pendergast, D.; Dewhurst, Y. Home economics and food literacy: An international investigation. *Int. J. Home Econ.* **2012**, *5*, 245–263.
32. Bellotti, B. Food literacy: Reconnecting the city with the country. *Agric. Sci.* **2010**, *22*, 29–34.
33. Bojang, K.P.; Manchana, V. Nutrition and healthy aging: A review. *Curr. Nutr. Rep.* **2023**, *12*, 369–375. [CrossRef]
34. Silva, P.; Araújo, R.; Lopes, F.; Ray, S. Nutrition and food literacy: Framing the challenges to health communication. *Nutrients* **2023**, *15*, 4708. [CrossRef] [PubMed]
35. Luta, X.; Hayoz, S.; Gréa Krause, C.; Sommerhalder, K.; Roos, E.; Strazzullo, P.; Beer-Borst, S. The relationship of health/food literacy and salt awareness to daily sodium and potassium intake among a workplace population in Switzerland. *Nutr. Metab. Cardiovasc. Dis.* **2018**, *28*, 270–277. [CrossRef] [PubMed]
36. Vidgen, H. *Food Literacy: Key Concepts for Health and Education*; Routledge: London, UK, 2016. [CrossRef]
37. Burlingame, B.; Dernini, S. Sustainable Diets and Biodiversity. 2010. Available online: https://www.fao.org/4/i3004e/i3004e.pdf (accessed on 16 June 2024).
38. Alsaffar, A.A. Sustainable diets: The interaction between food industry, nutrition, health and the environment. *Food Sci. Technol. Int.* **2016**, *22*, 102–111. [CrossRef] [PubMed]
39. Palumbo, R. Sustainability of well-being through literacy. The effects of food literacy on sustainability of well-being. *Agric. Agric. Sci. Procedia* **2016**, *8*, 99–106. [CrossRef]
40. Vettori, V.; Lorini, C.; Milani, C.; Bonaccorsi, G. Towards the implementation of a conceptual framework of food and nutrition literacy: Providing healthy eating for the population. *Int. J. Env. Res. Public Health* **2019**, *16*, 5041. [CrossRef]
41. Ellison, B.; Prescott, M.P. Examining nutrition and food waste trade-offs using an obesity prevention context. *J. Nutr. Educ. Behav.* **2021**, *53*, 434–444. [CrossRef]
42. Cullen, T.; Hatch, J.; Martin, W.; Higgins, J.W.; Sheppard, R. Food literacy: Definition and framework for action. *Can. J. Diet. Pract. Res.* **2015**, *76*, 140–145. [CrossRef]
43. Selçuk, K.T.; Çevik, C.; Baydur, H.; Meseri, M. Validity and reliability of the Turkish version of the self-perceived food literacy scale. *Prog. Nutr.* **2020**, *22*, 671–677. [CrossRef]
44. Poelman, M.P.; Coosje Dijkstra, S.; Sponselee, H.; Kamphuis, C.B.M.; Battjes-Fries, M.C.E.; Gillebaart, M.; Seidell, J.C. Towards the measurement of food literacy with respect to healthy eating: The development and validation of the self perceived food literacy scale among an adult sample in the Netherlands. *Int. J. Behav. Nutr. Phys. Act.* **2018**, *15*, 54. [CrossRef]
45. Thompson, C.; Byrne, R.; Adams, J.; Vidgen, H.A. Development, validation and item reduction of a food literacy questionnaire (IFLQ-19) with Australian adults. *Int. J. Behav. Nutr. Phys. Act.* **2022**, *19*, 113. [CrossRef]
46. Paynter, E.; Begley, A.; Butcher, L.M.; Dhaliwal, S.S. The validation and improvement of a food literacy behavior checklist for food literacy programs. *Int. J. Env. Res. Public Health* **2021**, *18*, 13282. [CrossRef] [PubMed]
47. Scarff, J.R. Orthorexia nervosa: An obsession with healthy eating. *Fed. Pr.* **2017**, *34*, 36.
48. Novara, C.; Pardini, S.; Maggio, E.; Mattioli, S.; Piasentin, S. Orthorexia Nervosa: Over concern or obsession about healthy food? *Eat. Weight. Disord.* **2021**, *26*, 2577–2588. [CrossRef] [PubMed]
49. Kabasakal-Cetin, A.; Aksaray, B.; Sen, G. The role of food literacy and sustainable and healthy eating behaviors in ultra-processed foods consumption of undergraduate students. *Food Qual. Prefer.* **2024**, *119*, 105232. [CrossRef]
50. Park, D.; Park, Y.K.; Park, C.Y.; Choi, M.K.; Shin, M.J. Development of a comprehensive food literacy measurement tool integrating the food system and sustainability. *Nutrients* **2020**, *12*, 3300. [CrossRef] [PubMed]
51. Lee, Y.; Kim, T.; Jung, H. Effects of university students' perceived food literacy on ecological eating behavior towards sustainability. *Sustainability* **2022**, *14*, 5242. [CrossRef]
52. Öztürk, E.E.; Özgen, L. Evaluation of the relationship between nutrition knowledge and sustainable food literacy. *J. Contemp. Med.* **2023**, *13*, 66–71. [CrossRef]

Disclaimer/Publisher's Note: The statements, opinions and data contained in all publications are solely those of the individual author(s) and contributor(s) and not of MDPI and/or the editor(s). MDPI and/or the editor(s) disclaim responsibility for any injury to people or property resulting from any ideas, methods, instructions or products referred to in the content.

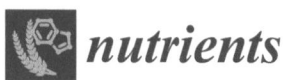 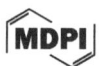

Article

Defatted Flaxseed Flour as a New Ingredient for Foodstuffs: Comparative Analysis with Whole Flaxseeds and Updated Composition of Cold-Pressed Oil

Diana Melo Ferreira [1], Susana Machado [1], Liliana Espírito Santo [1], Maria Antónia Nunes [1], Anabela S. G. Costa [1], Manuel Álvarez-Ortí [2], José E. Pardo [2], Rita C. Alves [1] and Maria Beatriz P. P. Oliveira [1,*]

[1] LAQV/REQUIMTE, Faculty of Pharmacy, University of Porto, Street of Jorge Viterbo Ferreira, 4050-313 Porto, Portugal; su_tche@hotmail.com (S.M.); lilianaespiritosanto81@gmail.com (L.E.S.); antonianunes.maria@gmail.com (M.A.N.); acosta@ff.up.pt (A.S.G.C.); rcalves@ff.up.pt (R.C.A.)

[2] Higher Technical School of Agricultural and Forestry Engineering, University of Castilla-La Mancha, Campus Universitario, s/n, 02071 Albacete, Spain; manuel.alvarez@uclm.es (M.Á.-O.); jose.pgonzalez@uclm.es (J.E.P.)

* Correspondence: beatoliv@ff.up.pt

Abstract: Background: Flaxseeds are functional foods popular in current diets. Cold-pressing is a solvent-free method to extract flaxseed oil, resulting in a by-product—defatted flour. Objectives/Methods: This study compared whole flaxseeds and defatted flour (proximate composition, fatty acids, vitamin E, total phenolics and flavonoids, antioxidant activity, amino acids, and protein quality) and updated the composition of cold-pressed oil (oxidative stability, peroxide value, UV absorbance, colour, fatty acids, vitamin E, total phenolics and flavonoids, and antioxidant activity) to assess the nutritional relevance and potential for food applications of these samples. Results: The flour had higher ash (6% vs. 4%), fibre (36% vs. 34%), protein (28% vs. 16%), phenolics (205 vs. 143 mg gallic acid equivalents/100 g), and antioxidant activity than seeds ($p < 0.05$), so it should be valued as a novel high-fibre food ingredient with high-quality plant-based protein, as it contains all essential amino acids (106 mg/g) and a high essential amino acids index (112%), with L-tryptophan as the limiting amino acid. The oil, while low in oxidative stability (1.3 h), due to its high polyunsaturated fatty acids sum (75%), mostly α-linolenic acid (57%), contains a significant amount of vitamin E (444 mg/kg), making it a specialty oil best consumed raw. Conclusions: The exploration of the flour as a minimally processed food ingredient highlights its role in supporting food security, circular economy, and sustainability goals, aligning with consumer preferences for natural, low-fat foods. Future research should investigate the bioactivity and shelf-life of the samples, as well as the bioavailability of compounds after digestion.

Keywords: *Linum usitatissimum* L.; food security; nutritional security; functional foods; cold pressing; minimal processing; sustainability; fatty acids; amino acids; antioxidants

Citation: Ferreira, D.M.; Machado, S.; Espírito Santo, L.; Nunes, M.A.; Costa, A.S.G.; Álvarez-Ortí, M.; Pardo, J.E.; Alves, R.C.; Oliveira, M.B.P.P. Defatted Flaxseed Flour as a New Ingredient for Foodstuffs: Comparative Analysis with Whole Flaxseeds and Updated Composition of Cold-Pressed Oil. *Nutrients* **2024**, *16*, 3482. https://doi.org/10.3390/nu16203482

Academic Editor: Maria Corbo

Received: 14 September 2024
Revised: 4 October 2024
Accepted: 8 October 2024
Published: 14 October 2024

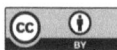

Copyright: © 2024 by the authors. Licensee MDPI, Basel, Switzerland. This article is an open access article distributed under the terms and conditions of the Creative Commons Attribution (CC BY) license (https://creativecommons.org/licenses/by/4.0/).

1. Introduction

The concept of food security includes access to sufficient, affordable, and nutritious food. However, nutritional security also incorporates access, availability, and affordability of foods that are safe, nutritious, align with food preferences, promote well-being, and prevent diseases [1]. Functional foods are foods that provide health benefits beyond basic nutrition, often due to the presence of bioactive compounds. These foods, which can include fortified, enriched, or natural foods, are designed to improve health and reduce the risk of disease. Functional foods play a crucial role in modern diets, as they offer an accessible way to enhance well-being through everyday eating habits [2]. Oilseeds have recently gained popularity due to their bioactive-rich composition, which can meet the global nutritional requirements of a growing population [3]. Examples of both functional foods and oilseeds include chia, sesame, and poppy seeds [4–7].

Flaxseeds (*Linum usitatissimum* L.), also known as linseeds, are another example. According to FAOSTAT, in 2022, flaxseed was mainly grown in the Russian Federation (almost 1.767 million tonnes), followed by Kazakhstan (almost 846 thousand tonnes), totalling almost 3.974 million tonnes worldwide [8].

Besides their rich nutritional content, flaxseeds have been recognized for their functional food properties, contributing to both human health and environmental sustainability [3,9]. The high levels of lignans (antioxidants) in these seeds are associated with potential anticancer properties, particularly in hormone-related cancers such as breast cancer [9,10]. Moreover, the dietary fibre found in flaxseeds is not only beneficial for digestive health and gut microbiota regulation [3,9] but also for regulating blood sugar levels, making it an important food for managing conditions like diabetes [9,11]. The global emphasis on plant-based diets has further highlighted the importance of flaxseeds as a sustainable source of essential nutrients, particularly in meeting the protein and n-3 FA requirements in populations with limited access to animal-based foods [9,12].

Cold-pressing, which relies on mechanical pressing, preserves the natural antioxidants that contribute to oil stability [13]. This is particularly important in oils rich in polyunsaturated fatty acids (PUFA), such as flaxseed oil, to prevent oxidation [14]. The by-products (defatted flours) resulting from oil extraction are generally considered wastes and should be further exploited by the food industry to prevent the depletion of the agricultural sector, while promoting sustainability and increasing food availability [5–7]. This approach is a step towards achieving the Sustainable Development Goal (SDG) 2 (zero hunger) [15].

Furthermore, the cold-pressing method is gaining attention not only for preserving the nutritional properties of the oil but also for its low environmental impact, aligning with broader goals of reducing carbon footprints in food production. The valorisation of by-products is a crucial step towards a circular economy, where waste materials are repurposed into valuable food ingredients, thus contributing to food security and sustainability purposes [5–7,16].

Recently, consumer demand for natural and minimally processed products with enhanced nutritional and healthy features has motivated cold-pressed oils as a food alternative. However, due to their high market price, they are susceptible to adulteration with cheaper and lower-quality refined oils [13]. Thus, one of the aims of this work was to update the physicochemical composition of cold-pressed flaxseed oil, while also discussing its food applications and potential functional and health-promoting traits. This will help to monitor its authenticity, regarding human health, consumer demand, and quality control.

This work also aimed to perform an overall chemical characterization of whole flaxseeds and their defatted flour (oil extraction by-product) and to compare them to assess their nutritional relevance. Moreover, the flour's potential as a novel food ingredient was explored, meeting current natural, minimal-processed, and low-fat diets. Also, valorising the flour for food purposes seems an important target to meet food security, nutritional security, circular economy, and sustainability goals. Additionally, an evaluation of the protein quality of the flour and seeds based on the amino acids (AAs) contents was conducted.

2. Materials and Methods

2.1. Chemicals

The chemicals used in this research were of analytical reagent grade. Boric acid was acquired from Labkem (Barcelona, Spain). Kjeldahl tablets, sodium sulphate, anhydrous sodium sulphate, and Folin–Ciocalteu reagent were acquired from Merck (Darmstadt, Germany). Sulfuric acid and methanol were from Honeywell Fluka™ (Düsseldorf, Germany). Petroleum ether and hydrochloric acid (1 M) were provided by CARLO ERBA Reagents (Val de Reuil Cedex, France). Sand, sodium hydroxide (1 M), and sodium dihydrogen phosphate were provided by VWR (Strasbourg, France). Ethanol (96%) was from AGA (Prior Velho, Portugal). Acetic acid (99–100%) was provided from Chem-Lab (Zedelgem, Belgium). A standard mixture (FAME 37) was obtained from Supelco (Bellefonte, PA, USA).

Total dietary fibre assay kit, celite, sodium carbonate, gallic acid, sodium nitrate, aluminium chloride, sodium acetate, ferric chloride, TPTZ (10 mM), ferrous sulphate, catechin, and HPLC-grade solvents were acquired from Sigma-Aldrich (St. Louis, MO, USA). Vitamin E standards (α, β, δ, γ-tocopherols and tocotrienols) were obtained from Calbiochem (La Jolla, CA, USA). The amino acids standards: L-aspartic acid (Asp, ≥99.5%), L-glutamic acid (Glu, ≥99.0%), L-asparagine (Asn, ≥99.0%), L-glutamine (Gln, ≥99.5%), L-alanine (Ala, ≥99.5%), L-arginine monohydrochloride (Arg, ≥99.0%), L-cystine (Cys, ≥99.0%), L-valine (Val, ≥99.0%), L-threonine (Thr, ≥99.0%), L-tyrosine (Tyr, ≥98.0%), L-leucine (Leu, ≥98.0%), L-tryptophan (Trp, ≥98.0%), L-lysine monohydrochloride (Lys, ≥99.0%), glycine (Gly, ≥99.0%), L-phenylalanine (Phe, ≥98.0%), L-serine (Ser, ≥99.0%), L-methionine (Met, ≥99.0%), L-isoleucine (Ile, ≥99.0%), trans-4-hydroxy-L-proline (Hyp, ≥99.0%), L-proline (Pro, ≥99.0%), and L-histidine mono-hydrochloride monohydrate (His, ≥99.0%) were purchased from Sigma-Aldrich (Darmstadt, Germany). Ultrapure water was obtained in a Milli-Q water purification system (Millipore, Bedford, MA, USA).

2.2. Samples and Sample Preparation

Golden flaxseeds were purchased in a Spanish supermarket. Oil and flour were obtained by cold-pressing 1 kg of flaxseeds using a screw press (Komet Oil Press CA59G, IBG Monforts Oekotec GmbH & Co. KG, Mönchengladbach, Germany). For the oil extraction, a nozzle with a 5 mm diameter was used. The barrel was preheated with a thermal ring until it reached 100 °C. Once the oil extraction process began, the thermal ring was removed, and extraction continued at room temperature (RT). The by-product obtained from cold-pressing the flaxseeds in the screw press was ground for homogenization (GM Grindomix 200, Retsch GmbH, Retsch-Allee, Haan, Germany) and used as the flour sample. The analyses began immediately after sample preparation. The oil was stored in the dark at 4 °C, while the flour and seeds were vacuum-sealed and kept at 4 °C in between analyses to minimize potential oxidative changes. The analysed samples are shown in Figure 1.

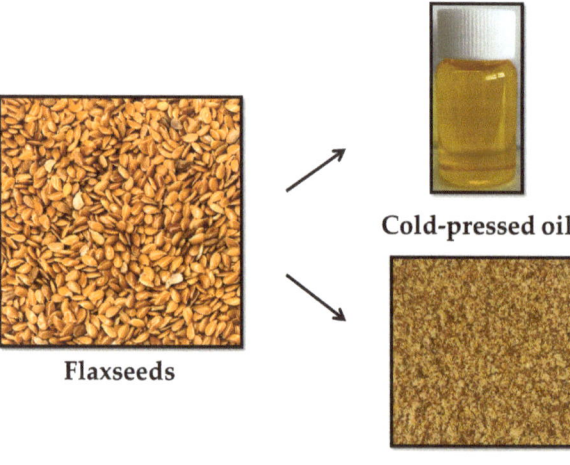

Figure 1. Analysed samples—golden flaxseeds, cold-pressed oil, and defatted flour.

2.3. Proximate Composition and Energy Values of Whole Flaxseeds and Defatted Flour

The proximate composition of the samples was determined using AOAC standard methods [17]. The moisture content was determined by drying (105 °C), using an infrared balance (model SMO01, Scaltec Instruments, GmbH, Goettingen, Germany). The ash content was determined by sample incineration (500 °C, method no. 920.153), using a muffle furnace (Thermolyne 48000, Thermo Fisher Scientific, Waltham, MA, USA). Total protein was calculated from the nitrogen content by Kjeldahl procedure (no. 978.04) with a nitrogen conversion factor of 6.25 [18], using a Buchi Digestion Unit K-424, a Scrubber B-414, and a KjelFlex K-360 (VELP Scientific, Usmate Velate, MB, Italy). Total fat was determined using a Soxhlet apparatus (method no. 991.36), a Huber Minichiller, and a P Selecta heating mantle (VELP Scientific, Usmate Velate, MB, Italy). Total dietary fibre and insoluble fibre were determined by enzymatic-gravimetric methods (no. 985.29), using a Multistirrer 6, a heating magnetic stirrer, a heated circulating bath, and a CSF 6 filtration system (VELP Scientific, Usmate Velate, MB, Italy). Soluble fibre and remaining carbohydrates were calculated by difference [18]. Energy values were calculated using the following estimates: fibre (2 kcal/g, 8 kJ/g), carbohydrates and protein (4 kcal/g, 17 kJ/g), and fat (9 kcal/g, 37 kJ/g) [19].

2.4. Fatty Acids (FA) of All Samples

The lipid fractions of the samples were extracted following the method described by Ferreira et al. [16]. FA were derivatized to fatty acids methyl esters (FAMEs) in accordance with ISO 12966-2:2017 [20]. FA were determined using a GC-2010 Plus gas chromatograph equipped with an AOC-20i automatic sampler and a split/splitless auto-injector (50:1 split ratio, 250 °C) and a flame ionization detector (270 °C) (Shimadzu, Tokyo, Japan). A CP-Sil 88 silica capillary column (50 × 250 m, 0.2 µm) (Varian, Middelburg, The Netherlands) was used for peak separation. Helium was the carrier gas (3.0 mL/min). The temperature programme was 120 °C held for 5 min, 2 °C/min to 160 °C held for 2 min, and 2 °C/min to 220 °C held for 10 min. The injection volume was 1.0 µL. Identification was achieved by comparison with a FAME 37 standard mix (Supelco, Bellefonte, PA, USA).

2.5. Vitamin E of All Samples

The lipid fractions of the samples were extracted following the method described by Ferreira et al. [16]. Vitamin E contents were determined using a HPLC system equipped with a MD-2015 multiwavelength diode array detector and a FP-2020 fluorescence detector (excitation at 290 nm and emission at 330 nm) (Jasco, Tokyo, Japan). A Supelcosil™ LC-SI column (75 × 3 mm, 3 µm) (Supelco, Bellefonte, PA, USA) was used for separation. The mobile phase consisted of 1.5% 1,4-dioxane in n-hexane (v/v) at a flow rate of 0.7 mL/min. The injection volume was 20 µL. Tocol (100 µg/mL, Matreya Inc., State College, PA, USA) was used as the internal standard.

2.6. Amino Acids (AAs) of Whole Flaxseeds and Defatted Flour

AA extraction and analysis were performed, according to Machado et al. [21], using a HPLC system equipped with MD-2015 Plus multiwavelength and FP-2020 Plus fluorescence detectors (Jasco, Tokyo, Japan) and a ZORBAX Eclipse Plus C18 column (40 °C, 4.6 × 250 mm, 5 µm, Agilent Technologies, Santa Clara, CA, USA). Alkaline (KOH 4M, 4 h, only for Trp) and acid hydrolysis (HCl 6M, 24 h) were performed in glass tubes using a heating block (110 °C, SBH130D/3, Stuart, Stafford, UK). Aliquots of hydrolysates were mixed with internal standard (L-norvaline, 2 mg/mL, Sigma-Aldrich, Darmstadt, Germany), and the mixtures were subjected to automatic online derivatization with OPA/3-MPA and FMOC in a AS-4150 autosampler. Fluorescence detection was monitored at λ_{exc} = 340 nm and λ_{em} = 450 nm (0–26.2 min) for OPA-derivatives and at λ_{exc} = 266 nm and λ_{em} = 305 nm (26.2–40 min) for FMOC-derivatives. OPA-derivatives were monitored at 338 nm and FMOC-derivatives at 262 nm. The gradient solvent system was (A) phosphate/borate buffer (ratio of 10 mM of Na_2HPO_4 to 10 mM of $Na_2B_2O_7$ [pH = 8.2] to 5 of mM NaN_3) and (B) MeOH:ACN:H_2O (45:45:10, $v/v/v$). The gradient program was as follows: 0.85 min, 2% B; 33.4 min, 57% B; 33.5 min, 85% B; 39.3 min, 85% B; 39.4 min, 2% B; and 40.0 min, 2% B. The flow rate was 1.5 mL/min. The injection volume was 3 µL.

2.7. Protein Quality of Whole Flaxseeds and Defatted Flour

The following equations were used to evaluate protein quality [22,23]:

2.7.1. Estimation of Amino Acid Chemical Score (AACS)

$$\mathrm{AACS}(\%) = \frac{\text{mg of AA in 1 g test protein}}{\text{mg of AA in 1 g requirement protein}} \times 100 \qquad (1)$$

AA—amino acid.

2.7.2. Estimation of Essential Amino Acids Index (EAAI)

$$\mathrm{EAAI}(\%) = n^{\log \mathrm{EAA}}, \text{ where } \log \mathrm{EAA} = \frac{1}{n}\left(\log\frac{100\ a1}{a1R} + \ldots + \log\frac{100\ an}{anR}\right) \qquad (2)$$

EAA—essential amino acid; n—number of amino acids (methionine and cysteine pairs count as 1); a—mg of amino acid per 1 g of protein in the food; and aR—mg of amino acid per 1 g of reference protein.

2.8. Total Phenolics and Total Flavonoids of All Samples

The extracts were prepared following the methods described by Melo et al. [5].

Total phenolics were determined according to Ferreira et al. [7]. In brief, 30 µL of each extract were mixed with 150 µL of Folin–Ciocalteu reagent and 120 µL of sodium carbonate (7.5%, m/V). The microplate was incubated at 45 °C (15 min), then cooled and protected from light (RT, 30 min). Absorbance was read at 765 nm using a microplate reader (Synergy HT GENS5, BioTek Instruments, Winooski, VT, USA). A calibration curve was generated with gallic acid (5–100 mg/mL, R^2 = 0.999). Results are expressed as gallic acid equivalents (GAEs).

Total flavonoids were also determined according to Ferreira et al. [7]. Briefly, 1 mL of each extract was mixed with 4 mL of distilled water and 300 µL of sodium nitrate (1%). After 5 min, 300 µL of aluminium chloride (5%) were added. After 1 min, 2 mL of sodium hydroxide (1 M) and 2.5 µL of distilled water were added. Absorbance was measured at 510 nm using a microplate reader (Synergy HT GENS5, BioTek Instruments, Winooski, VT, USA). A calibration curve was generated with epicatechin (0–400 µL/mL, R^2 = 0.999). Results are expressed as epicatechin equivalents (EE).

2.9. Ferric Reducing Antioxidant Power (FRAP) of All Samples

The extracts were prepared according to Melo et al. [5]. FRAP assay was determined according to Ferreira et al. [7]. In a microplate, 35 µL of each extract were mixed with 265 µL of FRAP reagent (0.3 M acetate buffer, 10 mM TPTZ solution, and 20 mM of ferric chloride) and incubated protected from light (37 °C, 30 min). Absorbance was measured at 595 nm. A calibration curve was prepared with ferrous sulphate (25–500 µmol/L, R^2 = 0.999). Results are expressed as ferrous sulphate equivalents (FSEs).

2.10. 2,2-Diphenyl-1-picrylhydrazyl Radical (DPPH•) Inhibition of All Samples

The extracts were prepared according to Melo et al. [5]. DPPH• inhibition assay was evaluated according to Ferreira et al. [7]. In a microplate, 30 µL of each extract were mixed with 270 µL of an ethanolic solution of DPPH•. Absorbance was measured at 525 nm, every 2 min, until 20 min, to observe the kinetics reaction. A calibration curve was prepared with Trolox (5.62–175.34 mg/L, R^2 = 0.998). Results are expressed as Trolox equivalents (TE).

2.11. Oxidative Stability of Cold-Pressed Flaxseed Oil

The oxidative stability was determined using the Rancimat method as described by Melo et al. [5]. Briefly, 3 g of oil were analysed, at 120 °C with an airflow rate of 20 L/h using a Rancimat apparatus (model 892, Metrohm Nordic ApS, Glostrup, Denmark). Results are expressed as oxidation induction time (h).

2.12. Peroxide Value of Cold-Pressed Flaxseed Oil

The peroxide value was determined according to NP-904:1987 [24]. Briefly, 0.5 g of sample, 10 mL of chloroform, 15 mL of glacial acetic acid, and 1 mL of saturated KI solution were mixed and stored in the dark (5 min). After that, 75 mL of deionized water were added, followed by titration with 0.01 N sodium thiosulfate and 1% starch solution.

2.13. UV Absorbance of Cold-Pressed Flaxseed Oil

The UV absorbance was determined following ISO 3656:2011 [25]. Primary and secondary oxidation products were read at 232 and 270 nm, respectively, using a Shimadzu UV Spectrophotometer UV-1800 (Shimadzu, Tokyo, Japan).

2.14. Colour of Cold-Pressed Flaxseed Oil

The colour was determined according to NP-937:1987 [26], at 445, 495, 560, 595, and 625 nm, using a Shimadzu UV Spectrophotometer UV-1800 (Shimadzu, Tokyo, Japan).

2.15. Statistical Analysis

Data were analysed with IBM SPSS Statistics (version 28, IBM Corp., Armonk, NY, USA). An independent samples t-test was applied to reveal significant differences between seeds and flour samples, with a 95% interval of confidence ($p < 0.05$). All determinations were performed in triplicate ($n = 3$).

3. Results

3.1. Comparative Analysis of Whole Flaxseeds and Defatted Flour

The results of the composition of flaxseeds and flour are presented in Table 1.

Table 1. Composition of whole flaxseeds and defatted flour.

Parameter	Seeds	Flour
Energy Value (kcal/100 g)	475 ± 1 [a]	314 ± 6 [b]
Energy Value (kJ/100 g)	1954 ± 5 [a]	1304 ± 26 [b]
Moisture (%)	8.42 ± 0.11 [b]	9.78 ± 0.13 [a]
Ash (%)	3.64 ± 0.02 [b]	5.64 ± 0.02 [a]
Total Protein (%)	16.07 ± 0.07 [b]	28.08 ± 0.82 [a]
Total Dietary Fibre (%)	33.73 ± 0.00 [b]	35.61 ± 0.00 [a]
Insoluble Fibre (%)	30.22 ± 0.00 [a]	25.66 ± 0.60 [b]
Soluble Fibre (%)	3.51 ± 0.00 [b]	9.96 ± 0.43 [a]
Remaining Carbohydrates (%)	0.03 ± 0.13 [b]	11.56 ± 0.56 [a]
Total Fat (%)	38.11 ± 0.04 [a]	9.33 ± 0.14 [b]
Fatty Acids (Relative %)		
C16:0 (Palmitic Acid)	5.06 ± 0.04 [b]	6.30 ± 0.07 [a]
C16:1c (Palmitoleic Acid)	0.06 ± 0.00 [b]	0.07 ± 0.00 [a]
C17:0 (Margaric Acid)	0.06 ± 0.00 [a]	0.05 ± 0.00 [b]
C18:0 (Stearic Acid)	3.35 ± 0.04 [a]	3.21 ± 0.15 [a]
C18:1n9c (Oleic Acid)	18.02 ± 0.09 [b]	18.28 ± 0.07 [a]
C18:2n6c (Linoleic Acid)	16.58 ± 0.08 [b]	17.07 ± 0.16 [a]
C18:3n3c (α-Linolenic Acid)	56.75 ± 0.19 [a]	54.88 ± 0.28 [b]
C20:0 (Arachidic Acid)	0.11 ± 0.00 [b]	0.13 ± 0.00 [a]
∑SFA (Saturated Fatty Acids)	8.59 ± 0.08 [b]	9.70 ± 0.15 [a]
∑MUFA (Monounsaturated Fatty Acids)	18.08 ± 0.09 [b]	18.35 ± 0.07 [a]
∑PUFA (Polyunsaturated Fatty Acids)	73.33 ± 0.13 [a]	71.95 ± 0.16 [b]
n-6/n-3	0.29 ± 0.00 [b]	0.31 ± 0.00 [a]

Table 1. *Cont.*

Parameter	Seeds	Flour
Total Vitamin E (mg/kg)	214.68 ± 9.34 [a]	48.49 ± 0.66 [b]
α-Tocopherol	73.67 ± 2.01 [a]	17.39 ± 0.14 [b]
γ-Tocopherol	141.01 ± 7.49 [a]	30.98 ± 0.53 [b]
Total Amino Acids (mg/g)	194.17 ± 8.92 [b]	314.18 ± 11.21 [a]
Asp	19.31 ± 0.90 [b]	31.31 ± 1.10 [a]
Glu	39.99 ± 1.99 [b]	64.94 ± 2.23 [a]
Ser	10.10 ± 0.48 [b]	16.14 ± 0.58 [a]
Gln	1.01 ± 0.09 [b]	2.03 ± 0.24 [a]
* His	6.24 ± 0.27 [b]	9.56 ± 0.27 [a]
Gly	12.42 ± 1.59 [b]	22.30 ± 0.92 [a]
* Thr	7.75 ± 0.35 [b]	12.15 ± 0.34 [a]
Arg	22.70 ± 1.18 [b]	36.59 ± 1.34 [a]
Ala	9.20 ± 0.43 [b]	14.90 ± 0.54 [a]
Tyr	4.33 ± 0.19 [b]	6.43 ± 0.25 [a]
* Val	9.55 ± 0.51 [b]	15.41 ± 0.51 [a]
* Met	2.80 ± 0.39 [b]	3.95 ± 0.16 [a]
* Trp	1.39 ± 0.03 [a]	1.47 ± 0.25 [a]
* Phe	9.75 ± 0.22 [b]	15.87 ± 1.87 [a]
* Ile	8.54 ± 0.48 [b]	12.94 ± 0.47 [a]
* Leu	11.83 ± 0.41 [b]	18.76 ± 0.77 [a]
* Lys	9.12 ± 0.92 [b]	15.98 ± 0.70 [a]
Hyp	1.50 ± 0.02 [b]	2.47 ± 0.07 [a]
Pro	6.63 ± 0.16 [b]	10.99 ± 0.30 [a]
Total Phenolics (mg GAE/100 g)	142.5 ± 7.2 [b]	204.9 ± 19.9 [a]
Total Flavonoids (mg EE/100 g)	53.9 ± 2.4 [b]	78.2 ± 4.5 [a]
FRAP (mmol FSE/100 g)	8.5 ± 0.4 [b]	14.3 ± 1.9 [a]
DPPH• Inhibition (mg TE/100 g)	57.2 ± 11.0 [b]	233.3 ± 22.6 [a]

* Essential amino acids. Results in fresh weight. Values presented as mean ± standard deviation ($n = 3$). Different small-case letters in the same row denote significant differences ($p < 0.05$). GAEs, gallic acid equivalents; EEs, epicatechin equivalents; FRAP, ferric reduction antioxidant power; FSEs, ferrous sulphate equivalents; DPPH•, 2,2-diphenyl-1-picrylhydrazyl; TE, Trolox equivalents.

The results from Table 1 indicate significant differences in the nutritional composition of whole flaxseeds and defatted flour. The energy value of whole seeds was higher, with 475 kcal/100 g (1954 kJ/100 g) compared to the flour's 314 kcal/100 g (1304 kJ/100 g). The flour had a slightly higher moisture content at 9.8% compared to the seeds' 8.4%. The ash content was also greater in the flour (5.6%) than in the seeds (3.6%). The flour had a higher protein content (28.1% vs. 16.1%) and total dietary fibre (35.6% vs. 33.7%), with more soluble fibre (10.0%) but less insoluble fibre (25.7%) compared to the seeds (3.5% soluble and 30.2% insoluble). The fat content was significantly reduced in the flour (9.3%) compared to the seeds (38.1%).

In terms of FA (Table 1), the flour showed higher percentages of palmitic acid (6.3% vs. 5.1%) and linoleic acid (17.1% vs. 16.6%), but a lower concentration of α-linolenic acid (54.9% vs. 56.8%). The flour also contained significantly less total vitamin E (48.5 mg/kg) than the whole seeds (214.7 mg/kg), along with lower levels of α-tocopherol (17.4 mg/kg vs. 73.7 mg/kg) and γ-tocopherol (31.0 mg/kg vs. 141.0 mg/kg).

However, the total AA content was much higher in the flour, with 314.2 mg/g compared to 194.2 mg/g in the seeds. Each AA, including essential ones like Lys (16.0 mg/g vs. 9.1 mg/g), Leu (18.8 mg/g vs. 11.8 mg/g), and Phe (15.9 mg/g vs. 9.8 mg/g), was more concentrated in the flour. Additionally, the flour had higher contents of total phenolics (205 mg GAE/100 g vs. 143 mg GAE/100 g) and total flavonoids (78 mg EE/100 g vs. 54 mg EE/100 g), and exhibited greater antioxidant activity, as indicated by FRAP (14 mmol

FSE/100 g vs. 9 mmol FSE/100 g) and DPPH• inhibition (233 mg TE/100 g vs. 57 mg TE/100 g) assays.

Overall, these results suggest that defatted flaxseed flour is a nutrient-dense ingredient, rich in protein, AAs, fibre, and antioxidants, making it a potentially valuable component for various food applications.

The results of the protein quality assessment are displayed in Table 2. Whole flaxseeds exhibited significantly higher levels of His, Ile, Leu, Phe + Tyr, Thr, and Trp compared to the flour. However, Met and Val levels did not show significant differences. Specifically, His content was 38.8 mg/g protein in seeds vs. 34.0 mg/g protein in flour, with corresponding AACSs of 258.7% and 226.9%, respectively. Ile was found at 53.1 mg/g protein in seeds compared to 46.1 mg/g protein in flour, yielding AACSs of 177.2% and 153.6%, respectively. Leu levels were 73.6 mg/g protein in seeds and 66.8 mg/g protein in flour, with AACSs of 124.8% and 113.3%, respectively. Lys content was nearly identical between seeds (56.8 mg/g protein) and flour (56.9 mg/g protein), and the AACSs were also comparable at 126.1% and 126.4%, respectively. Met levels were higher in seeds (17.4 mg/g protein) than in flour (14.1 mg/g protein), with AACSs of 109.0% and 88.0%, respectively. For Phe + Tyr, seeds had a content of 87.7 mg/g protein vs. 79.4 mg/g protein in flour, with AACSs of 230.7% and 209.0%, respectively. Thr levels were 48.2 mg/g protein in seeds compared to 43.3 mg/g protein in flour, with AACSs of 209.6% and 188.1%, respectively. Trp was significantly higher in seeds (8.7 mg/g protein) compared to flour (5.3 mg/g protein), with AACSs of 144.7% and 87.5%, respectively. Finally, Val content in seeds was 59.4 mg/g protein vs. 54.9 mg/g protein in flour, with AACSs of 152.4% and 140.7%, respectively. The limiting amino acid (LAA) was Met (109.0%) in seeds and Trp (87.5%) in flour. The EAAI was higher in seeds (129.5%) compared to the flour (111.8%).

Table 2. Protein quality of whole flaxseeds and defatted flour.

EAA	AA Estimates for Adults * (mg/g Protein)	Seeds (mg/g Protein)	Flour (mg/g Protein)	Seed AACS (%)	Flour AACS (%)
His	15	38.81 ± 1.68 [a]	34.04 ± 0.98 [b]	258.72 ± 11.19 [A]	226.90 ± 6.53 [B]
Ile	30	53.14 ± 2.98 [a]	46.08 ± 1.67 [b]	177.15 ± 9.95 [A]	153.59 ± 5.56 [B]
Leu	59	73.63 ± 2.53 [a]	66.82 ± 2.74 [b]	124.79 ± 4.28 [A]	113.25 ± 4.64 [B]
Lys	45	56.75 ± 5.75 [a]	56.89 ± 2.49 [a]	126.11 ± 12.78 [A]	126.43 ± 5.54 [A]
Met	16	17.44 ± 2.42 [a]	14.07 ± 0.56 [a]	109.03 ± 15.15 [A]	87.96 ± 3.47 [A]
Phe + Tyr	38	87.67 ± 2.54 [a]	79.44 ± 7.51 [a]	230.70 ± 6.69 [A]	209.04 ± 19.77 [A]
Thr	23	48.20 ± 2.18 [a]	43.26 ± 1.21 [b]	209.56 ± 9.46 [A]	188.10 ± 5.28 [B]
Trp	6	8.68 ± 0.16 [a]	5.25 ± 0.91 [b]	144.67 ± 2.66 [A]	87.50 ± 15.10 [B]
Val	39	59.42 ± 3.15 [a]	54.86 ± 1.81 [a]	152.36 ± 8.08 [A]	140.68 ± 4.63 [A]
LAA (%)	-	-	-	Met 109.03 ± 15.15 [A]	Trp 87.50 ± 15.10 [A]
EAAI (%)	-	129.45 ± 6.26 [a]	111.83 ± 2.23 [b]	-	-

* AA estimates for adults according to WHO/FAO/UNU (2007). Values presented as mean ± standard deviation ($n = 3$). Different small-case letters in the same row denote significant differences ($p < 0.05$). Different capital letters in the same row denote significant differences ($p < 0.05$). AA, amino acids; AACS, amino acid chemical score; EAA, essential amino acid; LAA, limiting amino acid; EAAI, essential amino acid index.

3.2. Cold-Pressed Flaxseed Oil

The results of the composition of the oil are presented in Table 3. The oxidative stability of the oil was measured at 1.3 h, indicating a relatively low resistance to oxidation. The peroxide value, a measure of primary oxidation products, was 2.4 meq O_2/kg, reflecting minimal initial oxidation. The oil exhibited low absorbance values at 232 nm ($K_{232} = 0.02$) and 270 nm ($K_{270} = 0.05$), which are indicative of minimal conjugated dienes and trienes, respectively. Chromatic coordinates were recorded as (x, y) = (0.475, 0.480), with a transparency of 65.8%. The dominant wavelength of 578 nm suggests a yellowish hue, typical for oils with a moderate level of pigmentation.

Table 3. Composition of cold-pressed flaxseed oil.

Parameter	Oil
Oxidative Stability (h)	1.3 ± 0.1
Peroxide Value (meq O_2/kg)	2.4 ± 0.0
K_{232nm}	0.016 ± 0.001
K_{270nm}	0.0500 ± 0.0005
Chromatic coordinates (x, y)	(0.4749, 0.4801)
Transparency (%)	65.8
Dominant wavelength (nm)	577.8
Purity	88.0
Fatty Acids (Relative %)	
C16:0 (Palmitic Acid)	4.81 ± 0.02
C18:0 (Stearic Acid)	3.18 ± 0.09
C18:1n9c (Oleic Acid)	18.47 ± 0.12
C18:2n6c (Linoleic Acid)	16.03 ± 0.08
C18:3n3c (α-Linolenic Acid)	57.51 ± 0.13
∑SFA (Saturated Fatty Acids)	7.99 ± 0.11
∑MUFA (Monounsaturated Fatty Acids)	18.47 ± 0.12
∑PUFA (Polyunsaturated Fatty Acids)	73.54 ± 0.21
n-6/n-3	0.28 ± 0.00
Total Vitamin E (mg/kg)	443.91 ± 6.23
α-Tocopherol	3.96 ± 0.10
α-Tocotrienol	3.68 ± 0.05
γ-Tocopherol	431.72 ± 6.39
δ-Tocopherol	4.55 ± 0.32
Total Phenolics (mg GAE/100 g)	2.3 ± 0.2
Total Flavonoids (mg EE/100 g)	0.4 ± 0.1
FRAP (µmol FSE/100 g)	96.0 ± 1.8
DPPH· Inhibition (mg TE/100 g)	0.2 ± 0.1

Results in fresh weight. Values presented as mean ± standard deviation ($n = 3$). K, extinction coefficient; GAEs, gallic acid equivalents; EEs, epicatechin equivalents; FRAP, ferric reduction antioxidant power; FSEs, ferrous sulphate equivalents; DPPH·, 2,2-diphenyl-1-picrylhydrazyl; TE, Trolox equivalents.

The FA profile of the oil (Table 3) shows a predominance of PUFAs, which constitute 73.5% of the total FA. The primary FAs include α-linolenic acid at 57.5%, oleic acid at 18.5%, and linoleic acid at 16.0%. The SFAs totalized 8.0%, while MUFAs account for 18.5%. The n-6/n-3 ratio is 0.3, indicating a higher concentration of n-3 FAs compared to n-6.

The oil contains a total vitamin E content of 443.9 mg/kg (Table 3). This includes α-tocopherol at 4.0 mg/kg, α-tocotrienol at 3.7 mg/kg, γ-tocopherol at 431.7 mg/kg, and δ-tocopherol at 4.6 mg/kg. Therefore, the predominant form of vitamin E in this oil is γ-tocopherol, which constitutes the majority of the total vitamin E content.

The oil's phenolics total was 2.3 mg GAE/100 g, while total flavonoids were found to be low (0.4 mg EE/100 g). The antioxidant activity, as assessed by the FRAP assay, was 96.0 µmol FSE/100 g. The DPPH• inhibition assay revealed a low antioxidant activity of 0.2 mg TE/100 g (Table 3).

4. Discussion

4.1. Comparative Analysis of Whole Flaxseeds and Defatted Flour

Energy used for metabolic homeostasis, thermoregulation, physical activity, and normal organ function is obtained from the oxidation of macronutrients [27].

The present study (Table 1) showed that flaxseeds revealed a significantly higher energy value than the flour (475 vs. 314 kcal/100 g, respectively) due to higher total fat content (38% vs. 9%, respectively) since this is the most energy dense macronutrient (9 kcal/g) [19]. Thus, flaxseed flour seems an interesting choice as a low-fat ingredient for the food industry, which will match current dietary trends focused on weight management and reduced fat intake.

Minerals are nutrients which sustain health, most of them function as cofactors for enzymes, biochemical substrates, and hormones [27].

Regarding the results of the proximate composition (Table 1), total ash content was significantly higher in flaxseed flour in comparison to flaxseeds (6% vs. 4%, respectively, Table 1). Another study reported the contents of individual minerals in flaxseed: K (831 mg/100 g), P (622 mg/100 g), Mg (431 mg/100 g), and Ca (236 mg/100 g) [28]. Thus, the flour becomes a higher source of total minerals in comparison to whole flaxseeds. It has been previously reported that the contents of Mg may help to enhance antioxidant capacity, while K and Ca contents may help to control high blood pressure [4].

The high-fibre contents (36% vs. 34% in flour and seeds, respectively, Table 1) besides providing nutritional value, can also provide gelling properties (e.g., water-holding and swelling capacity), functioning as a thickening and emulsifying agent—properties that can be helpful in developing new foodstuffs. Fibre ingestion can also help reduce glucose and cholesterol blood levels, ultimately decreasing the risk of heart disease and colon cancer. Moreover, flaxseed's fibre consumption has been associated with hunger suppression. Fibre also functions as a prebiotic stimulating the gut microbiota into producing small-chain FA (e.g., acetate, propionate, and butyrate), which can modulate important metabolic pathways in the organism [28–30].

Another study reported a higher fibre content in flaxseeds (soluble fibre at 10% and insoluble fibre at 30%, totalling 40% of dietary fibre), but the total fat content was similar (38.7%), even though moisture content was slightly lower (7%) [31].

Another research reported that flaxseed's fibre is present mostly in the hull, its soluble fibre was composed of acidic polysaccharides such as L-rhamnose (25%), L-galactose (12%), L-fructose (8%), and D-xylose (29%) and neutral polysaccharides such as L-arabinose (20%) and D-xylose-D-galactose (76%), while its insoluble fibre comprised cellulose (7–11%), lignin (2–7%), and acid detergent fibre (10–14%) [30].

Triglycerides are the main constituents of body fat, when FA are needed as an energy source the bound between the three FA and the glycerol is hydrolysed, the first are released into the blood stream and bound to albumin as free FA [27].

Flaxseeds presented a rich composition in fat, nevertheless cold-pressing the seeds revealed to be an effective method to reduce this high amount (seeds, 38%, vs. flour, 9%; Table 1). The obtained oil can have further applications, e.g., as a dietary supplement, as discussed below.

There are three main families of unsaturated FA—n-3, n-6, and n-9—classified according to the position of their first double bond, e.g., linoleic acid (LA, C18:2n6c, two double bonds) and arachidonic acid (C20:4n6c, four double bonds) are essential FA and precursors of compounds responsible for inflammation, coagulation, smooth muscle vasoconstriction, and vasodilation [27].

Diet-related noncommunicable diseases (NCDs), e.g., cardiovascular diseases (CVDs), diabetes, and cancer, are associated with major risk factors such as high ingestion of saturated fats (mostly from animal fats), leading to increased low-density lipoprotein (LDL) levels. Alternatively, unsaturated FA particularly oleic acid (OA, C18:1n9c), LA (C18:2n6c), and α-linolenic acid (ALA, C18:3n3c) are associated with NCD prevention [32].

Regarding the FAs profile (Table 1), flaxseeds and flour presented mostly ALA (57% vs. 55%, respectively), followed by OA (18%), and LA (17%), totalling high PUFA contents (seeds, 73%, vs. flour, 72%). These results are similar to those previously reported in another work: saturated fatty acids (SFAs, 8.9–12.7%), monounsaturated fatty acids (MUFAs, 16.1–20.5%), and PUFAs (69.0–73.7%) [32].

ALA (55–57%, Table 1) consumption was associated with lowering triglyceride and cholesterol levels, and blood pressure, as well as anti-inflammatory, antidiabetic, cardiac, and hepatic protective activities by redistributing lipids away from visceral fat and the liver. LA (17%, Table 1) can present inflammatory, hypertensive, and thrombotic activities if present in excessive quantity. A balanced n-6/n-3 ratio is vital for health and flaxseed samples' ratio was low (0.3, Table 1) which can compensate for the harmful effects of higher dietary consumption of SFA (in the present samples this sum was low: 8.6–9.7%; Table 1). However, in appropriate levels, LA has an important role in the formation of prostaglandins, leukotrienes, and thromboxane, which are key compounds in several processes in the organism, such as those previously mentioned [4,27].

Vitamin E is a liposoluble antioxidant which protects unsaturated fat from oxidation, especially in seeds. In humans, it presents anti-inflammatory activity, the prevention of neoplastic transformation, the protection of artery walls, and the prevention of LDL oxidation [33]. Particularly, α-tocopherol is a good chain-breaking and peroxyl radical scavenger (seeds, 74 mg/kg, vs. flour, 17 mg/kg; Table 1). γ-Tocopherol (seeds, 141 mg/kg, vs. flour, 31 mg/kg; Table 1) is more active against reactive nitrogen species [33]. Both vitamers were identified in flaxseed samples, γ-tocopherol was the predominant isomer, but seeds presented significantly more total vitamin E than the flour (215 mg/kg vs. 48 mg/kg, respectively; Table 1), probably due to their higher fat content (38% vs. 9%, respectively; Table 1) since this vitamin is liposoluble.

Unlike a previous study [34], the seeds and flour of this work did not present δ-tocopherol. However, as will be discussed later, the oil presented this isomer, but different conditions were applied to extract vitamin E, which could explain the different findings.

Proteins are constituted by chains of AAs linked by peptide bonds. AAs can be D- or L-isomers, with the latter being the naturally occurring form in proteins. There are 20 different AAs found in human proteins. Some are essential and must be obtained in the diet, while others are synthesized by the body (nonessential AAs). Some AAs play other roles besides protein structure, e.g., Tyr (4–6 mg/g, Table 1) is implicated in the formation of thyroid hormones, and Glu (40–65 mg/g, Table 1) is used in the synthesis of neurotransmitters [27].

Flaxseed flour presented a significantly higher total protein content (28%) in comparison to flaxseeds (16%), which was also reflected in the total AA content (314 vs. 194 mg/g, respectively; Table 1). The major AAs identified in the flour and seeds were Glu (65 vs. 40 mg/g, respectively; Table 1), Arg (37 vs. 23 mg/g, respectively; Table 1), and Asp (31 vs. 18 mg/g, respectively; Table 1). Glu was also a major AAs in other studies [31,34]. However, unlike reported by those authors, in the present study, Cys was not identified [31,34].

Recent data about Gln suggest that it plays a key role in cardiovascular health and CVD prevention. Indeed, this was the major AA found in the present samples (Table 1). This AA is a substrate for DNA, ATP, proteins, and lipid synthesis in vascular cells, influencing important processes such as proliferation, migration, and apoptosis. Moreover, it also presents potent antioxidant and anti-inflammatory activities in the circulation by promoting the expression of heme oxygenase-1, heat shock proteins, and glutathione. It is also an Arg precursor in nitric oxide synthesis, having an impact on several NCDs (e.g., hypertension, hyperlipidemia, glucose intolerance, obesity, and diabetes) [35].

Regarding the present results, all essential AAs (His, Thr, Val, Met, Trp, Phe, Ile, Leu, and Lys) were identified, totalling 106 vs. 67 mg/g in flaxseeds and flour, respectively (Table 1). Therefore, all branched-chain AAs (Val, Leu, and Ile) were present, totalling 47 vs. 30 mg/g, respectively (Table 1).

Regarding protein quality (Table 2), the AACS revealed that the LAA (which is the AA with lowest AACS) of flaxseeds was L-methionine (109%), and in the flour, it was L-tryptophan (87%). When comparing both samples, the scores were higher for the seeds in relation to the flour, except for Lys, Met, Phe + Tyr, and Val, which did not exhibit differences ($p < 0.05$). The EAAI was 129% for flaxseeds and 112% for the flour, revealing that both present a high-quality protein since the EAAI was higher than 90% [6], although the seeds presented a significantly higher index than the flour ($p < 0.05$). Overall, flaxseed flour's protein seems a cheaper source of high-quality protein in comparison to animal protein.

Phenolics are compounds with antioxidant activity which prevent and delay food deterioration, also helping to maintain their quality and nutritional value. In body tissues, they help to prevent damage from oxidative stress [5].

Flaxseeds are a natural source of phenolic compounds. Besides sesame seeds, flaxseeds are one of the major natural sources of lignans. These compounds are antioxidants known for their antidiabetic, antihypertensive, anti-inflammatory, and neuroprotective properties. This seed is the richest source of lignin precursors with possible biological benefits in reducing degenerative disease risk and opposing the lack of oestrogens. Moreover, lignans have been described as anti-carcinogenic compounds. In combination with their ALA content (55–57%, Table 1), these seeds may confer health benefits while allowing chemoprotection. Lignans' health benefits include lower CVD, osteoporosis, and breast cancer risk. After consumption, plant lignans are metabolized by gut bacteria into mammalian lignans that could prevent cancer [36–38].

Flaxseed flour was significantly richer in total phenolics in comparison to whole flaxseeds (205 mg of GAE/100 g vs. 142 mg of GAE/100 g, respectively; Table 1) which also occurred in total flavonoids (78.2 mg of EE/100 g vs. 53.9 mg of EE/100 g, respectively; Table 1). There were also significant differences in the FRAP assay (flour, 14.3 mmol FSE/100 g, vs. seeds, 8.5 mmol FSE/100 g; Table 1) and in the DPPH˙ inhibition assay (flour, 233.3 mg TE/100 g, vs. seeds, 57.2 mg TE/100 g; Table 1). Like macronutrient contents, phytochemical yields can vary due to different crops origins, plant genetics, and edaphoclimatic conditions [37].

Interestingly, the flour even with less oil displayed higher contents of the analysed phytochemicals and antioxidant activity, suggesting that these are probably present in flaxseeds' hulls, possibly as a protective response against environmental factors such as oxygen exposure. Therefore, it seems that the major protector of the oil is probably vitamin E (results discussed below).

Indeed, Bekhit et al. [33] also reported higher contents of total phenolic acids in the defatted extract (8440 mg/100 g) in comparison to the non-defatted extract (2767 mg/100 g), mainly p-hydroxybenzoic acid, followed by ferulic acid, coumaric acid, gallic acid, vanillin, sinapic acid, protocatechuic acid, and caffeic acid.

Another study obtained methanolic extracts from flaxseeds and flaxseed meal (2.7% fat), and similarly to the present findings, the obtained results were higher for the defatted meal. Total phenolics contents were 1538.7 µg/g for seeds and 1728.1 µg/g for the meal. Total flavonoids contents were 1.7 mg/g for seeds and 2.8 mg/g for the meal. FRAP assay results were 0.13 mmol TE/g for seeds and 1.09 mmol TE/g for the meal. DPPH• assay results were 0.12 mmol TE/g for seeds and 0.42 mmol TE/g for the meal [39].

Deme et al. [32] also analysed total phenolics (20.5–25.4 mg GAE/g) and FRAP (15.3–30.6 mmol Fe_2SO_4/100 g), but different extracting conditions were used (ethanol and ultrasonic bath), impairing direct comparisons with our results.

The bioavailability of the studied compounds after processing, cooking, and digestion should be evaluated in further studies.

When comparing the nutritional profiles of flaxseeds and their respective defatted flour (Table 1) with other popular seeds—sesame, poppy, and chia—notable differences emerge in the contents of macronutrients.

Sesame contains higher levels of ash, with 5% in seeds and 7% in cake, indicating greater mineral content. Additionally, sesame has slightly higher protein levels (19% in seeds and 30% in cake) and also has a higher fat content (53% in seeds and 32% in cake) than flax. However, regarding dietary fibre, flaxseeds excel, surpassing sesame which contains 20% in seeds and 25% in cake. Overall, while flax is richer in fibre, sesame offers more fat and minerals [5].

Poppy has an ash content of 7% in seeds and 10% in cake, indicating a higher mineral content, but contains lower protein levels (15% in seeds and 26% in cake) than flax. Poppy and flax present similar fat contents (39% in poppy seeds and 10% in poppy cake). Regarding dietary fibre, poppy contains lower levels (32% in seeds and 38% in cake). In summary, while flax tends to have higher fibre and protein contents, poppy is richer in minerals [6].

Chia has an ash content of 5% in seeds and 6% in cake, whereas flax exhibits lower ash levels. Both seeds are comparable in terms of protein (chia contains 18% in seeds and 27% in cake). Chia has a total fat content of 33% in seeds and 7% in cake. This indicates that flax is richer in fat compared to chia seeds. Regarding dietary fibre, chia seeds excel with a total dietary fibre content of 38% in seeds and 48% in cake, surpassing flaxseeds, which have 34% in seeds and 36% in flour. On the whole, while chia provides higher fibre and mineral contents, flax is richer in fat [7].

All of these seeds are in-demand in current diets because they have similar food applications and can provide several health benefits when consumed [4–7].

4.2. Defatted Flaxseed Flour as a New Ingredient for Foodstuffs

Defatted flaxseed flour provides new food options to consumers and manufacturers as a high-value by-product from oilseeds processing. It has potential for the R&D of new foodstuffs since it is a natural, minimally processed, functional ingredient, rich in dietary fibre and high-quality gluten-free protein [5–7]. It also contributes to the prevention of NCD because it is a low-fat ingredient since a high energy-dense and ultra-processed diet is known to induce obesity [40–42].

This by-product can be incorporated in novel foods as a functional ingredient such as bakery products, e.g., flaxseed flour (7.5%), was useful in producing fortified sourdough bread [43] and defatted flaxseed meal (5–10%) was used in toast and cake to partially substitute the wheat flour [44]. The use of this by-product for food purposes ensures food and nutritional security due to its complete composition in bioactive compounds, also promoting environmental sustainability with a zero-waste approach [1,45]. This approach also aligns with current food concerns, in particular to meet the SDG 2 [15].

Another study reported higher contents of total protein (35%) and fibre (37%) for flaxseed flour in relation to the present results, probably because of the lower total fat (2%) and moisture contents (6%) when compared to the present data. However, ash content was similar (6%). Like the present data, extracts showed a strong antioxidant activity against DPPH• [46].

4.3. Cold-Pressed Flaxseed Oil

Cold-pressed flaxseed oil presented a low oxidative stability (1.3 h, Table 3), which could be related to the high content of PUFAs (74%), mainly ALA (58%) and LA (16%). Both are valuable in diets since they are essential FAs that not synthesized in the body, so they must be obtained through food [32].

Another study reported a higher induction time (3.6 h), which decreased to 1.4 h in 6 months [13]. Unexpectedly, the latter value is closer to the present result (1.3 h). However, different conditions were used (110 °C, 10 L/h) in relation to the present study, in which a higher temperature (120 °C) and air flow rate (20 L/h) were used, which could have accelerated the oxidation process, explaining the lower induction period. Fortification with antioxidants or combining flaxseed oil with a more saturated oil could be strategies to achieve higher induction times [14]. Another approach to protect this oil from oxidation could be microencapsulation [47].

A higher n-6/n-3 ratio has been associated with the incidence of NCD [48]. However, flaxseed oil presented a low n-6/n-3 ratio (0.3, Table 3), which can counterbalance the harmful effects of higher dietary consumption of SFAs (8%) and LA (16%) in relation to ALA (58%).

MUFAs (18%) such as OA (18%) are recognized to reduce LDL levels, preventing atherosclerosis. Vegetable oils rich in unsaturated FA can easily suffer oxidation and produce toxic metabolites, especially with exposure to high temperatures. Nevertheless, antioxidants can improve oxidative stability [32].

Interestingly, another study reported a higher content of OA (23%), resulting in a lower PUFAs (66%) [49], which can be explained by different edaphoclimatic conditions or different origins of the seeds [37].

The vitamin E profile revealed α-tocotrienol and α-, γ-, and δ-tocopherols, totalling 444 mg/kg. This antioxidant appears to be the major contributor for oil protection since total phenolics (2.3 mg GAE/100 g) and total flavonoids (0.4 mg ECE/100 g) were low.

Another study with cold-pressed flaxseed oil found traces of α-tocopherol and contents of γ- and δ-tocopherols (35.3 mg/100 g and 0.2 mg/100 g, respectively), but did not identify α-tocotrienol, unlike the present data [49].

Although a high PUFA content (74%, Table 3) can present several health benefits, this oil presents low oxidative stability (1.3 h) and, consequently, low thermostability, which limits its use for cooking. If this oil presented higher contents of MUFAs (18%), its oxidative stability could be enhanced, resulting in better shelf-life since OA is known to promote stability in foodstuffs. However, its use in cooking has been recently recommended because of high lignin contents. The formation of oil blends with more SFA- and MUFA-rich oils can be proposed to increase stability [32,50,51].

Nevertheless, no products of primary oxidation (K_{232nm}) and secondary oxidation (K_{270nm}) were produced, and the peroxide value was low (2.4 meq O_2/kg, Table 3). However, these analyses were performed after oil extraction. The shelf-life period should be monitored to evaluate if these values increase with time. In another study, higher $K_{232\,nm}$ and K_{270nm} values were reported for this oil (1.50 and 0.24, respectively), although the peroxide value was lower 1.85 meq O_2/kg [52]. The use of amber containers for storage is recommended as light exposure can accelerate oxidation [50].

Therefore, this oil has the potential to be consumed raw, e.g., salad dressing, or used in the formulation of food supplements, contributing for the daily uptake of essential FAs, i.e., ALA (58%) and LA (16%), and antioxidants, i.e., vitamin E (444 mg/kg). Flaxseed oil's dietary supplementation had a positive effect in reducing type II diabetes due to inflammation reduction and changes in gut microbiota composition [51]. However, due to its expensive price, this oil is restricted to a niche market, being considered a specialty oil; therefore, it could have applications as a dietary supplement or in the paint and varnish industry [46].

Herchi et al. reported that DPPH˙ inhibition decreased from 65% to 50% during the heating of flaxseed oil, which can be explained by the decrease in total phenolics from 84 to 60 GAE, mg/100 g, and total flavonoids from 18 to 12 luteolin equivalents, mg/100 g, which also happened for carotenoid and chlorophyll contents [52].

The following phenolic compounds were reported in flaxseed oil: secoisolariciresinol, ferulic acid and its methyl ester, coumaric acid methyl ester, diphyllin, pinoresinol, matairesinol, p-hydroxybenzoic acid, vanillin, and vanillic acid [53]. Although the oil presented low total phenolics (2.3 mg, GAE/100 g) and total flavonoids (0.4 mg, ECE/100 g) and antioxidant activity (FRAP assay: 96.0 µmol, FSE/100 g; DPPH˙ inhibition: 0.2 mg, TE/100 g), it should be noted that the oil is protected inside the seed, where it is not exposed to environmental stresses; therefore, higher contents were obtained for flaxseeds and flour as discussed before.

4.4. Future Research

Regarding future research, the bioactivity of the seed, flour, and oil extracts should be further investigated by employing cellular assays (e.g., anti-diabetic, neuroprotective, anti-inflammatory potential, anti-allergic properties, and anti-microbial activity).

More research is also recommended to evaluate the shelf-life period and optimal storage conditions for these products to ensure their stability over time. This could involve studying the impact of different environmental factors, such as temperature, light, and humidity, on the degradation of bioactive compounds. Exploring novel preservation techniques, such as encapsulation or freeze-drying, may also enhance the longevity of these products.

Additionally, the bioavailability and metabolism of bioactive compounds after digestion could be assessed by the in vitro simulations of gastrointestinal digestion, so that food matrix interactions or the role of the gut microbiota and the outcomes on human health are better understood and validated.

5. Conclusions

There is a growing demand for functional foods containing bioactive compounds, such as flaxseeds. This study evaluated the chemical composition of flaxseeds to assess their nutritional relevance, highlighting that cold pressing is an effective method for oil extraction, yielding high-quality oil as well as defatted flour as a by-product. These products contained vitamin E and phenolic compounds, which appear to be the main contributors to the antioxidant properties of the samples.

Cold-pressed flaxseed oil has potential as a raw consumable, such as in salad dressings or nutraceuticals, due to its essential fatty acids (in particular LA, and predominantly ALA) and vitamin E content (α-tocotrienol and α-, γ-, and δ-tocopherols). Given its likely high market price, it can be considered a specialty oil, with potential applications as a dietary supplement.

Flaxseed flour, the by-product of oil extraction, should be valued and incorporated into the food industry, as it was found to be a richer source of total minerals, high-quality gluten-free protein, and high-fibre compared to whole flaxseeds. This makes it a valuable ingredient that can provide various functional properties to food products, aligning with goals for food and nutritional security, as well as circular economy and sustainability.

Although flaxseed products can offer significant nutritional benefits, they cannot compensate for poor dietary habits, such as the excessive consumption of saturated fats. Future research should focus on investigating bioactivity through cellular assays, evaluating shelf-life and storage conditions, and assessing bioavailability and metabolism after digestion to better understand and validate the health impacts of these products.

Author Contributions: Conceptualization, D.M.F., M.A.N., M.Á.-O. and M.B.P.P.O.; methodology, D.M.F., M.A.N., L.E.S., A.S.G.C. and S.M.; validation, M.A.N.; formal analysis, D.M.F.; investigation, D.M.F.; resources, J.E.P., R.C.A. and M.B.P.P.O.; data curation, D.M.F.; writing—original draft preparation, D.M.F.; writing—review and editing, R.C.A. and M.B.P.P.O.; visualization, D.M.F.; supervision, R.C.A., M.Á.-O. and M.B.P.P.O.; project administration, J.E.P.; funding acquisition, J.E.P. and M.B.P.P.O. All authors have read and agreed to the published version of the manuscript.

Funding: This research was funded by the Fundação para a Ciência e a Tecnologia/Ministério da Ciência, Tecnologia e Ensino Superior (FCT/MCTES)—Portugal (LA/P/0008/2020 [https://doi.org/10.54499/LA/P/0008/2020], UIDP/50006/2020 [https://doi.org/10.54499/UIDP/50006/2020], and UIDB/50006/2020 [https://doi.org/10.54499/UIDB/50006/2020]) and the FEDER Castilla-La Mancha Regional Government—Spain (SBPLY/19/180501/000047).

Institutional Review Board Statement: Not applicable.

Informed Consent Statement: Not applicable.

Data Availability Statement: All data are contained within the article.

Acknowledgments: D.M.F. is thankful for the PhD grant from FCT/MCTES (ref. 2022.13375.BD). L.E.S. is grateful to the Laboratório Associado para a Química Verde—Tecnologias e Processos Limpos—UIDB/50006/2020 for the grant REQUIMTE 2023-49. S.M. is grateful to the project PTDC/SAU-NUT/2165/2021-COBY4HEALTH funded by FCT for her research grant. R.C. Alves thanks FCT for funding through the Scientific Employment Stimulus—Individual Call (CEECIND/011 20/2017, https://doi.org/10.54499/CEECIND/01120/2017/CP1427/CT0001).

Conflicts of Interest: The authors declare no conflicts of interest.

References

1. Mozaffarian, D.; Fleischhacker, S.; Andrés, J.R. Prioritizing Nutrition Security in the US. *JAMA* **2021**, *325*, 1605–1606. [CrossRef] [PubMed]
2. Alongi, M.; Anese, M. Re-thinking functional food development through a holistic approach. *J. Funct. Foods* **2021**, *81*, 104466. [CrossRef]
3. Pareek, A.; Singh, N. Seeds as nutraceuticals, their therapeutic potential and their role in improving sports performance. *J. Phytol. Res.* **2021**, *34*, 127–138.
4. Melo, D.; Machado, T.B.; Oliveira, M.B.P.P. Chia seeds: An ancient grain trending in modern human diets. *Food Funct.* **2019**, *10*, 3068–3089. [CrossRef]
5. Melo, D.; Álvarez-Ortí, M.; Nunes, M.A.; Costa, A.S.G.; Machado, S.; Alves, R.C.; Pardo, J.E.; Oliveira, M.B.P.P. Whole or defatted sesame seeds (*Sesamum indicum* L.)? The effect of cold pressing on oil and cake quality. *Foods* **2021**, *10*, 2108. [CrossRef]
6. Melo, D.; Álvarez-Ortí, M.; Nunes, M.A.; Espírito Santo, L.; Machado, S.; Pardo, J.E.; Oliveira, M.B.P.P. Nutritional and Chemical Characterization of Poppy Seeds, Cold-Pressed Oil, and Cake: Poppy Cake as a High-Fibre and High-Protein Ingredient for Novel Food Production. *Foods* **2022**, *11*, 3027. [CrossRef]
7. Ferreira, D.M.; Nunes, M.A.; Santo, L.E.; Machado, S.; Costa, A.S.G.; Álvarez-Ortí, M.; Pardo, J.E.; Oliveira, M.B.P.P.; Alves, R.C. Characterization of Chia Seeds, Cold-Pressed Oil, and Defatted Cake: An Ancient Grain for Modern Food Production. *Molecules* **2023**, *28*, 723. [CrossRef] [PubMed]
8. FAOSTAT. Food and Agriculture Organisation of the United Nations. Available online: https://www.fao.org/faostat/en/#data/QCL/visualize (accessed on 21 August 2024).
9. Nowak, W.; Jeziorek, M. The Role of Flaxseed in Improving Human Health. *Healthcare* **2023**, *11*, 395. [CrossRef]
10. Calado, A.; Neves, P.M.; Santos, T.; Ravasco, P. The Effect of Flaxseed in Breast Cancer: A Literature Review. *Front. Nutr.* **2018**, *5*, 4. [CrossRef]
11. Villarreal-Renteria, A.I.; Herrera-Echauri, D.D.; Rodríguez-Rocha, N.P.; Zuñiga, L.Y.; Muñoz-Valle, J.F.; García-Arellano, S.; Bernal-Orozco, M.F.; Macedo-Ojeda, G. Effect of flaxseed (*Linum usitatissimum*) supplementation on glycemic control and insulin resistance in prediabetes and type 2 diabetes: A systematic review and meta-analysis of randomized controlled trials. *Complement. Ther. Med.* **2022**, *70*, 102852. [CrossRef]
12. Saini, R.K.; Prasad, P.; Sreedhar, R.V.; Akhilender Naidu, K.; Shang, X.; Keum, Y.-S. Omega−3 Polyunsaturated Fatty Acids (PUFAs): Emerging Plant and Microbial Sources, Oxidative Stability, Bioavailability, and Health Benefits—A Review. *Antioxidants* **2021**, *10*, 1627. [CrossRef]
13. Durazzo, A.; Fawzy Ramadan, M.; Lucarini, M. Cold Pressed Oils: A Green Source of Specialty Oils. *Front. Nutr.* **2022**, *8*, 836651. [CrossRef] [PubMed]
14. Grajzer, M.; Szmalcel, K.; Kuźmiński, Ł.; Witkowski, M.; Kulma, A.; Prescha, A. Characteristics and Antioxidant Potential of Cold-Pressed Oils—Possible Strategies to Improve Oil Stability. *Foods* **2020**, *9*, 1630. [CrossRef] [PubMed]
15. Nations, U. Goal 2: Zero Hunger. Available online: https://www.un.org/sustainabledevelopment/hunger/ (accessed on 28 August 2024).
16. Ferreira, D.M.; Barreto-Peixoto, J.; Andrade, N.; Machado, S.; Silva, C.; Lobo, J.C.; Nunes, M.A.; Álvarez-Rivera, G.; Ibáñez, E.; Cifuentes, A.; et al. Comprehensive analysis of the phytochemical composition and antitumoral activity of an olive pomace extract obtained by mechanical pressing. *Food Biosci.* **2024**, *61*, 104759. [CrossRef]
17. AOAC. *Official Methods of Analysis*, 21st ed.; Association of Official Analytical Chemists: Arlington, VA, USA, 2019.
18. Tontisirin, K. *Chapter 2: Methods of food analysis. Food Energy: Methods of Analysis and Conversion Factors: Report of a Technical Workshop*; Food and Agriculture Organization of the United Nations: Rome, Italy, 2003.
19. European Commission. Regulation (EU) No 1169/2011 of the European Parliament and of the Council of 25 October 2011 on the provision of food information to consumers. *Off. J. Eur. Union* **2011**, *54*, 18–61.
20. *ISO 12966*; Animal and Vegetable Fats and Oils—Gas Chromatography of Fatty Acid Methyl Esters: Part 2: Preparation of Methyl Esters of Fatty Acids. ISO: Geneva, Switzerland, 2017.
21. Machado, S.; Costa, A.S.G.; Pimentel, F.B.; Oliveira, M.B.P.P.; Alves, R.C. A study on the protein fraction of coffee silverskin: Protein/non-protein nitrogen and free and total amino acid profiles. *Food Chem.* **2020**, *326*, 126940. [CrossRef] [PubMed]
22. WHO/FAO/UNU. *Protein and Amino Acid Requirements in Human Nutrition*; WHO: Geneva, Switzerland, 2007; pp. 93–102, ISSN 0512-3054.
23. Oser, B.L. *An Integrated Essential Amino Acid Index for Predicting the Biological Value of Proteins. Protein and Amino Acid Nutrition*; Elsevier: Amsterdam, The Netherlands, 1959; Volume 281.
24. *NP 904*; Edible Fats and Oils—Determination of Peroxide Value. ISO: Geneva, Switzerland, 1987; Volume 904.
25. *ISO 3656*; Animal and Vegetable Fats and Oils—Determination of Ultraviolet Absorbance Expressed as Specific UV Extinction. ISO: Geneva, Switzerland, 2011.
26. *NP 937*; Edible Fats and Oils—Oils Colour Determination and Their Chromatic Characteristics. ISO: Geneva, Switzerland, 1987.
27. Costa-Pinto, R.; Gantner, D. Macronutrients, minerals, vitamins and energy. *Anaesth. Intensive Care Med.* **2020**, *21*, 157–161. [CrossRef]
28. Bernacchia, R.; Preti, R.; Vinci, G. Chemical composition and health benefits of flaxseed. *Austin J. Nutri. Food Sci.* **2014**, *2*, 1045.

29. Devi, R.; Bhatia, M. Thiol functionalization of flaxseed mucilage: Preparation, characterization and evaluation as mucoadhesive polymer. *Int. J. Biol. Macromol.* **2019**, *126*, 101–106. [CrossRef]
30. Parikh, M.; Netticadan, T.; Pierce, G.N. Flaxseed: Its bioactive components and their cardiovascular benefits. *Am. J. Physiol. Heart Circ. Physiol.* **2018**, *314*, H146–H159. [CrossRef]
31. Shim, Y.Y.; Gui, B.; Arnison, P.G.; Wang, Y.; Reaney, M.J.T. Flaxseed (*Linum usitatissimum* L.) bioactive compounds and peptide nomenclature: A review. *Trends Food Sci. Technol.* **2014**, *38*, 5–20. [CrossRef]
32. Deme, T.; Haki, G.; Retta, N.; Woldegiorgis, A.; Geleta, M. Fatty Acid Profile, Total Phenolic Content, and Antioxidant Activity of Niger Seed (*Guizotia abyssinica*) and Linseed (*Linum usitatissimum*). *Front. Nutr.* **2021**, *8*, 674882. [CrossRef] [PubMed]
33. Bekhit, A.E.-D.A.; Shavandi, A.; Jodjaja, T.; Birch, J.; Teh, S.; Mohamed Ahmed, I.A.; Al-Juhaimi, F.Y.; Saeedi, P.; Bekhit, A.A. Flaxseed: Composition, detoxification, utilization, and opportunities. *Biocatal. Agric. Biotechnol.* **2018**, *13*, 129–152. [CrossRef]
34. Mannucci, A.; Castagna, A.; Santin, M.; Serra, A.; Mele, M.; Ranieri, A. Quality of flaxseed oil cake under different storage conditions. *LWT* **2019**, *104*, 84–90. [CrossRef]
35. Durante, W. The Emerging Role of l-Glutamine in Cardiovascular Health and Disease. *Nutrients* **2019**, *11*, 2092. [CrossRef]
36. Landete, J.M. Plant and mammalian lignans: A review of source, intake, metabolism, intestinal bacteria and health. *Food Res. Int.* **2012**, *46*, 410–424. [CrossRef]
37. Garros, L.; Drouet, S.; Corbin, C.; Decourtil, C.; Fidel, T.; Lebas de Lacour, J.; Leclerc, E.A.; Renouard, S.; Tungmunnithum, D.; Doussot, J.; et al. Insight into the Influence of Cultivar Type, Cultivation Year, and Site on the Lignans and Related Phenolic Profiles, and the Health-Promoting Antioxidant Potential of Flax (*Linum usitatissimum* L.) Seeds. *Molecules* **2018**, *23*, 2636. [CrossRef] [PubMed]
38. Rodríguez-García, C.; Sánchez-Quesada, C.; Toledo, E.; Delgado-Rodríguez, M.; Gaforio, J.J. Naturally Lignan-Rich Foods: A Dietary Tool for Health Promotion? *Molecules* **2019**, *24*, 917. [CrossRef] [PubMed]
39. Quezada, N.; Cherian, G. Lipid characterization and antioxidant status of the seeds and meals of *Camelina sativa* and flax. *Eur. J. Lipid Sci. Technol.* **2012**, *114*, 974–982. [CrossRef]
40. Fardet, A. Characterization of the Degree of Food Processing in Relation With Its Health Potential and Effects. *Adv. Food Nutr. Res.* **2018**, *85*, 79–129. [CrossRef]
41. Hall, K.D.; Ayuketah, A.; Brychta, R.; Cai, H.; Cassimatis, T.; Chen, K.Y.; Chung, S.T.; Costa, E.; Courville, A.; Darcey, V.; et al. Ultra-Processed Diets Cause Excess Calorie Intake and Weight Gain: An Inpatient Randomized Controlled Trial of Ad Libitum Food Intake. *Cell Metab.* **2019**, *30*, 67–77.e63. [CrossRef] [PubMed]
42. Guiné, R.; Florença, S.; Barroca, M.; Anjos, O. foods The Link between the Consumer and the Innovations in Food Product Development. *Foods* **2020**, *9*, 1317. [CrossRef] [PubMed]
43. Sanmartin, C.; Taglieri, I.; Venturi, F.; Macaluso, M.; Zinnai, A.; Tavarini, S.; Botto, A.; Serra, A.; Conte, G.; Flamini, G.; et al. Flaxseed Cake as a Tool for the Improvement of Nutraceutical and Sensorial Features of Sourdough Bread. *Foods* **2020**, *9*, 204. [CrossRef] [PubMed]
44. Mostafa, M.K.; Selim, K.A.-H.; Mahmoud, A.A.-T.; Ali, R.A. Effect of bioactive compounds of defatted flaxseed meal on rheological and sensorial properties of toast and cake. *J. Food Sci. Technol.* **2019**, *4*, 707–719. [CrossRef]
45. Poppy, G.M.; Jepson, P.C.; Pickett, J.A.; Birkett, M.A. Achieving food and environmental security: New approaches to close the gap. *Philos. Trans. R. Soc. Lond. B Biol. Sci.* **2014**, *369*, 20120272. [CrossRef]
46. Herchi, W.; Arráez-Román, D.; Trabelsi, H.; Bouali, I.; Boukhchina, S.; Kallel, H.; Segura-Carretero, A.; Fernández-Gutierrez, A. Phenolic compounds in flaxseed: A review of their properties and analytical methods. An overview of the last decade. *J. Oleo Sci.* **2014**, *63*, 7–14. [CrossRef]
47. Kaushik, P.; Dowling, K.; McKnight, S.; Barrow, C.J.; Adhikari, B. Microencapsulation of flaxseed oil in flaxseed protein and flaxseed gum complex coacervates. *Food Res. Int.* **2016**, *86*, 1–8. [CrossRef]
48. Zhuang, P.; Wang, W.; Wang, J.; Zhang, Y.; Jiao, J. Polyunsaturated fatty acids intake, omega-6/omega-3 ratio and mortality: Findings from two independent nationwide cohorts. *Clin. Nutr.* **2019**, *38*, 848–855. [CrossRef]
49. Tańska, M.; Mikołajczak, N.; Konopka, I. Comparison of the effect of sinapic and ferulic acids derivatives (4-vinylsyringol vs. 4-vinylguaiacol) as antioxidants of rapeseed, flaxseed, and extra virgin olive oils. *Food Chem.* **2018**, *240*, 679–685. [CrossRef]
50. Zeb, A. A comprehensive review on different classes of polyphenolic compounds present in edible oils. *Food Res. Int.* **2021**, *143*, 110312. [CrossRef]
51. Rabail, R.; Shabbir, M.A.; Sahar, A.; Miecznikowski, A.; Kieliszek, M.; Aadil, R.M. An Intricate Review on Nutritional and Analytical Profiling of Coconut, Flaxseed, Olive, and Sunflower Oil Blends. *Molecules* **2021**, *26*, 7187. [CrossRef] [PubMed]
52. Herchi, W.; Ben Ammar, K.; Bouali, I.; Bou Abdallah, I.; Guetat, A.; Boukhchina, S. Heating effects on physicochemical characteristics and antioxidant activity of flaxseed hull oil (*Linum usitatissimum* L.). *Food Sci. Technol.* **2016**, *36*, 97–102. [CrossRef]
53. Herchi, W.; Sawalha, S.; Arráez-Román, D.; Boukhchina, S.; Segura-Carretero, A.; Kallel, H.; Fernández-Gutierrez, A. Determination of phenolic and other polar compounds in flaxseed oil using liquid chromatography coupled with time-of-flight mass spectrometry. *Food Chem.* **2011**, *126*, 332–338. [CrossRef]

Disclaimer/Publisher's Note: The statements, opinions and data contained in all publications are solely those of the individual author(s) and contributor(s) and not of MDPI and/or the editor(s). MDPI and/or the editor(s) disclaim responsibility for any injury to people or property resulting from any ideas, methods, instructions or products referred to in the content.

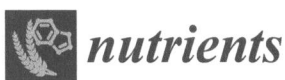

Article

Nutritional Education Needs and Preferences of Sports Volunteers: Access, Expectations, and Forms of Support

Mateusz Rozmiarek

Department of Sports Tourism, Faculty of Physical Culture Sciences, Poznan University of Physical Education, 61-871 Poznan, Poland; rozmiarek@awf.poznan.pl

Abstract: The aim of this study was to analyze the needs and preferences of sports volunteers regarding nutritional education, with particular emphasis on the availability of educational materials and expectations towards event organizers. The methodology was grounded in a qualitative approach, employing detailed individual interviews (IDIs) with seventeen volunteers (n = 17) who were actively involved in various sporting events, including races, triathlons, and athletic competitions at local, national, and international levels. This sample size was justified as it was sufficient to achieve data saturation, meaning no new significant themes emerged after these interviews. The results indicate that most participants feel a lack of access to reliable information about nutrition, with 70% (n = 12) indicating a need for educational materials, which limits their ability to make informed dietary decisions. Volunteers expect event organizers to provide educational materials and prefer a variety of practical forms of education, such as interactive workshops and accessible online resources. While the volunteers expressed a desire for improved nutritional education, further investigation is needed to establish a direct link between this education and potential enhancements in their performance and well-being. For this reason, greater attention should be paid to the nutritional education of volunteers, which is a key element of their preparation to work in high-stress and physically intense conditions.

Keywords: volunteering; sport; nutrition; volunteer management; sports event management; dietary preferences; diet; nutritional education; qualitative research; interviews

Citation: Rozmiarek, M. Nutritional Education Needs and Preferences of Sports Volunteers: Access, Expectations, and Forms of Support. *Nutrients* **2024**, *16*, 3568. https://doi.org/10.3390/nu16203568

Academic Editors: Ariana Saraiva and António Raposo

Received: 2 October 2024
Revised: 17 October 2024
Accepted: 18 October 2024
Published: 21 October 2024

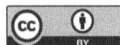

Copyright: © 2024 by the author. Licensee MDPI, Basel, Switzerland. This article is an open access article distributed under the terms and conditions of the Creative Commons Attribution (CC BY) license (https://creativecommons.org/licenses/by/4.0/).

1. Introduction

Sports volunteering is an integral part of organizing sporting events, both at the local and international levels [1–3]. Volunteers support various aspects of event organization, ranging from logistics to athlete care and technical support [4,5]. Their role in the functioning of such events is invaluable, and their presence often determines the logistical success of the entire undertaking. Volunteering in sports activities typically occurs during two main situations: the duration of championships and training or preparation sessions. The nature of the volunteer work can vary significantly depending on the duration and intensity of the event, the specific demands of the sport, and whether the activities take place indoors or outdoors. Nevertheless, despite the crucial contribution of volunteers, their specific needs, especially those related to nutrition, remain largely neglected. Given the increasing demands associated with the intensity of work, long hours, and the activities undertaken, it is worth considering how proper nutrition could influence the performance and overall condition of volunteers.

From the perspective of the scientific literature, the area of athlete nutrition is well-researched [6–9]. Studies on the physiology of physical exertion clearly indicate that a properly balanced diet is a key factor influencing the recovery capabilities, muscle strength, and mental resilience of athletes [10]. Undeniably, what an athlete consumes directly affects their ability to maintain a high level of performance during competitions [11–13]. However, despite certain similarities between the intensity of sports volunteers' work and the physical challenges faced by athletes, the nutritional needs of the former have not received similar attention in research and contain fundamental differences. Understanding the specific nutritional needs of sports volunteers is crucial for their performance during sporting events. The work of a volunteer, often performed under significant physical and mental stress, requires maintaining stable energy levels and adequate recovery [14]. Unlike athletes, who benefit from the care of dietitians and have access to carefully designed nutritional plans, volunteers do not need to present maximized fitness levels but only an individual level of fitness sufficient to perform their tasks. A diet that is too poor or inappropriate can contribute to decreased performance and even weaken the body's immune system, which in the long run may lead to fatigue or exhaustion [15].

One of the key issues faced by volunteers is the limited access to reliable information about nutrition [16]. Although modern technologies offer broad access to content related to a healthy lifestyle, the quality of this information can be questionable [17,18]. Many blogs, websites, and social media profiles promote content that may be fragmented, unverified, or based on trendy yet not always scientifically supported nutritional theories [19,20]. For volunteers who lack specialized knowledge, this can lead to nutritional decisions that do not support their optimal condition and health.

An important area to explore in the context of sports volunteers is their awareness of how diet affects both physical and mental health. Although the topic of healthy eating is increasingly present in public debate [21,22], not everyone has access to reliable educational materials, especially when they are delivered in a complicated or impractical manner. For volunteers who operate under stress and time pressure, such as those involved in sporting events, the nutritional choices they make can be significantly compromised. Inadequate nutrition can lead to decreased performance, fatigue, and impaired mental health, which in turn can affect their overall satisfaction and motivation. Therefore, nutrition education should be tailored to their specific needs in order to realistically improve their performance and well-being during these high-pressure situations. This is particularly important given that previous research on volunteer satisfaction and motivation [23–30], which has been the most extensively studied element of their functioning, has not explored this aspect. Addressing the challenges posed by inadequate nutrition education is urgent, as reliable and accessible resources could make a significant difference in the effectiveness of sports volunteers.

The role of event organizers in supporting volunteers should, therefore, also include issues related to their nutrition. Organizers, who are responsible for ensuring the working and resting conditions for volunteers, have the opportunity to provide them with educational materials about healthy eating, which would help volunteers better understand how diet affects their performance and how they should plan their meals before, during, and after sporting events. Many volunteers already possess some level of nutritional knowledge due to their involvement in physical activities; however, this knowledge can vary widely among individuals. The introduction of such support could improve not only their well-being but also their engagement and effectiveness during work.

Preferences regarding forms of nutrition education may vary depending on various factors such as age, level of education, experience in volunteering, and availability of technology. While it is true that many volunteers are likely to have some background in nutrition, particularly those actively participating in sports, there is still a notable gap in tailored educational resources that address the specific needs of volunteers across different sports and roles. Younger volunteers may prefer modern solutions, such as mobile applications or interactive online courses, while older individuals may prefer more traditional forms, such as printed materials or direct workshops. Importantly, access to nutrition education and materials supporting healthy eating may also be limited by various barriers. Not only can a lack of time or an overload of responsibilities on the part of event organizers be problematic, but financial barriers, technological limitations, or a lack of awareness among organizers can also contribute to a low level of nutritional knowledge among volunteers. These barriers highlight the need for structured programs that can systematically address these gaps, ensuring all volunteers, regardless of their background, receive adequate nutrition education.

The objective of this study is to determine the needs and preferences of sports volunteers regarding nutrition education, with a particular focus on the availability of educational materials, expectations of event organizers, and preferred forms of support. Specifically, this study examined the availability of educational materials (e.g., information on the quality of meals, their energy value, the role of hydration, and meal timing), methods of knowledge delivery (e.g., workshops, online resources, printed materials), and the relevance of the information provided in the context of the volunteers' specific roles and activities. To better understand these issues, two research hypotheses were formulated:

Hypothesis 1. *Volunteers expect that event organizers will provide access to educational materials on healthy eating.*

Hypothesis 2. *Sports volunteers prefer diverse forms of nutrition education.*

This study aims to investigate these issues through in-depth interviews with sports volunteers to better understand their experiences, needs, and preferences regarding nutrition education.

2. Materials and Methods

The research methodology is based on a qualitative approach utilizing in-depth interviews (IDIs) [31]. The IDI is considered one of the most effective methods for gaining profound insights into individuals and examining various topics [32]. Thanks to the individual approach to respondents, as opposed to methods such as focus groups, it allows for more detailed results and greater engagement in discussions on sensitive or personal topics [33].

2.1. Sample Selection

This study involved 17 sports volunteers, including nine women (designated as V3-4, V7, V10, V12-14, V16-17) and eight men (V1-2, V5-6, V8-9, V11, V15). The volunteers participated in the organization of different sporting events, such as races of different distances, triathlons, and athletic competitions. As part of the study, interviews were conducted regarding the volunteers' expectations for access to educational materials on healthy eating as well as their preferences regarding forms of support. The aliases of the participants, along with their ages, are presented in Table 1. All participants were of legal age and had experience working at various sports events organized in the past two years. The sample was selected through purposive sampling, meaning that participants were chosen based on specific criteria. The key requirements were: (1) active participation in sports volunteering for at least two years—ongoing collaboration with organizations responsible for volunteer management at sporting events, ensuring the continuous presence of volunteers at sporting events; (2) experience gained at sports events at the local, national, and international levels. Participants who were not of legal age and those who did not meet the required criteria outlined in the key requirements were excluded from the study. Participants held diverse roles in volunteering, which allowed for the collection of varied perspectives on the dietary requirements and habits related to their roles.

Table 1. Table of participants.

Male Volunteers		Female Volunteers	
Alias	Age	Alias	Age
V1	25	V3	20
V2	19	V4	18
V5	22	V7	18

Table 1. *Cont.*

Male Volunteers		Female Volunteers	
Alias	Age	Alias	Age
V6	20	V10	23
V8	24	V12	19
V9	21	V13	25
V11	28	V14	18
V15	23	V16	19
		V17	20

2.2. Justification for Sample Size

The sample size was defined according to qualitative research principles, which dictate that the number of participants is typically established based on the point of data saturation. Achieving saturation means that subsequent interviews do not yield new significant themes or information that could meaningfully affect the comprehension of the studied topic. In the case of this research, data saturation was achieved after conducting seventeen interviews, demonstrating that the sample was adequate for obtaining complete and thorough information. Such a sample size is also supported in the literature on qualitative research methodology [34,35].

2.3. Procedure

The investigation was performed through semi-structured interviews, allowing participants to freely express their thoughts in open-ended questions. This methodology enabled more detailed responses and the discovery of unexpected themes regarding the needs and preferences of sports volunteers in the field of nutrition education. The interviews focused on three key areas: volunteers' expectations of event organizers concerning access to educational materials, their preferences for different forms of support, and the barriers associated with the availability of nutrition education. This approach facilitated an understanding of the volunteers' attitudes toward learning about nutrition, taking into account their individual needs.

Conversations with participants took place from 1 July to 15 August 2023. Each interview lasted approximately 90 min and addressed various issues related to nutrition within the realm of sports volunteering, with an emphasis on the availability of educational materials and preferred forms of support. The interviews were captured with the participants' permission.

The entire research procedure was in accordance with ethical scientific standards. Participants were fully briefed on the study's goals, its nature, and the voluntary aspect of their involvement. Each respondent gave informed consent to take part in the study and for the recording of the interviews. Anonymity and confidentiality were ensured, and the collected data were presented in a manner that prevented the identification of participants.

2.4. Data Analysis

The information gathered from the interviews underwent analysis following a four-step thematic analysis process: (1) Transcribing the recordings and preliminary familiarization with the collected material; (2) classifying participants' responses and identifying common themes; (3) organizing the classifications into wider thematic categories; (4) analyzing the results and deriving conclusions from the recognized themes. Each of these stages was conducted following the established guidelines for the rigor of qualitative research, ensuring high reliability and adequacy of the obtained conclusions.

To increase the transparency and thoroughness of the analysis, a multi-phase and iterative approach to thematic analysis was adopted. Following the initial transcription of the interviews, the transcripts were reviewed multiple times to thoroughly grasp the participants' statements. Data coding occurred at two levels: (1) Open coding, which revealed potentially significant themes, and (2) axial coding, which clustered thematic connections and enabled the recognition of key motifs. This process was facilitated by analytical tools like NVivo (version number 12), which guaranteed a systematic coding approach.

All codes were subsequently compared and organized to refine the thematic categories. The analysis results were compared with the scarce existing research in related thematic fields, enabling the conclusions to be placed within a wider context. The author used a meticulous method for coding and classifying the data. To decrease subjectivity and increase the objectivity of the results, the researcher frequently reassessed the identified motifs and compared them with the original codes to ensure consistent interpretation.

3. Results

Below are the key findings that emerged from discussions, supported by quotes from the participants.

3.1. Expectations of Volunteers Regarding Access to Educational Materials on Healthy Eating

In the conducted study, the vast majority (n = 12) indicated a lack of access to educational materials on healthy eating during organized events. V2 stated, "We didn't have any materials; it wasn't even mentioned". Similar feelings were echoed by V3, who noted, "The organizers didn't provide us with any information or resources on nutrition. Do I think they should? I think it wouldn't hurt". V8 also pointed out this issue, saying, "I don't recall any educational materials. However, I think they could be useful".

Other volunteers confirmed these observations, emphasizing that the lack of access to information limited their abilities. V12 stated, "One time, one of the women felt unwell. I thought maybe she was low on sugar and suggested she eat a candy bar I had with me, but I really don't know if that was the right thing to do or if I harmed her". V5 shared similar sentiments, saying, "In my opinion, the organizers should at least inform us on a basic level about the role of nutrition so that we have at least a fundamental understanding of it". V6 added, "I understand that these are sporting events and not directly related to nutrition, but the organizers didn't show any interest at all, and they should have". Another volunteer, V16, emphasized, "I didn't receive any information. If I had materials, my knowledge would certainly be greater". V4 stated, "Generally, during the volunteering, I don't pay much attention to this and just do my job, but having any access to additional knowledge would always be valuable". V10 added, "I have never had any meetings during sporting events where healthy eating was discussed. And there are always many briefings with volunteers before the event, so there was room for that". V9 presented a similar position: "We meet so many times and share our responsibilities, but to hold some training or provide us with printed information on nutrition education, that never happened". V15 emphasized categorically: "We never received any information. I feel that the organizers do not realize how important this is". V17 agreed, saying, "I think the organizers do not understand how important educational materials on various topics are for us, not only in terms of nutrition but also comprehensive knowledge about the sports that are organized during the events we support. Without this, we cannot operate effectively".

Several volunteers (n = 4) shared their experiences related to limited access to materials. V13 said, "Having participated in volunteering for several years, I have heard something about healthy eating a few times, but it was only during meetings and not in the form of materials". V7 added, "I know it could be done better. We always said we wanted more information, but we never received a response". V11 noted, "There were a few cases where we had access to such materials, but it was definitely not regular". V14 criticized the regular lack of education, saying, "Discussions on this topic are definitely irregular and thus insufficient".

Finally, one of the volunteers (n = 1), V1, had slightly different experiences. He said, "I had the opportunity to use educational materials a few times, and I was very satisfied with that. It increased my awareness of nutrition and expanded my knowledge, which is useful in everyday life". His positive experience is an exception that seems to highlight the need for greater availability and regularity in providing materials on healthy eating by event organizers. In light of the collected opinions, it can be concluded that the research hypothesis is confirmed, and volunteers expect more care from the organizers to ensure the appropriate educational resources.

3.2. Preferences for Forms of Nutritional Education

In the conducted study, opinions were gathered regarding their preferences for forms of nutrition education. Two individuals (n = 2) emphasized that it is crucial for them that educational materials are easily accessible and practical. V2 stated, "I value forms of education that I can have on hand at all times. The easier the materials are to access, the better I can use them". A similar opinion was expressed by V14, who said, "I'm interested in short instructional videos that I can watch in my free time. Such materials are the most practical for me". Another group of volunteers (n = 3) pointed out the need for interactive and engaging forms of education. V3 said, "I like workshops where I can learn something new and immediately try it out. Theoretical approaches don't work for me". V4 emphasized, "Interactive sessions with experts make sense. When I can ask questions and discuss, I absorb knowledge much better". V6 agreed, stating, "Practical group activities would probably be the best. We learn from each other, which increases our motivation".

Further volunteers (n = 4) highlighted the importance of available online resources. V7 stated, "I appreciate the ability to use mobile apps that offer recipes and nutrition advice. It's very convenient. Of course, the organizers of sporting events don't promote them, but I think that's a mistake. I try to use the Fitatu app, although I'm probably doing it incorrectly since I've never been shown how to use it". V12 added, "Webinars are a great learning format for me. I can participate from anywhere, which is nice, and it makes me feel like I'm expanding my knowledge". V17 noted, "The availability of materials in PDF format that I can download and review at my convenience would be pleasant". This group also included V15, who added, "Practical guides in PDF format or even infographics would make sense".

Some volunteers (n = 3) also emphasized that nutrition education should be tailored to their specific needs. V16 said, "I would like nutrition education to be more personalized. I often feel that general advice doesn't fit everyone". V9 added, "Knowledge about appropriate meals before and after physical activity would be very useful for preparing adequately for tasks. When I know I'll be working physically, I will certainly prepare myself better with that knowledge". In a similar tone, V13 noted, "It would be good to have access to materials that take different activities into account. Not everyone has the same nutritional needs".

Among the volunteers, there were also individuals (n = 3) who expressed a desire to utilize traditional forms of education. V11 stated, "I believe that well-organized seminars or classes in classrooms are valuable. I just want to hear information from an expert to be sure that it is reliable". V8 added, "Some of the more formal education methods can also be effective, especially when the topic is comprehensive". V10 noted, "Maybe it would be worth combining traditional methods with modern ones to reach a broader audience".

The last two individuals (n = 2) in the group of volunteers highlighted additional aspects of nutrition education. V5 said, "Sometimes I lack materials that are tailored to current nutrition trends. I would like to know what is currently in vogue". V1 added, "It is important to me that education is dynamic and changes with new research. I'm curious how new information can influence nutritional decisions".

4. Discussion

This study was conducted based on the methodology of in-depth individual interviews. The choice of this method stems from the desire to understand not only the basic behaviors of sports volunteers in the context of their nutritional choices but also their expectations regarding nutrition education. The method enabled a detailed examination of the needs, preferences, and obstacles that volunteers encounter concerning nutrition education issues. The qualitative approach enabled the questions to be adapted flexibly to the unique experiences of the respondents, capturing subtle differences in expectations regarding nutrition education.

The results of the conducted study reveal a serious problem regarding the lack of access to educational materials on healthy nutrition among sports volunteers. The vast majority of participants indicated that event organizers did not provide them with appropriate informational resources. A significant aspect is that a lack of knowledge about healthy eating can not only affect the well-being of volunteers but also impact the effectiveness of their actions during events. According to previous research conducted by Rozmiarek [16], the majority of sports volunteers do not focus on their diet, leading to random food choices that may negatively affect their performance. The study results also indicate the necessity of nutrition education among sports volunteers and promoting the utilization of trustworthy sources of information regarding healthy eating.

In light of these findings, event organizers could enhance nutrition education through several specific strategies. One potential approach is forming partnerships with certified nutritionists to develop tailored educational materials or hold workshops focused on healthy eating habits for volunteers. Additionally, event organizers could create online resources, such as interactive platforms or mobile applications, to provide volunteers with easy access to up-to-date nutritional guidelines. These strategies could facilitate continuous learning, providing volunteers with the necessary knowledge and tools to make informed dietary choices before, during, and after sports events.

It should be noted that the lack of access to educational materials regarding nutrition can result in decisions being made based on insufficient or inaccurate information. Previous studies highlight that improper dietary decisions can result not only in poor well-being but also in an increased risk of injuries and health problems [36–40]. Organizers should be aware that nutrition education is a key element not only for volunteers but also for event participants, who may be exposed to various health situations. Having the right information about nutrition can influence the overall safety and comfort of all individuals involved in the event. Therefore, it is worth considering the introduction of training and workshops that present the basic principles of healthy eating in an accessible way to enhance the competencies of volunteers and event participants in this field.

Volunteer preferences regarding forms of education are also crucial for understanding their expectations of organizers. The study results indicate the need for diverse and interactive forms of teaching, reflecting the changing approach to adult education. Contemporary research shows that active teaching methods, such as workshops or discussion sessions, are more effective compared to traditional lectures [41,42]. Therefore, event organizers should invest in educational forms that not only engage participants but also facilitate better knowledge absorption. Offering practical experiences where volunteers can acquire new skills and knowledge interactively will contribute to increasing their motivation and involvement.

The issue of personalizing nutrition education is another key aspect that requires attention. The study results indicate the need to tailor educational materials to the specific needs of volunteers, which can be especially crucial given the variety of events they participate in. Personalizing nutrition education can contribute to increasing its effectiveness and participant satisfaction, as each form of activity has its own unique nutritional requirements. Event organizers should consider collaborating with nutrition experts to develop materials tailored to different disciplines, allowing for more precise and effective preparation of volunteers for their roles.

It is also essential to consider how the Polish cultural context may influence the applicability of these findings to other countries or settings. Poland's specific dietary customs, public health priorities, and volunteer management practices may shape volunteers' expectations and behaviors in ways that differ from those in other regions. For example, the availability of local nutritional education resources and cultural attitudes toward healthy eating may vary, potentially limiting the direct transferability of the results. Future studies should address these cultural differences to provide insights that are more universally applicable.

The final aspect to emphasize is the importance of updating educational materials in the context of the dynamic development of knowledge about nutrition. Research shows that as new discoveries and dietary trends emerge, it is crucial for educational materials to be continuously adjusted to current recommendations and standards [43]. Volunteers highlighted that they want to stay informed about the latest information, which is especially important in light of changes in nutrition science. To effectively support volunteers, event organizers should implement mechanisms for monitoring and updating materials, ensuring that they provide knowledge that is not only current but also relevant to their needs and expectations.

5. Strengths and Limitations

A strength of the conducted study was the use of individual interviews, which allowed for a detailed examination of the individual experiences and preferences of volunteers regarding nutrition education. This approach provided rich, multifaceted data that facilitated an understanding of expectations concerning access to educational materials and support forms in the context of their engagement in sports volunteering. The interviews also enabled an analysis of participants' nutritional awareness, allowing for the identification of differences in the perception of nutrition education and the obstacles they encounter in accessing information and materials on the subject.

However, this study has specific limitations that could influence the ability to generalize the findings. Firstly, the research was carried out in Poland, which may limit the relevance of the findings to a wider population of sports volunteers in other countries. Poland's cultural context, including local dietary preferences, health education systems, and attitudes toward volunteering, may affect the applicability of the results to other regions. Differences in access to nutrition education resources across countries should be considered when interpreting the study's findings. To gain a deeper understanding of the influence of various factors, such as cultural variations and levels of education, additional research involving a larger and more diverse participant group is essential.

Furthermore, the use of interviews might introduce subjectivity into the responses, especially regarding the assessment of one's own educational preferences and needs. This subjectivity could potentially limit the reliability of the findings, as respondents may not always have a clear or accurate understanding of their needs. In the future, it would be worthwhile to consider utilizing quantitative methods, such as surveys or analyses of the availability of educational materials, to gather more impartial data. Quantitative methods enable more accurate results and enable the analysis of a broader dataset, which increases the reliability of the conclusions drawn. For instance, future research could aim to measure the nutritional knowledge of a larger and more diverse group of volunteers through surveys, assessing the effectiveness of existing educational resources across different sports and cultural contexts.

Such an approach can also help identify trends and correlations that could be difficult to discern in qualitative research. The introduction of these methods could greatly improve the quality of future research on nutrition education among sports volunteers and provide more relevant and universal conclusions. A possible research question for future studies could focus on the relationship between volunteers' nutritional knowledge and their performance at events, exploring how enhanced education impacts their effectiveness and well-being.

Additionally, it is important to consider the feasibility of incorporating nutrition education into the structure of sporting events, as organizers may face budget or time constraints. While the recommendation to include nutrition education is valid, these practical limitations might affect its implementation. To address this, event organizers could explore cost-effective solutions, such as incorporating brief digital resources or collaborating with external sponsors or nutrition experts, which would allow for the dissemination of educational content without significantly increasing the logistical or financial burden. This approach would help ensure that nutrition education can be integrated into sporting events in a realistic and sustainable manner.

6. Conclusions

The results of the conducted study clearly indicate a significant gap in access to nutrition education for sports volunteers, which has a substantial impact on their performance and overall well-being during sports events. Although volunteers recognize the need to expand their knowledge about healthy eating, event organizers rarely provide them with appropriate educational materials. By enhancing nutrition education through various forms of support, such as interactive workshops or access to practical online resources, not only can volunteer engagement be increased, but it can also contribute to their better physical and mental condition.

To make a meaningful impact, event organizers could implement specific programs, such as partnering with certified nutritionists to conduct regular workshops focused on healthy eating habits or creating comprehensive online platforms where volunteers can access tailored nutritional resources. Successful examples include initiatives that provide meal plans and nutrition guides tailored to different types of events, ensuring that volunteers are well-informed about their dietary needs. A key step toward improving the working conditions for volunteers should, therefore, be the incorporation of nutritional aspects into the organization of sports events, which will allow for better utilization of their capabilities and aid in the overall success of the initiatives.

Improving volunteers' nutrition education can directly influence their energy levels, focus, and stamina during events, which are critical factors in ensuring their efficiency and ability to perform assigned tasks effectively. Well-nourished volunteers are less likely to experience fatigue, dehydration, or lack of concentration, which in turn reduces the likelihood of mistakes or underperformance. As a result, their enhanced physical and mental condition can improve the overall coordination and flow of the event, contributing to its success by minimizing disruptions, ensuring smooth operations, and fostering a positive experience for both participants and organizers. Additionally, well-informed volunteers can act as ambassadors for healthy living, further reinforcing the event's reputation and its alignment with promoting wellness.

Funding: This research received no external funding.

Institutional Review Board Statement: This research carried out with sports volunteers followed the principles outlined in the Declaration of Helsinki despite not needing approval from an Ethics Committee. This study utilized in-depth interviews, which did not impact participants' health or involve any experimental procedures. All participants gave informed consent, ensuring complete respect for their autonomy and privacy. Furthermore, participants' personal information was safeguarded in accordance with current privacy regulations, and the results analysis relied on anonymous data, fully adhering to confidentiality and participant protection requirements.

Informed Consent Statement: Informed consent was obtained from all subjects involved in the study.

Data Availability Statement: The original contributions presented in the study are included in the article; further inquiries can be directed to the corresponding author.

Conflicts of Interest: The author declares no conflicts of interest.

References

1. Baum, T.G.; Lockstone, L. Volunteers and Mega Sporting Events: Developing a Research Framework. *Int. J. Event Manag. Res.* **2007**, *3*, 29–41.
2. Okada, A.; Ishida, Y.; Yamauchi, N.; Grönlund, H.; Zhang, C.; Krasnopolskaya, I. Episodic Volunteering in Sport Events: A Seven-Country Analysis. *Voluntas* **2021**, *33*, 459–471. [CrossRef] [PubMed]
3. Ringuet-Riot, C.; Cuskelly, G.; Auld, C.; Zakus, D.H. Volunteer Roles, Involvement and Commitment in Voluntary Sport Organizations: Evidence of Core and Peripheral Volunteers. In *Sport and the Communities*; Routledge: New York, NY, USA, 2016; pp. 116–133.

4. Schulz, J.; Nichols, G.; Auld, C. Issues in the Management of Voluntary Sport Organizations and Volunteers. In *Routledge Handbook of Sports Development*; Routledge: Abingdon, UK, 2010; pp. 437–450.
5. Wicker, P. Volunteerism and Volunteer Management in Sport. *Sport Manag. Rev.* **2017**, *20*, 325–337. [CrossRef]
6. Jenner, S.L.; Buckley, G.L.; Belski, R.; Devlin, B.L.; Forsyth, A.K. Dietary Intakes of Professional and Semi-Professional Team Sport Athletes Do Not Meet Sport Nutrition Recommendations—A Systematic Literature Review. *Nutrients* **2019**, *11*, 1160. [CrossRef]
7. Vázquez-Espino, K.; Rodas-Font, G.; Farran-Codina, A. Sport Nutrition Knowledge, Attitudes, Sources of Information, and Dietary Habits of Sport-Team Athletes. *Nutrients* **2022**, *14*, 1345. [CrossRef]
8. Miškulin, I.; Šašvari, A.; Dumić, A.; Bilić-Kirin, V.; Špiranović, Ž.; Pavlović, N.; Miškulin, M. The general nutrition knowledge of professional athletes. *Hrana U Zdr. I Boles. Znan.-Stručni Časopis Za Nutr. I Dijetetiku* **2019**, *8*, 25–32.
9. Cotugna, N.; Vickery, C.E.; McBee, S. Sports nutrition for young athletes. *J. Sch. Nurs.* **2005**, *21*, 323–328. [CrossRef]
10. Przewłócka, K.; Korewo-Labelle, D.; Berezka, P.; Karnia, M.J.; Kaczor, J.J. Current Aspects of Selected Factors to Modulate Brain Health and Sports Performance in Athletes. *Nutrients* **2024**, *16*, 1842. [CrossRef]
11. Economos, C.D.; Bortz, S.S.; Nelson, M.E. Nutritional Practices of Elite Athletes: Practical Recommendations. *Sports Med.* **1993**, *16*, 381–399. [CrossRef]
12. Maughan, R. The Athlete's Diet: Nutritional Goals and Dietary Strategies. *Proc. Nutr. Soc.* **2002**, *61*, 87–96. [CrossRef]
13. Castillo, M.; Lozano-Casanova, M.; Sospedra, I.; Norte, A.; Gutiérrez-Hervás, A.; Martínez-Sanz, J.M. Energy and Macronutrients Intake in Indoor Sport Team Athletes: Systematic Review. *Nutrients* **2022**, *14*, 4755. [CrossRef] [PubMed]
14. O'Brien, L.; Townsend, M.; Ebden, M. 'Doing something positive': Volunteers' experiences of the well-being benefits derived from practical conservation activities in nature. *Volunt. Int. J. Volunt. Nonprofit Organ.* **2010**, *21*, 525–545. [CrossRef]
15. Schmidt, M.A. *Tired of Being Tired: Overcoming Chronic Fatigue and Low Vitality*; Frog Books: Berkeley, CA, USA, 1995.
16. Rozmiarek, M. The Role of Nutrition in Maintaining the Health and Physical Condition of Sports Volunteers. *Nutrients* **2024**, *16*, 3336. [CrossRef] [PubMed]
17. Cline, R.J.; Haynes, K.M. Consumer Health Information Seeking on the Internet: The State of the Art. *Health Educ. Res.* **2001**, *16*, 671–692. [CrossRef]
18. Eysenbach, G.; Powell, J.; Kuss, O.; Sa, E.R. Empirical Studies Assessing the Quality of Health Information for Consumers on the World Wide Web: A Systematic Review. *JAMA* **2002**, *287*, 2691–2700. [CrossRef]
19. Vasconcelos, C.; Costa, R.L.D.; Dias, Á.L.; Pereira, L.; Santos, J.P. Online Influencers: Healthy Food or Fake News. *Int. J. Internet Mark. Advert.* **2021**, *15*, 149–175. [CrossRef]
20. Castellini, G.; Savarese, M.; Graffigna, G. Online Fake News about Food. Self-Evaluation, Social Influence, and the Stages of Change Moderation. *Int. J. Environ. Res. Public Health* **2021**, *18*, 2934. [CrossRef]
21. Vettori, V.; Lorini, C.; Milani, C.; Bonaccorsi, G. Towards the Implementation of a Conceptual Framework of Food and Nutrition Literacy: Providing Healthy Eating for the Population. *Int. J. Environ. Res. Public Health* **2019**, *16*, 5041. [CrossRef]
22. Höijer, K.; Lindö, C.; Mustafa, A.; Nyberg, M.; Olsson, V.; Rothenberg, E.; Sepp, H.; Wendin, K. Health and Sustainability in Public Meals—An Explorative Review. *Int. J. Environ. Res. Public Health* **2020**, *17*, 621. [CrossRef]
23. Johnston, M.E.; Twynam, G.D.; Farrell, J.M. Motivation and Satisfaction of Event Volunteers for a Major Youth Organization. *Leis. Loisir* **1999**, *24*, 161–177. [CrossRef]
24. Bang, H.; Chelladurai, P. Motivation and Satisfaction in Volunteering for 2002 World Cup in Korea. In Proceedings of the Conference of the North American Society for Sport Management, Ithaca, NY, USA, 30 May–5 June 2003.
25. Reeser, J.C.; Berg, R.L.; Rhea, D.; Willick, S. Motivation and Satisfaction Among Polyclinic Volunteers at the 2002 Winter Olympic and Paralympic Games. *Br. J. Sports Med.* **2005**, *39*, e20. [CrossRef] [PubMed]
26. Bang, H.; Ross, S.D. Volunteer Motivation and Satisfaction. *J. Venue Event Manag.* **2009**, *1*, 61–77.
27. Love, A.; Hardin, R.; Koo, W.; Morse, A.L. Effects of Motives on Satisfaction and Behavioral Intentions of Volunteers at a PGA Tour Event. *Int. J. Sport Manag.* **2011**, *12*, 86–101. [CrossRef]
28. Wang, C.; Wu, X. Volunteers' Motivation, Satisfaction, and Management in Large-Scale Events: An Empirical Test from the 2010 Shanghai World Expo. *Voluntas Int. J. Volunt. Nonprofit Organ.* **2014**, *25*, 754–771. [CrossRef]
29. Ma, X.; Draper, J. Motivation and Satisfaction of Marathon Volunteers: How Important Is Volunteers' Level of Running Experience? *J. Conv. Event Tour.* **2017**, *18*, 41–59. [CrossRef]
30. Vetitnev, A.; Bobina, N.; Terwiel, F.A. The Influence of Host Volunteer Motivation on Satisfaction and Attitudes Toward Sochi 2014 Olympic Games. *Event Manag.* **2018**, *22*, 333–352. [CrossRef]
31. Milena, Z.R.; Dainora, G.; Alin, S. Qualitative Research Methods: A Comparison Between Focus-Group And In-Depth Interview. *Ann. Univ. Oradea Econ. Sci.* **2008**, *4*, 1279–1283.
32. Fontana, A.; Frey, J.H. The interview. From structured questions to negotiated text. In *Handbook of Qualitative Research*, 2nd ed.; Lincoln, Y.S., Denzin, N.K., Eds.; Sage: Thousand Oaks, CA, USA, 2000; pp. 645–672.
33. Kaplowitz, M.D. Statistical analysis of sensitive topics in group and individual interviews. *Qual. Quant.* **2000**, *34*, 419–431. [CrossRef]
34. Hennink, M.; Kaiser, B.N. Sample Sizes for Saturation in Qualitative Research: A Systematic Review of Empirical Tests. *Soc. Sci. Med.* **2022**, *292*, 114523. [CrossRef]
35. Boddy, C.R. Sample Size for Qualitative Research. *Qual. Mark. Res.* **2016**, *19*, 426–432. [CrossRef]
36. Robbins, J. *Diet for a New America: How Your Food Choices Affect Your Health*; HJ Kramer: Tiburon, CA, USA, 2012.

37. Carlisle, S.; Hanlon, P. Connecting Food, Well-being and Environmental Sustainability: Towards an Integrative Public Health Nutrition. *Crit. Public Health* **2014**, *24*, 405–417. [CrossRef]
38. Lane, M.M.; Gamage, E.; Travica, N.; Dissanayaka, T.; Ashtree, D.N.; Gauci, S.; Lotfaliany, M.; O'Neil, A.; Jacka, F.N.; Marx, W. Ultra-Processed Food Consumption and Mental Health: A Systematic Review and Meta-Analysis of Observational Studies. *Nutrients* **2022**, *14*, 2568. [CrossRef] [PubMed]
39. Grajek, M.; Krupa-Kotara, K.; Białek-Dratwa, A.; Sobczyk, K.; Grot, M.; Kowalski, O.; Staśkiewicz, W. Nutrition and Mental Health: A Review of Current Knowledge About the Impact of Diet on Mental Health. *Front. Nutr.* **2022**, *9*, 943998. [CrossRef] [PubMed]
40. Gheonea, T.C.; Oancea, C.-N.; Mititelu, M.; Lupu, E.C.; Ioniță-Mîndrican, C.-B.; Rogoveanu, I. Nutrition and Mental Well-being: Exploring Connections and Holistic Approaches. *J. Clin. Med.* **2023**, *12*, 7180. [CrossRef]
41. Preszler, R.W. Replacing Lecture with Peer-Led Workshops Improves Student Learning. *CBE—Life Sci. Educ.* **2009**, *8*, 182–192. [CrossRef]
42. Lenz, P.H.; McCallister, J.W.; Luks, A.M.; Le, T.T.; Fessler, H.E. Practical Strategies for Effective Lectures. *Ann. Am. Thorac. Soc.* **2015**, *12*, 561–566. [CrossRef]
43. Contento, I.R. *Nutrition Education: Linking Research, Theory, and Practice*; Jones & Bartlett Publishers: Burlington, MA, USA, 2016.

Disclaimer/Publisher's Note: The statements, opinions and data contained in all publications are solely those of the individual author(s) and contributor(s) and not of MDPI and/or the editor(s). MDPI and/or the editor(s) disclaim responsibility for any injury to people or property resulting from any ideas, methods, instructions or products referred to in the content.

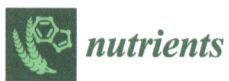 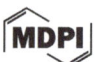

Article

Mediterranean Food Pattern Adherence in a Female-Dominated Sample of Health and Social Sciences University Students: Analysis from a Perspective of Sustainability

Leandro Oliveira [1,*], Ariana Saraiva [2], Maria João Lima [3], Edite Teixeira-Lemos [3], Jwaher Haji Alhaji [4], Conrado Carrascosa [5] and António Raposo [1,*]

[1] CBIOS (Research Center for Biosciences and Health Technologies), Universidade Lusófona de Humanidades e Tecnologias, Campo Grande 376, 1749-024 Lisboa, Portugal
[2] Research in Veterinary Medicine (I-MVET), Faculty of Veterinary Medicine, Lisbon University Centre, Lusófona University, Campo Grande 376, 1749-024 Lisboa, Portugal; ariana.saraiva@ulusofona.pt
[3] CERNAS Research Centre, Polytechnic University of Viseu, 3504-510 Viseu, Portugal; mjoaolima@esav.ipv.pt (M.J.L.); etlemos3@gmail.com (E.T.-L.)
[4] Department of Health Sciences, College of Applied Studies and Community Service, King Saud University, P.O. Box 2455, Riyadh 11451, Saudi Arabia; jalhejjy@ksu.edu.sa
[5] Department of Animal Pathology and Production, Bromatology and Food Technology, Faculty of Veterinary, Universidad de Las Palmas de Gran Canaria, Trasmontaña s/n, 35413 Arucas, Spain; conrado.carrascosa@ulpgc.es
* Correspondence: leandroliveira.nut@gmail.com (L.O.); antonio.raposo@ulusofona.pt (A.R.)

Abstract: Background/Objectives: The goal of this pilot study is to evaluate adherence to the Mediterranean Food Pattern (MFP) in a self-selected sample of university students, addressing a perspective of food sustainability. In addition, it seeks to relate adherence to MFP with sociodemographic characteristics and nutritional status. Methods: This is a cross-sectional pilot study whose data collection was carried out by an online questionnaire between January and April 2023. Results: Two hundred and forty-eight students participated—most of them were female (78.2%), had a median of 22 (20; 30) years, resided in the central region of Portugal (42.3%), and were pursuing a degree (73.4%) in a public higher education institution (66.5%). The prevalence of overweight (overweight and obesity) found was 33.1%. Females predominantly used olive oil as their main source of fat (95.9%, $p = 0.009$) and had a higher consumption of sugary drinks (81.4%, $p = 0.004$) compared to males, who reported usage rates of 85.2% and 63.0%, The median score of the Mediterranean Diet Adherence Screener was 7 points, presented with an interquartile range (Q1: 6, Q3: 8), indicating moderate adherence. The analysis showed no differences between the sexes ($p = 0.087$). There was also a negative correlation between adherence to the MFP and the body mass index ($p = 0.007$; r = −0.171). In addition, adherence to the MFP was associated with the area of study and the course attended, with students in health-related fields showing higher adherence. Conclusions: These findings underscore the necessity for targeted interventions aimed at promoting adherence to the MFP among university students, which could contribute to improved health outcomes and enhanced environmental sustainability.

Keywords: food sustainability; mediterranean diet; sustainable diets; university students

Citation: Oliveira, L.; Saraiva, A.; Lima, M.J.; Teixeira-Lemos, E.; Alhaji, J.H.; Carrascosa, C.; Raposo, A. Mediterranean Food Pattern Adherence in a Female-Dominated Sample of Health and Social Sciences University Students: Analysis from a Perspective of Sustainability. *Nutrients* 2024, *16*, 3886. https://doi.org/10.3390/nu16223886

Received: 13 October 2024
Revised: 28 October 2024
Accepted: 12 November 2024
Published: 14 November 2024

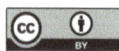

Copyright: © 2024 by the authors. Licensee MDPI, Basel, Switzerland. This article is an open access article distributed under the terms and conditions of the Creative Commons Attribution (CC BY) license (https://creativecommons.org/licenses/by/4.0/).

1. Introduction

Food sustainability refers to the ability to meet current dietary needs without compromising the ability of future generations to meet theirs. It involves practices that conserve natural resources, reduce waste, and prioritize foods with a lower environmental impact. This is an increasing concern in public health, as it aims to ensure the availability of healthy foods for all while protecting the environment [1]. The processes of food production, processing, distribution, and consumption have implications for both human health and the environment. Moreover, food production inevitably contributes to harmful environmental effects, particularly through factors related to climate, land use, water consumption, and gas emissions. Greenhouse gasses (GHGs) such as carbon dioxide (CO_2), methane (CH_4), and nitrous oxide (N_2O) are known contributors to global warming [2].

In this context, the Mediterranean Food Pattern (MFP) can play a critical role in mitigating climate change effects, as it is recognized as a dietary model that supports health, environmental sustainability, sociocultural values, and economic stability [3]. The MFP is commonly adhered to by populations living in countries bordering the Mediterranean Sea or those influenced by the region. In the 1960s, Ancel Keys first defined the MFP as a low-fat diet rich in vegetable oils, based on the traditional dietary habits of the 20th century in places such as Crete, various regions of Greece, and southern Italy. This diet is characterized by a high consumption of plant-based foods such as cereals, fruits, vegetables, nuts, seeds, and olives. Additionally, it includes a moderate to high consumption of fish and seafood, a moderate intake of eggs, poultry, and dairy products (such as cheese, milk, and yogurt), and a low consumption of red meat. Extra virgin olive oil is the primary source of added fat in this dietary pattern [1,4]. The MFP is continuously evolving, with various adaptations that reflect the diverse food cultures of the Mediterranean region.

According to the National Food and Physical Activity Survey (IAN-AF 2015–2016) [5], there has been a notable deviation from the MFP among the Portuguese population. This shift is reflected in the increased consumption of meat, fish, eggs, dairy products, and cereals, while the intake of vegetables and legumes has declined. Additionally, ultra-processed foods such as cookies, cakes, sweets, salty snacks, pizza, alcoholic beverages, and non-alcoholic beverages (excluding water) now contribute significantly to the diet, accounting for 29% of total consumption [5]. These dietary changes not only deviate from the health-promoting characteristics of the MFP but also pose a challenge to food sustainability. An increased consumption of resource-intensive foods like meat, coupled with a reduced intake of plant-based foods, significantly enlarges the environmental footprint of the Portuguese diet, further straining natural resources and contributing to unsustainable food systems.

A 2020 report from the General Health Directorate [6] revealed that only 26% of the Portuguese population closely adheres to the MFP, with adherence rates even lower among university students [7,8]. The reduced adherence to the MFP correlates with increased dietary practices that demand more natural resources and contribute to environmental degradation. A recent study [8] involving higher education students and researchers in Portugal found that only 8.2% showed high adherence to the MFP. Given the MFP's recognition for its lower environmental impact compared to other dietary patterns, assessing adherence to the MFP provides insights into the sustainability of food choices among university students. As the MFP is based on the consumption of plant-based foods and limits the intake of resource-intensive foods, a decrease in adherence directly impacts both health outcomes and environmental sustainability.

Entering higher education represents a critical life transition, during which students are exposed to new environments, stress, and often changes in socioeconomic conditions [9]. These factors can lead to the adoption of less healthy and less sustainable eating habits, such as an increased consumption of foods high in sugar, fat, and salt, and a decreased consumption of vegetables [9]. These behaviors further deviate from the MFP and contribute to less sustainable dietary practices.

Therefore, the aim of this pilot study is to evaluate the adherence to the MFP among a sample of university students, with a particular focus on sustainability. By analyzing MFP adherence through the lens of sustainability, the study provides a comprehensive understanding of the relationship between dietary patterns, sociodemographic characteristics, and nutritional status. This pilot study also explores how sociodemographic factors, such as gender, age, and educational background, influence both adherence to the MFP and the broader implications for food sustainability.

Based on the existing literature regarding the relationship between adherence to the MFP, sociodemographic factors, and nutritional status, this study formulates the following hypotheses:

H1: *There are significant differences in the consumption of foods associated with the Mediterranean Food Pattern among university students based on sociodemographic factors.*

H2: *Students enrolled in non-health-related courses exhibit lower adherence to the MFP compared to students in health-related fields.*

H3: *Students with a higher Body Mass Index (BMI) are likely to demonstrate a lower adherence to the MFP.*

H4: *High adherence to the Mediterranean Food Pattern is associated with lower BMI among university students.*

2. Materials and Methods

2.1. Study Design and Data Collection

This is a cross-sectional pilot study targeting higher education students in Portugal. Data collection took place between January and April 2023, a period chosen to avoid potential seasonal biases in eating habits. This timeframe was selected as it spans across different months, capturing dietary behaviors during both winter and early spring. This ensures a more representative snapshot of students' food consumption patterns, minimizing the impact of seasonal variations, such as holiday-specific dietary changes or shifts in food availability. An email was distributed to 50 higher education institutions in Portugal, inviting them to share the questionnaire with their students. The distribution request was made through general communication channels, either by sending the survey request to the institution's main contact email or, when applicable, to the communication office. Only 5 of the 50 institutions contacted agreed to disseminate the questionnaire among their students. Additionally, five institutions responded that they do not disseminate external surveys, while the remaining institutions did not provide any response.

The inclusion criteria for this study were being a higher education student in Portugal and being over 18 years old. Aside from not consenting to participate in the study, no exclusion criteria were established. Data collection was conducted using an online questionnaire through the Google Forms® platform, with all data being self-reported. The questionnaire consisted of four sections: sociodemographic characterization (gender, age, course, and institution attended, course area, anthropometric data), adherence to the MFP, and e-health literacy.

Responses were classified as invalid if participants submitted incomplete questionnaires, particularly if key sections were left unanswered.)

Only the sections related to sociodemographic characterization and adherence to the MFP will be analyzed in this study.

The BMI was calculated using the equation: BMI = weight (kg)/height^2 (m), utilizing the self-reported weight and height of the participants [10]. The BMI values were then classified according to the World Health Organization's criteria [11].

Adherence to the Mediterranean Food Pattern was assessed using the Mediterranean Diet Adherence Screener (MEDAS) tool [12], which has been validated for the Portuguese population [13]. This tool comprises 14 questions regarding the consumption or frequency of consumption of foods characteristic of the Mediterranean diet. The final score is obtained by summing the scores of all responses, with a possible range of 0 to 14. Adherence is classified as low ($\leq$5 points), moderate (6 to 9 points), or high ($\geq$10 points) [12,13].

The classification of responses as valid or invalid was based on predefined criteria. A response was deemed invalid if it was incomplete or contained inconsistent information. For example, responses that provided descriptions of foods instead of the requested number of portions were categorized as invalid. The questionnaire was intentionally designed to be straightforward and focused, which helped reduce the likelihood of collecting irrelevant or incomplete data. Additionally, it incorporated a mandatory response mechanism that alerted participants if they attempted to submit the survey without answering all required questions.

While the questionnaire did not include a formal attention-check mechanism, its logical structure and consistency checks facilitated the effective identification and filtering of invalid samples.

2.2. Ethical Considerations

This study was conducted in accordance with the ethical standards outlined in the 1964 Declaration of Helsinki and its subsequent comparable ethical guidelines [14]. All relevant information was thoroughly communicated to the study participants. They received informed consent forms detailing the study's purpose and procedures. Participants were also assured of the confidentiality of their data and informed that the study received approval from the Ethics Commission of the School of Health Sciences and Technologies (P10-22, 7 December 2022).

2.3. Statistical Analysis

The statistical analysis was conducted using the Statistical Package for the Social Sciences (SPSS), version 26.0, for Windows. Descriptive statistics were used to provide a comprehensive overview of the participants' sociodemographic characteristics and nutritional status. These analyses included calculating means, median, and interquartile range (Q1, Q3), and determining the absolute (n) and relative (%) frequencies.

The normality of the distribution of quantitative variables was assessed using the Shapiro–Wilk test, as it is more sensitive to deviations from normality, especially in smaller sample sizes.

Inferential statistical methods were applied to examine the association between variables. Fisher's exact test or the chi-square test was used to assess the independence between pairs of categorical variables, allowing for the evaluation of associations within the data. The Mann–Whitney U Test or Kruskal–Wallis Test was employed to compare median ranks between independent samples when the variables were continuous and did not follow a normal distribution. Additionally, the Spearman Correlation Coefficient (r) was utilized to evaluate the strength and direction of the linear relationship between pairs of continuous variables.

To evaluate the factors associated with adherence to the MFP, a multinomial logistic regression analysis was conducted. The dependent variable was categorized into three groups: low, moderate, and high adherence to the MFP. The independent variables included the following: sex, area of residence, type of higher education institution, undergoing course, and area of course. The covariables included BMI, and age. The fit of the final model was assessed using the log-likelihood statistic. The overall significance of the model was evaluated through the chi-square test, which compared the log-likelihood of the final model against a null model. Additionally, Pseudo R^2 values (Cox and Snell, Nagelkerke, and McFadden) were calculated to evaluate the explanatory power of the model. The results were reported as odds ratios (Exp(B)) with 95% confidence intervals to provide insight into the effects of the independent variables on the likelihood of belonging to each adherence category.

The criterion for rejecting the null hypothesis was set at $p < 0.05$. Therefore, when the *p*-value was less than 0.05, the result was considered statistically significant, indicating a meaningful association or difference between the variables under analysis. These methodologies align with those applied in similar recent studies that assessed the same target population, ensuring the robustness and reliability of the findings [15,16].

3. Results

Among the five universities that agreed to collaborate, a total of 257 questionnaires were collected. However, nine of these were excluded due to invalid responses, resulting in a final sample comprising 248 participants.

The sociodemographic characteristics of these participants are summarized in Table 1. The majority of participants were female (78.2%), with a median age of 22 years (20; 30). Most participants resided in the Centro region of Portugal (42.3%), were enrolled in undergraduate degree programs (73.4%), and attended public higher education institutions (66.5%). The majority of participants are from health-related courses (39.1%), followed by those from social sciences and humanities (22.6%), exact and life sciences (13.7%), engineering and architecture (8.9%), and the arts (4.8%). Additionally, 10.9% of respondents either did not specify their course area or belong to unspecified fields. The prevalence of overweight (including pre-obesity and obesity) among the sample was 33.1%.

Table 1. The sociodemographic characterization of the respondents (n = 248).

	n (%)		n (%)
Sex		Area of the course	
Female	194 (78.2)	Health	97 (39.1)
Male	54 (21.8)	Exact and life sciences	34 (13.7)
Age		Engineering and Architecture	22 (8.9)
Median (P25; P75)	22 (20; 30)	Social Sciences and Humanities	56 (22.6)
Area of residence		Arts	12 (4.8)
North	41 (16.5)	Unknown or unspecified	27 (10.9)
Center	105 (42.3)	Type of Higher Education Institution	
Lisbon Metropolitan Area	62 (25.0)	Public-State	165 (66.5)
Alentejo	9 (3.6)	Public-Non-state	5 (2.0)
Algarve	5 (2.0)	Private	78 (31.5)
Autonomous Region of the Azores	24 (9.7)	Nutritional state [a]	
Autonomous Region of Madeira	2 (0.8)	Low weight	16 (6.5)
Undergoing course		Normal weight	150 (60.5)
Professional Superior Technical Course	6 (2.4)	Pre-obesity	58 (23.4)
Graduation	182 (73.4)	Obesity	24 (9.7)
Master or Integrated Master	51 (20.6)		
Doctorate	6 (2.4)		
Postgraduate	3 (1.2)		

[a] Calculated through the body mass index and classified according to the criteria of the World Health Organization [11].

In terms of adherence to the MFP (see Table 2), the majority of participants reported using olive oil as their primary cooking fat (93.5%), with 77.4% consuming fewer than one sugary or carbonated drink per day and 64.5% eating pastry products or sweets less than three times a week. Additionally, 74.2% preferred poultry or rabbit over red meats, and around 90% consumed two or more servings of vegetables, pasta, or rice at least twice weekly.

However, the adherence was lower in other areas: only 16.9% consumed three or more portions of oilseeds weekly, and 23.8% had less than one portion of red or processed meat per day. Moreover, 25.4% reported consuming fewer than four tablespoons of olive oil daily, 31.0% had fewer than three pieces of fruit daily, 39.9% consumed less than three portions of fish or seafood weekly, and 40.3% ate fewer than two portions of vegetables daily. These findings confirmed H1, highlighting significant sociodemographic differences in consumption patterns related to the MFP. Females were more likely to use olive oil as their primary fat source ($p = 0.009$) but also consumed sugary drinks more frequently ($p = 0.004$). Furthermore, students in health-related fields demonstrated better adherence to the MFP compared to their peers in non-health-related courses ($p = 0.001$).

Table 2. Adherence to the Mediterranean Food Pattern according to the MEDAS and sex comparison ($n = 248$).

Mediterranean Diet Adherence Screener	Criteria for 1 Point	Total n (%)		Female n (%)		Male n (%)		p
		0 Points	1 Point	0 Points	1 Point	0 Points	1 Point	
1. Do you use olive oil as the main cooking fat?	Yes	16 (6.5)	232 (93.5)	8 (4.1)	186 (95.9)	8 (14.8)	46 (85.2)	0.009 *a
2. How much olive oil do you consume in one day (including use for frying, seasoning, salads, meals away from home, etc....)?	≥4 tablespoons	185 (74.6)	63 (25.4)	146 (75.3)	48 (24.7)	39 (72.2)	15 (27.8)	0.650 b
3. How many portions of vegetable products do you consume per day?	≥2	148 (59.7)	100 (40.3)	114 (58.8)	80 (41.2)	34 (63.0)	20 (37.0)	0.578 b
4. How many fruit pieces (including natural fruit juices) do you consume a day?	≥3	171 (69.0)	77 (31.0)	139 (71.6)	55 (28.4)	32 (59.3)	22 (40.7)	0.082 b
5. How many portions of red meat, hamburger or meat products (ham, sausage, etc....) do you consume a day?	<1	189 (76.2)	59 (23.8)	144 (74.2)	50 (25.8)	45 (83.3)	9 (16.7)	0.165 b
6. How many portions of butter, margarine or cream do you consume per day?	<1	139 (56.0)	109 (44.0)	105 (54.1)	89 (45.9)	34 (63.0)	20 (37.0)	0.247 b
7. How many sugary or carbonated drinks do you consume a day?	<1	56 (22.6)	192 (77.4)	36 (18.6)	158 (81.4)	20 (37.0)	34 (63.0)	0.004 *b
8. How many glasses of wine do you drink a week?	≥7 cups	242 (97.6)	6 (2.4)	191 (98.5)	3 (1.5)	51 (94.4)	3 (5.6)	0.119 a
9. How many portions of pulses do you consume per week?	≥3	133 (53.6)	115 (46.4)	103 (53.1)	91 (46.9)	30 (55.6)	24 (44.4)	0.748 b
10. How many portions of fish or seafood do you consume per week?	≥3	149 (60.1)	99 (39.9)	116 (59.8)	78 (40.2)	33 (61.1)	21 (38.9)	0.861 b
11. How many times a week do you consume pastry products or commercial sweets (not homemade), such as cakes, cookies?	<3	88 (35.5)	160 (64.5)	67 (34.5)	127 (65.5)	21 (38.9)	33 (61.1)	0.554 b
12. How many portions of oilseeds (walnuts, almonds, including peanuts) do you consume per week?	≥3	206 (83.1)	42 (16.9)	162 (83.5)	32 (16.5)	44 (81.5)	10 (18.5)	0.726 b
13. Do you prefer to consume chicken, turkey, or rabbit instead of cow, pork, hamburger, or sausage?	Yes	64 (25.8)	184 (74.2)	46 (23.7)	148 (76.3)	18 (33.3)	36 (66.7)	0.153 b
14. How many times a week do you consume vegetables, pasta, rice, or other dishes made with a braised (tomato, onion, leeks or garlic and olive oil)?	≥2	22 (8.9)	228 (91.1)	15 (7.7)	179 (92.3)	7 (13.0)	47 (87.0)	0.277 a
Total Score-Median (P25; P75)	--------	7 (6; 8)		7 (6; 8)		6 (5; 8)		0.087 c

* $p < 0.05$; [a] Fisher's exact test; [b] chi-square test; [c] Mann–Whitney test.

Another factor negatively influencing adherence to the MFP is that 97.6% of participants reported consuming fewer than seven glasses of wine per week. Analysis indicated that females were more likely than males to use olive oil as their primary fat source ($p = 0.009$) and to consume more sugary drinks ($p = 0.004$). The median MEDAS score was 7 (Q1: 6; Q3: 8), reflecting moderate adherence, with no significant differences between genders (see Table 3). The results supported H2, as students enrolled in non-health-related courses demonstrated significantly lower adherence to the MFP compared to those in health-related fields ($p = 0.001$). Additionally, a significant negative correlation was found between adherence to the MFP and BMI ($r = -0.171$; $p = 0.007$), providing partial support for H3, since students with higher BMI were generally less likely to adhere to the MFP. This correlation further supports H4, as those with higher adherence to the MFP typically had lower BMI values.

Table 3. Relationship between adherence to the Mediterranean Food Pattern according to the MEDAS and sociodemographic characteristics ($n = 248$).

	Adherence to the Mediterranean Dietary Pattern			p
	Low	Moderate	High	
Sex				
Female	42 (21.6)	138 (71.1)	14 (7.2)	0.087 [a]
Male	19 (35.2)	33 (61.1)	2 (3.7)	
Area of residence				
North	14 (34.1)	24 (58.5)	3 (7.3)	0.337 [b]
Center	18 (17.1)	79 (75.2)	8 (7.6)	
South	19 (25.0)	53 (69.7)	4 (5.3)	
Islands (Azores and Madeira)	10 (38.5)	15 (57.7)	1 (3.8)	
Undergoing course				
Professional Superior Technical Course or Graduation	51 (27.1)	126 (67.0)	11 (5.9)	0.103 [a]
Integrated Masters or Postgraduation	10 (16.7)	45 (75.0)	5 (8.3)	
Area of the course				
Health	13 (13.4)	75 (77.3)	9 (9.3)	0.001 *[a]
Non-health	48 (31.8)	96 (63.6)	7 (4.6)	
Type of Higher Education Institution				
Public	44 (26.7)	110 (66.7)	11 (6.7)	0.212 [a]
Private	17 (20.5)	61 (73.5)	5 (6.0)	
Nutritional state				
Low weight/normal weight	36 (21.7)	118 (71.1)	12 (7.2)	0.007 *[c]
Overweight (pre-obesity and obesity)	25 (30.5)	53 (64.6)	4 (4.9)	$r: -0.171$
Age	---------------------------------------			0.201 [c] $r: 0.081$
Total	61 (24.6)	171 (69.0)	16 (6.5)	-----

* $p < 0.05$; [a] Mann–Whitney test; [b] Kruskal–Wallis test; [c] Spearman Correlation.

Note: Statistical tests considered sociodemographic characteristics (categorical variables) versus the MEDAS (continuous variables). Age and nutritional status (body mass index) were considered continuous variables.

The multinomial logistic regression analysis was conducted to evaluate the factors associated with the adherence to the MFP. The final model demonstrated a log-likelihood of -344.979, yielding a chi-square statistic of 40.983 with a $p < 0.002$, indicating that the model fits the data significantly well. The Pseudo R^2 values were assessed as follows: Cox and Snell (0.152), Nagelkerke (0.193), and McFadden (0.106), suggesting a moderate explanatory power of the model in describing the adherence to the MFP.

Table 4 presents the coefficients from the multinomial logistic regression, analyzing factors associated with low and moderate adherence to the MFP in comparison to high adherence.

Table 4. Multinomial logistic regression, analyzing factors associated with low and moderate adherence to the MFP in comparison to high adherence.

Adherence to the Mediterranean Dietary Pattern Classes	B	Standard Error	Wald	df	p *	Exp(B)	95% Confidence Interval for Exp(B)	
							Lower Limit	Upper Limit
Low Adherence to the Mediterranean dietary pattern								
Intercept	−2.055	2.227	0.851	1	0.356			
BMI	0.145	0.079	3.397	1	0.065	1.157	0.991	1.350
Age	−0.063	0.037	2.834	1	0.092	0.939	0.872	1.010
Sex (Male)	0.768	0.874	0.771	1	0.380	2.155	0.388	11.952
Area of residence								
Autonomous Region of the Azores/Madeira	0.113	1.308	0.007	1	0.931	1.120	0.086	14.546
North	0.292	0.998	0.086	1	0.770	1.339	0.189	9.477
Center	−1.010	0.807	1.565	1	0.211	0.364	0.075	1.773
Type of Higher Education Institution								
Private	0.203	0.759	0.071	1	0.789	1.225	0.277	5.428
Area of the course								
Non-Health	1.858	0.694	7.171	1	0.007 *	6.408	1.645	24.957
Undergoing course								
Professional Superior Technical Course/Graduation	0.680	0.769	0.783	1	0.376	1.974	0.437	8.912
Moderate Adherence to the Mediterranean dietary pattern								
Intercept	0.017	2.015	0.000	1	0.993			
BMI	0.079	0.074	1.158	1	0.282	1.083	0.937	1.251
Age	−0.002	0.032	0.002	1	0.962	0.998	0.938	1.062
Sex (Male)	0.203	0.831	0.059	1	0.807	1.225	0.240	6.242
Area of residence								
Autonomous Region of the Azores/Madeira	−0.042	1.251	0.001	1	0.974	0.959	0.083	11.148
North	−0.132	0.932	0.020	1	0.888	0.877	0.141	5.443
Center	−0.280	0.728	0.148	1	0.700	0.755	0.181	3.145
Type of Higher Education Institution								
Private	0.359	0.689	0.271	1	0.603	1.432	0.371	5.524
Area of the course								
Non-Health	0.631	0.617	1.047	1	0.306	1.880	0.561	6.300
Undergoing course								
Professional Superior Technical Course/Graduation	0.359	0.672	0.285	1	0.593	1.432	0.384	5.344

* $p < 0.05$.

Reference categories: For the adherence to the Mediterranean dietary pattern classes, the reference category is "High"; for area of residence, the reference category is "Lisbon

Metropolitan Area/Alentejo/Algarve"; for area of the course, it is "Health"; and for type of higher education institution, it is "Public".

95% CI: Confidence intervals for Exp(B) indicate the range in which the true effect size may lie.

The analysis revealed significant associations with adherence levels. For low adherence, a positive relationship with BMI was observed (B = 0.145; p = 0.065), suggesting that higher BMI may be linked to lower adherence, though this was not statistically significant. Additionally, students enrolled in non-health-related courses showed a significant positive effect (B = 1.858; p = 0.007), indicating a higher likelihood of low adherence to the MFP among these students.

In contrast, none of the factors related to moderate adherence, including BMI, age, gender, area of residence, or type of educational institution, demonstrated significant associations, suggesting that these variables did not strongly influence moderate adherence to the MFP. The findings supported H2, as students in non-health-related courses had significantly lower adherence to the MFP compared to their counterparts in health-related fields. The multinomial logistic regression results confirmed this association (B = 1.858; p = 0.007). While the data provided partial confirmation for H3, the association between higher BMI and low adherence, although indicative, was not statistically significant (B = 0.145; p = 0.065).

4. Discussion

This cross-sectional pilot study aimed to evaluate the adherence of university students to the MFP, with a particular focus on food sustainability. Additionally, the study sought to investigate potential associations between adherence to the MFP, sociodemographic characteristics, and the nutritional status of the participants. Overall, the study found a high prevalence of overweight (33.1%) and moderate adherence to the MFP (69.0%), with only 6.5% of students showing high adherence.

These results align with the existing literature, particularly regarding nutritional status. The majority of students in this study had a normal weight (60.5%), which is higher than the figures reported for the general population. In contrast, 34.8% of the Portuguese population is classified as pre-obese, and 22.3% as obese, meaning fewer than 50% of the population is within the normal weight range [5]. However, the prevalence of normal weight among students in this study is lower than that reported in studies conducted with higher education students in Ecuador [17] and Portugal [18], both of which found a prevalence greater than 70%.

These differences may be explained by the dietary habits of higher education students. Several studies, including this one, have reported a negative association between adherence to the MFP and BMI [19,20]. In our analysis, a negative correlation was initially observed, indicating that higher adherence to the MFP was associated with lower BMI values. However, this association dissipated following the application of the multinomial logistic regression model, suggesting that the relationship between adherence to the MFP and BMI may be confounded by other variables not considered in the model, such as physical activity level, total caloric intake, nutritional knowledge, lifestyle habits, and psychological factors. As reported by the Directorate-General for Health in 2020 [6], only 26% of the Portuguese population shows high adherence to the MFP. In this study, the prevalence of high adherence was lower than in several studies involving higher education students in Portugal [7,8,21]. For instance, in Almeida's study [21], which included 759 students from the University of Porto, 21.3% showed high adherence to the MFP. Similarly, Graça et al. [8] found a prevalence of 8.2% among higher education students and researchers in Portugal. Another study with 305 students from Lusófona University (Lisbon) reported a high adherence rate of 12.5% [7]. On a national scale, a study that included 480 students from higher education institutions and adults from the general population indicated a prevalence of 11% for high adherence to the MFP.

Internationally, a study of 584 Spanish university students reported a prevalence of 36.4% for high adherence to the MFP, with findings differing from this study, as females consumed fewer sugary drinks and more alcoholic beverages than males [22]. In the present study, low wine consumption was recorded, which negatively impacted adherence scores. While this may seem positive given Portugal's high levels of alcohol consumption [23], it should be interpreted cautiously due to the potential consumption of other alcoholic beverages. A study at a university in Peru reported a high adherence prevalence of 14.2% [19], while a study at a university in Lebanon indicated a 41.0% prevalence of high adherence to the MFP. The Lebanese study also revealed a low consumption of vegetables, fish, and nuts, alongside a preference for white meats and refined products [24], patterns similar to those found in the present study.

Our study provided evidence that gender differences exist in sugary drink consumption among university students in Portugal, with females consuming more sugary drinks than males. This finding is consistent with data from the 2019 National Health Survey conducted by the National Institute of Statistics (Portugal), which also identified variations in sugary drink consumption based on gender, showing that women reported a higher frequency of consumption compared to men among the population aged 15 years and older [25].

In relation to dietary preferences, the living situation of students plays a crucial role in their adherence to the MFP. The transition from living with family to independent living often introduces changes in food choices, with convenience foods becoming more prominent [26,27]. These foods, characterized by their affordability, quick preparation time, and appealing sensory properties, tend to replace traditional, home-cooked meals that align more closely with the MFP. As a result, there is a shift in eating habits towards less healthy, more processed foods, particularly among students living independently. Comparative studies highlight this divergence, showing that students who remain at home maintain healthier eating habits, such as a higher intake of fruits, vegetables, legumes, and fish—staples of the MFP—whereas those who live independently tend to adopt less balanced diets [26–29].

Another key factor influencing dietary preferences among students is the quality of meals offered in university canteens [29]. There have been several reports criticizing university canteens for providing meals that are low in nutritional quality. Studies have found that these meals often contain excessive amounts of protein, fat, and salt, which are inconsistent with the principles of the MFP. Given that the MFP promotes a diet rich in plant-based foods, lean proteins, and moderation in fat and salt consumption, the disparity in the nutritional content of canteen meals may discourage students from adhering to MFP guidelines. This, in turn, contributes to lower overall adherence to the MFP among university students, as canteens are a primary food source for many students [30].

4.1. Adherence to the Mediterranean Food Pattern and Sustainability

The literature indicates that individuals with higher adherence to the MFP are more likely to meet nutritional recommendations. The MFP is plant-based, providing essential nutrients, dietary fiber, and bioactive compounds that contribute to overall well-being, satiety, and the maintenance of a healthy diet [1]. This dietary pattern has demonstrated beneficial effects on lipoprotein levels, endothelial function, insulin resistance, metabolic syndrome, antioxidant capacity, and has shown reductions in myocardial and cardiovascular mortality, as well as cancer incidence, particularly in those who have experienced acute myocardial infarction [1]. Consequently, the MFP has been linked to numerous health benefits, particularly in preventing non-communicable chronic diseases such as cardiovascular disease, obesity, diabetes, and cancer [4].

A study conducted in Tunisia [31], utilizing mathematical diet optimization models, demonstrated that a nutritionally adequate eating pattern that does not consider environmental impact can increase land use and negatively affect biodiversity and soil quality, as well as water consumption. In this context, changes in eating patterns that reduce the intake of animal products—identified as having a greater environmental impact—by replacing them with plant-based foods, can lead to positive environmental effects [32].

Several studies have confirmed that the MFP has a lower environmental impact compared to other dietary patterns [2,4], largely due to its emphasis on plant-based foods and the limited consumption of animal products. This results in reduced land use, lower water consumption, and fewer greenhouse gas emissions compared to other dietary patterns [30,33]. However, given the MFP's reliance on vegetables, it is essential to prioritize crops with lower water demands to mitigate water resource consumption [32].

From a sociocultural perspective, the MFP is deeply ingrained in the lifestyles of Mediterranean populations and has evolved over centuries, influenced by diverse customs, religious practices, and cultural beliefs, as well as the succession of various dominant civilizations in the region. Frugality, a core principle of the MFP, emphasizes careful food preparation, moderate portion sizes, and the avoidance of waste. These principles are closely tied to the cultural, social, and economic values associated with meals in Mediterranean societies [4]. In these cultures, food transcends mere physiological needs, and communal meals are seen as opportunities for social interaction, pleasure, and enjoyment. They represent daily moments for bonding and shared experiences. Thus, the MFP is not only a reflection of dietary habits but also a manifestation of the rich diversity of Mediterranean food cultures, considered synonymous with the cultural and culinary heritage of the region [3]. Recognizing its significance, UNESCO designated the MFP as an Intangible Cultural Heritage of Humanity in 2010, underscoring its value as a model to be preserved and promoted [4].

Economically, the MFP promotes the preservation and growth of traditional activities by respecting local particularities, thereby fostering a balance between land and society [1]. Given its global visibility, the MFP can play a pivotal role in the sustainable development of small rural Mediterranean areas, particularly by valuing traditional and regional food products [3]. Achieving this objective requires emphasizing local food products and empowering local producers. This necessitates increased transparency and the protection of traditional Mediterranean food products through labeling, adherence to quality standards, and the clear identification of product origins. Furthermore, it is crucial to harmonize tradition, innovation, and sustainability in order to drive the economic and cultural development of Mediterranean regions [3].

From a practical standpoint, adherence to the MFP presents challenges for university students, primarily due to the convenience and accessibility of processed foods, which often come at the expense of environmental sustainability [34]. The shift towards these dietary patterns not only undermines adherence to the MFP but also contributes to increased waste and resource inefficiency. The convenience and accessibility of processed and ready-made foods, combined with a lack of food preparation skills or limited financial resources, often lead to a derivation from the MFP [35]. To improve adherence, interventions targeting university canteens, as well as educational programs promoting the benefits of the MFP and sustainable eating practices, could be beneficial.

This way, while the MFP offers significant health and environmental advantages, its practical implementation among university students faces barriers related to lifestyle changes, economic factors, and institutional food quality [36]. Addressing these barriers requires a multi-faceted approach that promotes both the health and sustainability benefits of the MFP. This includes advocating for public policies that improve food quality in university canteens, implementing educational campaigns to inform students about sustainable eating practices, and addressing economic constraints that limit access to healthier food options. Such interventions are crucial for fostering a culture of sustainability within student populations in Portugal.

4.2. Study Limitations and Future Directions

Like all studies, this one has some limitations. It is a cross-sectional pilot study, which does not allow us to determine associations' temporal direction or generalize the results. Another limitation arises from using a non-probabilistic, non-representative sample of university students, as the participants were self-selected. This self-selection occurs because individuals choose to participate in the study based on their own initiative after receiving the invitation. This may lead to biases, as those who choose to respond may possess different characteristics, motivations, or dietary habits compared to those who do not participate. Therefore, the findings may not accurately reflect the overall population of university students in Portugal.

The gender disproportion in our study may be attributed to the fact that our sample is predominantly composed of students from health and social sciences, fields in which there is a higher representation of females. It is worth noting that in Portugal, approximately 54% of higher education students are female, with even higher rates of feminization in fields such as health and social protection (76.8%), education (76.6%), and social sciences, journalism, and information (65.8%). This suggests that while our sample shows a gender imbalance, it aligns with the trends observed in certain fields of study. Additionally, the sample showed a skewed gender distribution, with 78% of participants identifying as female. This imbalance raises concerns about the representativeness of the sample, as it may not reflect the true gender proportions within the university student population. However, it is worth noting that in Portugal (2023), approximately 60% of higher education students are female [37], indicating that while our sample is skewed, it is not entirely unrepresentative.

Additionally, all data were self-reported rather than independently measured; therefore, there may be discrepancies due to the underestimation or overestimation of variables that could be objectively measured, such as weight and height.

Furthermore, although non-parametric tests such as the Mann–Whitney and Kruskal–Wallis tests are appropriate for analyzing non-normally distributed data, they come with certain limitations. While these tests can effectively identify significant differences between groups, they provide less detailed insights into the underlying distribution of the data compared to parametric tests. As a result, caution is warranted when interpreting p-values derived from these analyses, as subtler variations within the data may remain undetected. In this study, the non-parametric analyses were supplemented by a multinomial logistic regression model, enabling a more comprehensive exploration of the relationships among various factors influencing adherence to the Mediterranean Food Pattern (MFP). This multifaceted approach aimed to strengthen the robustness of the findings and highlights the importance of employing diverse analytical methods to achieve a thorough understanding of the dietary habits and associated outcomes of higher education students.

A strength of this study is the use of the MEDAS, a validated tool widely applied in studies across Portugal and the Mediterranean region. This allows for direct comparisons of our results with other population groups within Portugal and internationally.

For future research, several directions should be explored. First, expanding the sample size and diversity is essential to strengthen the robustness of the analyses. A larger dataset would facilitate the examination of more complex relationships, such as interactions between sociodemographic factors and dietary adherence, potentially providing deeper insights into student eating behaviors.

Although we chose not to implement fuzzy set qualitative comparative analysis (fsQCA) in this pilot study, future research with a larger and more diverse sample could benefit from this approach. fsQCA could offer a more systematic understanding of the configurational relationships between factors like lifestyle, socioeconomic background, and health outcomes, contributing to a more comprehensive analysis of MFP adherence. Incorporating fsQCA in future studies may provide a richer, more nuanced understanding of how various factors interact to influence dietary patterns and sustainability practices.

Additionally, future studies should aim to conduct a more representative analysis of university students. It would also be advantageous to explore the relationship between MFP adherence and perceptions of sustainability, incorporating additional variables such as residential area and the distinction between urban and rural environments.

5. Conclusions

In this pilot study, the prevalence of overweight exceeding 30% was identified among university students. Approximately 7% of participants demonstrated high adherence to the MFP, while about 25% exhibited low adherence. Students enrolled in health-related courses showed greater adherence to the MFP compared to their peers in other disciplines. Additionally, a negative correlation was initially identified between adherence to the MFP and BMI, suggesting that higher adherence to the MFP was associated with lower BMI values. However, this association diminished after applying the multinomial logistic regression model. This finding indicates that the relationship between MFP adherence and BMI may be influenced by other confounding variables accounted for in the model. Participants primarily used olive oil as their main source of fat and reported consuming fewer sugary drinks daily compared to their counterparts. However, there was also a high consumption of red meat and a low intake of vegetables.

As a pilot study, these findings highlight the importance of developing targeted interventions specifically aimed at university students to promote adherence to the MFP. Such interventions are crucial not only for improving health outcomes associated with this dietary approach but also for encouraging more environmentally sustainable eating habits, with a focus on plant-based foods.

Author Contributions: Conceptualization, L.O.; methodology, L.O.; software, L.O.; validation, L.O. and A.R.; formal analysis, L.O.; investigation, L.O., A.S., M.J.L., E.T.-L., J.H.A. and C.C.; resources, L.O.; data curation, L.O.; writing—original draft preparation, L.O.; writing—review and editing, L.O., A.S., M.J.L., E.T.-L., J.H.A., C.C. and A.R.; visualization, L.O. and A.R.; supervision, A.R.; project administration, A.R.; funding acquisition, A.S., M.J.L., E.T.-L., J.H.A., C.C. and A.R. All authors have read and agreed to the published version of the manuscript.

Funding: Researchers Supporting Project Number (RSPD2024R1013), King Saud University, Riyadh, Saudi Arabia.

Institutional Review Board Statement: This study was conducted in accordance with the ethical principles stipulated in the 1964 Helsinki Declaration and its subsequent amendments, as well as in accordance with comparable ethical norms. Informed consent was obtained, where the study's procedures and objectives were explained in detail. Approval was obtained for the study by the Ethics Commission of the School of Health Sciences and Technologies of the Lusófona University (P10-22, 7 December 2022).

Informed Consent Statement: Informed consent was obtained from all subjects involved in the study.

Data Availability Statement: Data are contained within the article.

Acknowledgments: The authors would like to express their thanks to all participants, and to all those who shared the online questionnaire. Furthermore, the authors extend their appreciation to the Researchers Supporting Project Number (RSPD2024R1013), King Saud University, Riyadh, Saudi Arabia.

Conflicts of Interest: The authors declare no conflicts of interest.

References

1. Serra-Majem, L.; Ortiz-Andrellucchi, A. The Mediterranean diet as an example of food and nutrition sustainability: A multidisciplinary approach. *Nutr. Hosp.* **2018**, *35*, 96–101. [PubMed]
2. Alsaffar, A.A. Sustainable diets: The interaction between food industry, nutrition, health and the environment. *Food Sci. Technol. Int.* **2016**, *22*, 102–111. [CrossRef] [PubMed]
3. Dernini, S.; Berry, E.M.; Serra-Majem, L.; La Vecchia, C.; Capone, R.; Medina, F.X.; Aranceta-Bartrina, J.; Belahsen, R.; Burlingame, B.; Calabrese, G.; et al. Med Diet 4.0: The Mediterranean diet with four sustainable benefits. *Public Health Nutr.* **2017**, *20*, 1322–1330. [CrossRef] [PubMed]
4. Serra-Majem, L.; Tomaino, L.; Dernini, S.; Berry, E.M.; Lairon, D.; Ngo de la Cruz, J.; Bach-Faig, A.; Donini, L.M.; Medina, F.X.; Belahsen, R.; et al. Updating the Mediterranean Diet Pyramid Towards Sustainability: Focus on Environmental Concerns. *Int. J. Environ. Res. Public Health* **2020**, *17*, 8758. [CrossRef]
5. Lopes, C.; Torres, D.; Oliveira, A.; Severo, M.; Alarcão, V.; Guiomar, S.; Mota, J.; Teixeira, P.; Rodrigues, S.; Lobato, L.; et al. *Inquérito Alimentar Nacional e de Atividade Física, IAN-AF 2015-2016: Relatório de resultados*; Universidade do Porto: Porto, Portugal, 2017.

6. Gregório, M.J.; Sousa, S.; Chkoniya, V.; Graça, P. *Estudo de Adesão AO Padrão Alimentar Mediterrânico*; Direção-Geral da Saúde: Lisboa, Portugal, 2020.
7. Ferreira-Pêgo, C.; Rodrigues, J.; Costa, A.; Sousa, B. Adherence to the Mediterranean diet in Portuguese university students. *Biomed. Biopharm. Res.* **2019**, *16*, 41–49. [CrossRef]
8. Graça, T.; Bôto, J.; Almeida-de-Souza, J.; Rodrigues, N.; Ferro-Lebres, V.; Meireles, M. Consumo de azeite e adesão ao Padrão Alimentar Mediterrânico entre académicos de origem lusófona. *RevSALUS* **2022**, *4*, 1–11.
9. Buyuktuncer, Z.; Ayaz, A.; Dedebayraktar, D.; Inan-Eroglu, E.; Ellahi, B.; Besler, H.T. Promoting a Healthy Diet in Young Adults: The Role of Nutrition Labelling. *Nutrients* **2018**, *10*, 1335. [CrossRef]
10. World Health Organization. *Obesity: Preventing and Managing the Global Epidemic: Report of a WHO Consultation*; World Health Organization: Geneva, Switzerland, 2000.
11. Weir, C.B.; Jan, A. *BMI Classification Percentile and Cut Off Points*; StatPearls: Treasure Island, FL, USA, 2023.
12. Schröder, H.; Fitó, M.; Estruch, R.; Martínez-González, M.A.; Corella, D.; Salas-Salvadó, J.; Lamuela-Raventós, R.; Ros, E.; Salaverría, I.; Fiol, M.; et al. A short screener is valid for assessing Mediterranean diet adherence among older Spanish men and women. *J. Nutr.* **2011**, *141*, 1140–1145. [CrossRef]
13. Gregório, M.J.; Rodrigues, A.M.; Salvador, C.; Dias, S.S.; de Sousa, R.D.; Mendes, J.M.; Coelho, P.S.; Branco, J.C.; Lopes, C.; Martínez-González, M.A.; et al. Validation of the Telephone-Administered Version of the Mediterranean Diet Adherence Screener (MEDAS) Questionnaire. *Nutrients* **2020**, *12*, 1511. [CrossRef]
14. World Medical Association. World Medical Association Declaration of Helsinki: Ethical principles for medical research involving human subjects. *JAMA* **2013**, *310*, 2191–2194. [CrossRef]
15. Oliveira, L.; Raposo, A. Factors That Most Influence the Choice for Fast Food in a Sample of Higher Education Students in Portugal. *Nutrients* **2024**, *16*, 1007. [CrossRef] [PubMed]
16. Oliveira, L.; BinMowyna, M.N.; Alasqah, I.; Zandonadi, R.P.; Teixeira-Lemos, E.; Chaves, C.; Alturki, H.A.; Albaridi, N.A.; Alribdi, F.F.; Raposo, A. A Pilot Study on Dietary Choices at Universities: Vending Machines, Canteens, and Lunch from Home. *Nutrients* **2024**, *16*, 1722. [CrossRef] [PubMed]
17. Hernández Gallardo, D.; Arencibia, R.; Linares-Girela, D.; Murillo-Plúa, D.; Bosques-Cotelo, J.; Manrique, M. Condición nutricional y hábitos alimentarios en estudiantes universitarios de Manabí, Ecuador. *Rev. Española Nutr. Comunitaria* **2021**, *27*, 13.
18. Fernandes, J.D. *Estudo Comparativo Dos Níveis de Atividade Física, Comportamento Sedentário E Hábitos Alimentares de Estudantes Do Ensino Superior*; Universidade Lusófona de Humanidades e Tecnologias: Lisboa, Portugal, 2016.
19. Vera-Ponce, V.J.; Guerra Valencia, J.; Torres-Malca, J.R.; Zuzunaga-Montoya, F.E.; Zeñas-Trujillo, G.Z.; Cruz-Ausejo, L.; Loayza-Castro, J.A.; De La Cruz-Vargas, J.A. Factors associated with adherence to the Mediterranean diet among medical students at a private university in Lima, Peru. *Electron. J. Gen. Med.* **2023**, *20*, em483. [CrossRef]
20. Dominguez, L.J.; Veronese, N.; Di Bella, G.; Cusumano, C.; Parisi, A.; Tagliaferri, F.; Ciriminna, S.; Barbagallo, M. Mediterranean diet in the management and prevention of obesity. *Exp. Gerontol.* **2023**, *174*, 112121. [CrossRef]
21. Almeida, S. *Adesão AO Padrão Alimentar de Tipo Mediterrânico Em Estudantes Da Universidade Do Porto: Estudo Dos Fatores Associados*; Universidade do Porto: Porto, Portugal, 2020.
22. López-Moreno, M.; Garcés-Rimón, M.; Miguel, M.; Iglesias López, M.T. Adherence to Mediterranean Diet, Alcohol Consumption and Emotional Eating in Spanish University Students. *Nutrients* **2021**, *13*, 3174. [CrossRef] [PubMed]
23. OECD. *Preventing Harmful Alcohol Use*; OECD: Paris, France, 2021.
24. Karam, J.; Bibiloni, M.d.M.; Serhan, M.; Tur, J.A. Adherence to Mediterranean Diet Among Lebanese University Students. *Nutrients* **2021**, *13*, 1264. [CrossRef]
25. Antonopoulou, M.; Mantzorou, M.; Serdari, A.; Bonotis, K.; Vasios, G.; Pavlidou, E.; Trifonos, C.; Vadikolias, K.; Petridis, D.; Giaginis, C. Evaluating Mediterranean diet adherence in university student populations: Does this dietary pattern affect students' academic performance and mental health? *Int. J. Health Plan. Manag.* **2020**, *35*, 5–21. [CrossRef]
26. Instituto Nacional de Estatística. *População Residente Com 15 E Mais Anos de Idade (N.º) Por Local de Residência (NUTS-2013), Sexo, Grupo Etário E Frequência Do Consumo de Refrigerantes açucarados*; Quinquenal. Instituto Nacional de Estatística: Lisboa, Portugal, 2020. Available online: https://www.ine.pt/xportal/xmain?xpid=INE&xpgid=ine_indicadores&indOcorrCod=0010111&c (accessed on 11 November 2024).
27. Papadaki, A.; Hondros, G.; Scott, J.A.; Kapsokefalou, M. Eating habits of university students living at, or away from home in Greece. *Appetite* **2007**, *49*, 169–176. [CrossRef]
28. Bernardo, G.L.; Jomori, M.M.; Fernandes, A.C.; RPDC, P. Food intake of university students. *Rev. Nutr.* **2017**, *30*, 847–865. [CrossRef]
29. Franchini, C.; Biasini, B.; Sogari, G.; Wongprawmas, R.; Andreani, G.; Dolgopolova, I.; Gómez, M.I.; Roosen, J.; Menozzi, D.; Mora, C.; et al. Adherence to the Mediterranean Diet and its association with sustainable dietary behaviors, sociodemographic factors, and lifestyle: A cross-sectional study in US University students. *Nutr. J.* **2024**, *23*, 56. [CrossRef] [PubMed]
30. Fernandes, D.; Cantinas universitárias falham na higiene e qualidade alimentar. Publico. 3 October 2002. Available online: https://www.publico.pt/2002/10/03/sociedade/noticia/cantinas-universitarias-falham-na-higiene-e-qualidade-alimentar-186749 (accessed on 11 November 2024).

31. Perignon, M.; Sinfort, C.; El Ati, J.; Traissac, P.; Drogué, S.; Darmon, N.; Amiot, M.-J.; Achir, N.; Alouane, L. How to meet nutritional recommendations and reduce diet environmental impact in the Mediterranean region? An optimization study to identify more sustainable diets in Tunisia. *Glob. Food Secur.* **2019**, *23*, 227–235. [CrossRef]
32. Tepper, S.; Kissinger, M.; Avital, K.; Shahar, D.R. The Environmental Footprint Associated with the Mediterranean Diet, EAT-Lancet Diet, and the Sustainable Healthy Diet Index: A Population-Based Study. *Front. Nutr.* **2022**, *9*, 870883. [CrossRef] [PubMed]
33. Castaldi, S.; Dembska, K.; Antonelli, M.; Petersson, T.; Piccolo, M.G.; Valentini, R. The positive climate impact of the Mediterranean diet and current divergence of Mediterranean countries towards less climate sustainable food consumption patterns. *Sci. Rep.* **2022**, *12*, 8847. [CrossRef] [PubMed]
34. Aguirre Sánchez, L.; Roa-Díaz, Z.M.; Gamba, M.; Grisotto, G.; Moreno Londoño, A.M.; Mantilla-Uribe, B.P.; Méndez, A.Y.R.; Ballesteros, M.; Kopp-Heim, D.; Minder, B.; et al. What Influences the Sustainable Food Consumption Behaviours of University Students? A Systematic Review. *Int. J. Public Health* **2021**, *66*, 1604149. [CrossRef]
35. da Rocha, B.R.S.; Rico-Campà, A.; Romanos-Nanclares, A.; Ciriza, E.; Barbosa, K.B.F.; Martínez-González, M.; Martín-Calvo, N. Adherence to Mediterranean diet is inversely associated with the consumption of ultra-processed foods among Spanish children: The SENDO project. *Public Health Nutr.* **2021**, *24*, 3294–3303. [CrossRef]
36. Wongprawmas, R.; Sogari, G.; Menozzi, D.; Mora, C. Strategies to Promote Healthy Eating Among University Students: A Qualitative Study Using the Nominal Group Technique. *Front. Nutr.* **2022**, *9*, 821016. [CrossRef]
37. Fernandes, A.M.; Marvão, L.; Miguel, S. *Igualdade de Género Em Portugal—Boletim Estatístico 2023*; Comissão para a Cidadania e a Igualdade de Género (CIG)/Direção de Serviços de Apoio à Estratégia e ao Planeamento (DSAEP)/Divisão de Comunicação, Informação e Documentação (DCID): Lisbon, Portugal, 2023.

Disclaimer/Publisher's Note: The statements, opinions and data contained in all publications are solely those of the individual author(s) and contributor(s) and not of MDPI and/or the editor(s). MDPI and/or the editor(s) disclaim responsibility for any injury to people or property resulting from any ideas, methods, instructions or products referred to in the content.

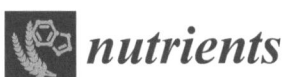

Article

Food Security in the Rural Mapuche Elderly: Analysis and Proposals

Angélica Hernández-Moreno [1], Olga Vásquez-Palma [2,*], Leonardo Castillo-Cárdenas [3], Juan Erices-Reyes [3], Alexsa Guzmán-Jiménez [4], Carlos Domínguez-Scheid [5], María Girona-Gamarra [6], Marco Cáceres-Senn [7] and Jorge Hochstetter-Diez [8]

[1] Departamento de Salud Pública, Facultad de Medicina, y Centro de Estudios y Promoción de los Derechos Humanos, Universidad de La Frontera, Temuco 4811240, Chile; angelica.hernandez@ufrontera.cl
[2] Departamento de Procesos Terapéuticos, Universidad Católica de Temuco, Temuco 4813302, Chile
[3] Departamento de Ciencias Jurídicas, Facultad de Ciencias Jurídicas y Empresariales, Temuco 4811240, Chile; leonardo.castillo@ufrontera.cl (L.C.-C.)
[4] Centro de Estudios del Desarrollo, Providencia 7500026, Chile; alexsa.guzman@gmail.com
[5] Doctorado en Derecho, Ciencia Política y Criminología, Universidad de Valencia, 46010 Valencia, Spain; dominguezscheid@gmail.com
[6] Escuela de Nutrición, Departamento de Nutrición Básica, Universidad de la República, Montevideo 11600, Uruguay; mgirona@nutricion.edu.uy
[7] Carrera de Ingeniería Informática, Facultad de Ingeniería y Ciencias, Universidad de La Frontera, Temuco 4811240, Chile; m.caceres04@ufromail.cl
[8] Departamento de Ciencias de La Computación e Informática, Facultad de Ingeniera y Ciencias, Universidad de la Frontera, Temuco 4811240, Chile; jorge.hochstetter@ufrontera.cl
* Correspondence: ovasquez@uct.cl

Abstract: Background: The increase in population longevity often occurs in contexts of inequity and relative poverty, accompanied by economic deterioration. This becomes a social determinant that has a direct impact on food security. This phenomenon particularly affects certain groups and territories, although there is still a lack of disaggregated references. Intersections between factors such as being a rural inhabitant, Indigenous, woman, or elderly person are observed in relation to food security, which forces us to pay greater attention to gaps that have remained invisible for years. Objective: The objective of this study is to analyze the main factors that affect the food security of Mapuche men and women over 60 years of age living in the rural area of Temuco, Chile. Method: Qualitative, descriptive, and interpretative research was carried out, observing the process from the interpretative symbolic paradigm and the complexity approach. Results: The data are made up of the discourses of these subjects, whose analysis allowed for the identification of results. These results show that producing their own food enables rural Mapuche elders to achieve food security. The cultural food heritage preserved by Mapuche elders, especially women, acts as a facilitating factor, as do community spaces that reinforce their culture. Among the obstacles to food security are migration to the city for work, pathological aging, and the limited production of culturally healthy foods (affected by environmental problems, cultural changes, the destabilization of group identity, and public policies that are incongruent with the territorial worldview). Conclusions: While rural Mapuche elders retain valuable practices for their food security, inadequate policies, migration and environmental degradation present significant challenges.

Keywords: right to food; Mapuche elders; food security; rurality; public policies

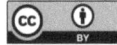

1. Introduction

One of the United Nations (UN) Sustainable Development Goals (SDGs), which seems far from being achieved, is to end hunger by 2023. Despite the fact that, as the Food and Agriculture Organization of the United Nations (FAO) points out, there is an excess of food produced, one in seven people in the world still go hungry [1]. This is primarily due to famine on the African continent, which is largely caused by frequent and worsening droughts that are becoming more common across all continents [2,3]. This is leading to greater inequality in access to healthy food. Another significant factor lies in the market, such as the sharp rise in agrifood prices, which mainly affects food-importing countries. This situation is exacerbated by the high concentration of natural resources under corporate control and the severe precarization of the peasantry [1].

The global disparities in access to healthy food represent a dehumanizing reality [4]. In other words, those responsible for these disparities deny the humanity of those affected. Therefore, it is essential to exert ethical pressure on governments and international organizations to eradicate these inequalities.

A total of 29.6% of the world's population experiences moderate or severe levels of food insecurity, meaning they do not have access to adequate food [5]. This issue particularly affects vulnerable groups such as women, children, rural communities, Indigenous peoples, the elderly, and migrants [6].

The new United Nations report, Panorama of Food and Nutritional Security 2022, states that 22.57% of people in Latin America and the Caribbean do not have sufficient means to access a healthy diet. In the Caribbean, 52% of the population has been affected by this situation; in Mesoamerica, this number reaches 27.8%, and in South America, 18.4%. It was reported that 131.3 million people in the region could not afford a healthy diet in 2020. This represents an increase of 8 million with respect to 2019 and is due to the higher average daily cost of this type of diet in Latin America and the Caribbean compared to the rest of the world's regions, reaching the Caribbean value of USD 4.23, followed by South America and Mesoamerica with USD 3.61 and USD 3.47, respectively [5].

In this paper, we will refer to a specific segment of the vulnerable groups, which are the rural Indigenous elderly. In this context, Chile presents an accelerated population aging process; 19.7% of its population was over 60 years old in 2020, being one of the four Latin American countries in an advanced stage of aging, and in 2050, it will be one of the most aged countries in the region, with 30.6%. In La Araucanía, this corresponds to 21.6% of the population [7]. Although this increased longevity is associated with improved living conditions, the extension of this stage is also accompanied by a rapid decline and deficits in access to basic social benefits, considering the lack of equity and economic precariousness of the aging population, which is an important social determinant that influences food security.

Addressing the aging of marginalized groups requires understanding its magnitude and implications, which is not always feasible due to the information gap regarding specific groups, such as the rural population, as highlighted in the literature review [8]. This study seeks to address this gap by investigating the perspectives of rural Mapuche elders on their food security in relation to culture, public policies, and implemented systems, and their role as either facilitating or limiting factors in the development of food security.

Aging and the inequalities that have become a pandemic pose enormous challenges for laws and public policies aimed at strengthening rights related to human welfare, especially within the framework of the Inter-American Convention on the Protection of the Human Rights of Older Persons, ratified by Chile [9]. In order to evaluate the effectiveness of these initiatives, it is necessary to have references that facilitate the planning of legislation and policies that account for the diverse realities of this population group. However, as previously mentioned, there is a lack of data on sensitive geographic areas, showing intersections between being a rural inhabitant, an Indigenous person, a woman, and an elderly person with respect to food insecurity. This highlights the need to focus more on the gaps that have been overlooked for years.

In this context, the increase in the age of inhabitants and the search for opportunities outside the territory have contributed to the problems faced by peasant and Indigenous family farming, making it difficult for them to continue to exist. Even though this sector has received very little support from public policies, it has contributed to a greater diversity of food for humans [10]. Today, young people migrate to big cities, and the elderly do their best to continue producing their own food, as they are practically discarded by the system. This has a negative impact on the life role of adults, the elderly, and rural woman, which is closely related to traditional agriculture, which provides sustenance to the family [11]. In addition, this undermines the right of the elderly to an adequate and varied diet. This is a matter of concern due to the importance of nutrition in this stage of life, which promotes better health, mental health, integration, and autonomy [12]. Studies in Latin America indicate that Indigenous food systems are based on the broad biodiversity of their ecosystems for food production and harvesting, which is related to cultural heritage and the reaffirmation of identities [13] and, on the other hand, that human groups with the lowest welfare conditions, Indigenous and rural populations, are more food insecure [14].

The objective of this study is to analyze the main factors affecting the food and nutritional security of Mapuche men and women over 60 years of age living in the rural area of Temuco in the years 2022 and 2023. Our contribution consists of gathering sensitive information regarding the perception of this age and ethnic group of rural inhabitants on the state of their food security and the factors that influence it.

2. Background

Food security is a multidisciplinary problem at the national and international levels, and in many countries it is a priority line of action, being an elementary condition for the welfare of the population, a point of support for strategic processes of participation, personal growth, education, determinant of nutritional status, and general health of a person, which in turn influences the physiological processes in general or the competence of people as workers, producers, and consumers; not to mention its influence on the economic, political, sociological, and environmental factors [15].

Food security was initially defined at the World Food Conference in 1974, relating it to the supply of basic foods at all times for the growing population, and this concept was later defined as food availability. Over time, it has become more complex. For example, in the Rome Declaration of 1996, the dimensions of people's access to food and its biological utilization in the human body were incorporated. Later, in 2009, the dimension of stability of the previously mentioned factors was added, followed by cultural adequacy. In recent decades, the condition of sustainability has been included, referring to the ecosystem impacts of agriculture [16].

Likewise, its presence is measured by the distribution and income of sufficient, safe, varied, equitable, and apt food for consumption, immersed within an environment that guarantees the tranquility of the population to have access to it. But, from the point of view of epidemiology and public health, its definition is associated with the absence of disease or contamination with pathogenic organisms that cause structural or physiological complications at the systemic level [16]. Food security is understood to be achieved when people's need for sufficient and safe food is satisfied. Initially, food security did not address the means or methods to achieve it, but concern has been growing about the environmental problems caused by food production within the framework of global challenges [16].

According to the World Health Organization (WHO), older adults are those who are 60 years of age or older. Globally, it is projected that this population sector will continue to grow and will exceed two billion by the year 2050. According to recent research on aging in Latin America, the average growth rate of older adults living in the countries of this region is 3.4 percent per year. This figure is growing faster than the number of children, underscoring the importance of aging as a social phenomenon. Older age by itself need not be synonymous with declining health [17]. Global aging has implied new, more integrative and multidimensional approaches, highlighting the context in which people age and focusing efforts on the basis of positive aging, on the maintenance of the physical, cognitive, social, and productive functions of the elderly [18].

On the other hand, 38.5% of Chile's senior citizens (MS) state that their monthly income is less than CLP 200,000 [19], with 66% of this value being women; they suffer lower incomes due to longer life expectancy [20], a situation aggravated by the conditions imposed by the Chilean pension system [21]. One in three elderly people state that their income does not allow them to meet their basic needs, and 19% of elderly-only households are permanently worried about not having enough food [19]. The precariousness triggered by the COVID-19 emergency we are experiencing has focused on specific sectors and human groups. In the country, 10.8% of the population suffers from poverty, which increases to 13.8% in the rural sector, 13.2% in the Indigenous population, and 5.6% in the elderly, increasing multidimensional poverty to 22.1% [22].

In La Araucanía, one of Chile's poorest regions, 17.4% of elderly people are in this condition, as are 37.3% of households with an elderly head of household [23]. These averages reflect realities in a country whose macroeconomic indicators appear to be one of the best in the region. In addition to the above, there is a strong and misguided tendency to approach this age group as if it corresponded to a homogeneous category that shares the same problems, attributes, and needs [24]. This greatly limits the possibilities to diversify and profile interventions according to personal resources, culture, territory, and specific needs.

3. Materials and Methods

Qualitative, descriptive, and interpretative research was carried out, observing the process from the interpretative symbolic paradigm [25] and the complexity approach [26]. Both theoretical places allow the observation and analysis of the subjectivity expressed by people to answer the research question: what are the factors that affect the food security of Mapuche people over 60 years old, particularly inhabitants of the rural area of Temuco?

This research was approved by the Scientific Ethics Committee of the Universidad de La Frontera in Evaluation Act N°075/22, dated 3 August 2022. Subsequently, fieldwork was carried out with a qualitative methodology with ethnographic support, with convenience sampling according to the objectives, which allowed the selection and participation of members of the territory. The methodology is divided into four stages (see Figure 1).

(i) Stage 1: Contact with the territory. This was carried out through the Boyeco Territorial Roundtable. A meeting was held with leaders, after which the communities were informed of the project in an extended territorial meeting. To define the study participants, the territory was spatially divided into four segments (mapping), in which the communities to be intervened and the potential participants were identified.

(ii) Stage 2: Fieldwork and study participants. Fieldwork was conducted in nine Mapuche communities in Boyeco, Temuco, in the Araucanía Region of Chile. The people interviewed were men and women over 60 years of age, as well as leaders from the mentioned territory. The type of instrument applied was an ethnographic interview (Geertz, 2012), adapted to the subject and their contextual conditions, guided by the research objective. The richness of this type of interview is associated with its flexibility and the opportunity it provides participants to clearly and deeply express their ideas. For this reason, questions are approached based on the conceptual themes suggested by the objectives, and no closed or repetitive questions are pre-formulated for each interviewee. Eleven open interviews were conducted, each lasting an average of an hour and a half. As a complementary technique, two focus groups were conducted, each consisting of at least ten people, including both men and women who were members of Indigenous community organizations from the same territory. The duration of these sessions was approximately two hours. Both instruments were applied in different communities within the same territory.

(iii) Stage 3: Analysis of results. To obtain the results, an intersectional analysis of the data was carried out based on the grounded theory [27]. The process begins by linking the research objectives with the discourse obtained through interviews and focus groups and selecting relevant quotes. Emerging conceptual categories were constructed based on the discourse of the interviewees, considering their meanings and their particular worldviews in response to the objectives explored. Subsequently, more abstract ideas were developed and associated with existing theory, leading to the construction of conceptual networks (Figures 2–4). This was supported by the Atlas/ti 22 software.

(iv) Stage 4: Communication of results. The results were presented to the participating communities and validated by them.

For the validity and limit of the application of the data construction techniques, we resorted to the application of the saturation phenomenon [28,29] and triangulation by the author and technique [30]. The research was carried out within a framework of ethical protection in accordance with bioethical deontological principles and current legislation in Chile.

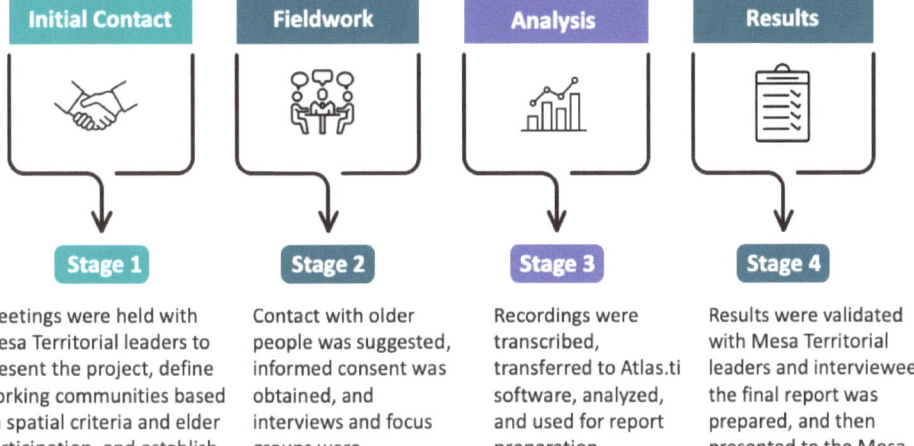

Figure 1. Work methodology.

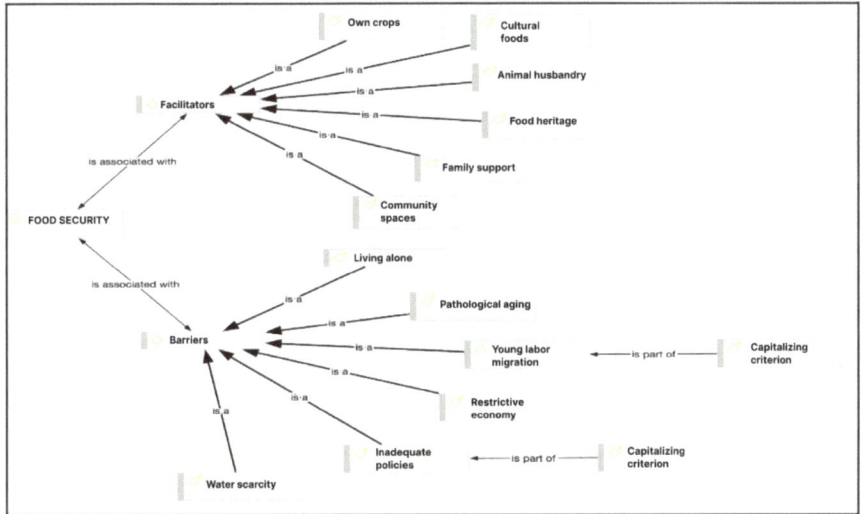

Figure 2. Barriers and facilitators of food security for Mapuche elderly in rural Temuco.

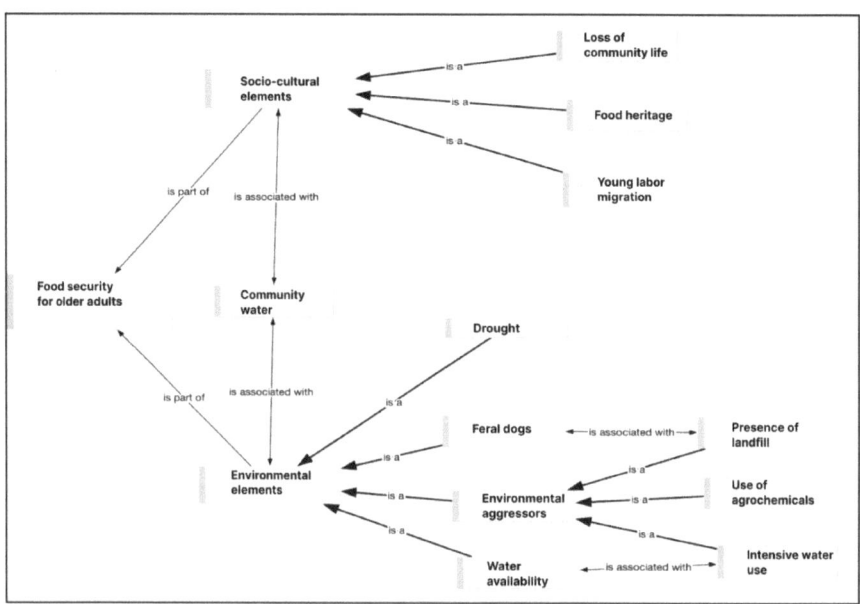

Figure 3. Sociocultural and environmental elements that affect food security among rural Mapuche older people in Temuco.

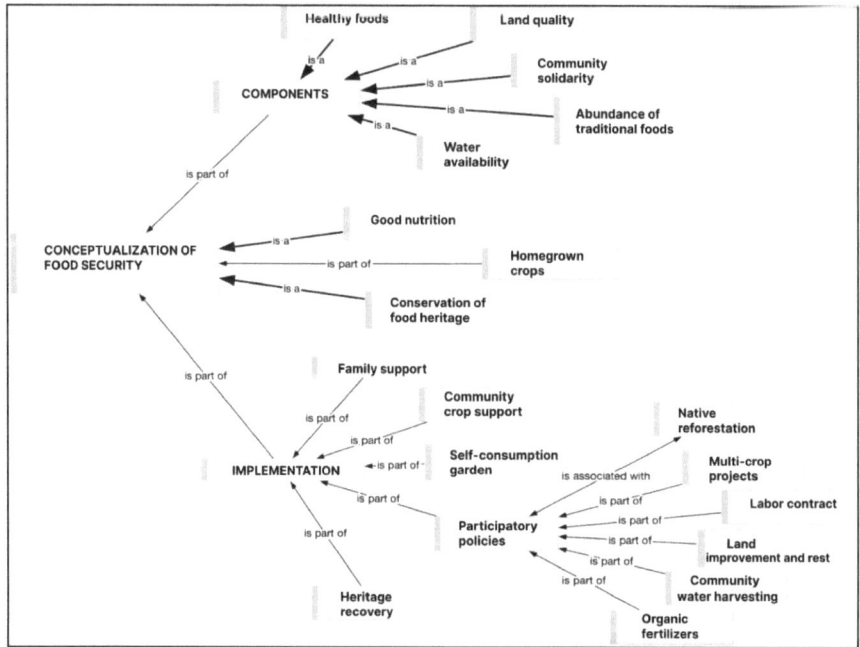

Figure 4. Conceptualization and components of food security and its implementation in rural areas.

4. Results

The results obtained in relation to each of the specific objectives proposed are presented below.

4.1. Food Safety Enablers and Barriers

Figure 2 presents the results regarding the facilitators and barriers to food security from the perspective of rural Mapuche elders interviewed. In the own crops code, they state that having the possibility of cultivating their fields and producing their own food allows them to have food security (quote interview 4, in Table 1).

Regarding so-called "cultural foods", they state that growing foods with which they grew up and which were validated by their culture of origin are recognized as nutritious. This makes them feel that they have food security. Therefore, the lack of them generates a feeling of scarcity and food insecurity (quote from community leader 1, in Table 1).

Poultry and animal husbandry are equally important for the elderly. The raising of chickens of various breeds has been largely maintained in the communities, but animal husbandry has been significantly impacted by the emergence of packs of feral dogs, which attack birds, sheep, and calves. As a result, many families have chosen to stop raising animals (citation focus group 1, in Table 1).

Food heritage, understood as the knowledge and practices related to the production, collection, preparation, and consumption of food within Mapuche culture, is considered a facilitating factor, as this knowledge is still preserved. Older women are the ones who re-signify food heritage, noting that young women have discontinued this role, both in feeding their families and in educating their children. Likewise, institutions do not take responsibility for preserving this type of heritage knowledge either (quote from community leader 3, in Table 1). Family support is essential for older adults, but this does not mean they are unable to engage in activities related to their food sustenance. Having family support helps them maintain their food production units (quote from interview 2, in Table 1).

Community spaces are also important places for Mapuche culture. They are cultural territories where people can meet, carry out their domestic chores, and keep their livestock. They are spaces where water was frequently found and was accessible to all because the sites were not fenced. In these places, people conversed, played, and generated bonds of trust, in addition to the aforementioned tasks (multiple interview quote 1, in Table 1).

Table 1. Identification of food safety enablers.

Participants	Testimonials
Interview 4	"If they are cultivating in their fields they have the possibility of growing their own food, which is like the culture they grew up with, the food like the cereals that they sowed in the houses, the legumes, the vegetables, in that I think they do tell me security".
Community leader 1	"The food is mainly soup, that's like good food, lots of toasted flour, seasonal vegetables".
Focus group 1	"It was also necessary to lock them up early, I left them and it was dark, and that was it! and of course the dogs got into the woods there and caught the sheep cornered, and they killed three sheep, they left in a shot".
Community leader 3	"but there is also no accompaniment, so to speak, as to what food they can prepare with what they have in their homes, with what they can produce, or what they know culturally".
Interview 2	"Before, life in the countryside was more relaxed, it was somehow more bearable. One did not live in this tension of having to fulfill schedules, we had more time to be able to dedicate to the old people, but not now poh, now the person who works has to be leaving already at 6 in the morning in the bus some 7 in the morning at least 7: 30 in the morning he or she has to be out of the house, so that means that the grandmother or grandfather has to get up alone in the morning and has to struggle alone and if he or she has little mobility then he or she will no longer be able to go to the garden to look for a product to make something healthy, but will have to eat what they left or what was left from the previous day".
multiple interviews 1	"Before, it was nice to wash in the marshes because you washed and sometimes your clothes would come off, the streams like that, you don't know that the only thing left there was the broom, or it was a bit funny to go far away to fetch water in a bucket or to go there to wash. I knew that the ladies would get married later (everyone laughs), not nowadays, nowadays everyone has a house so they can't even go out to the countryside (laughs)".

Family food production is considered essential for food security, as it ensures the availability of food defined as culturally healthy and accessible to families. The vegetable garden emerges as both a practical and symbolic element of great significance, directly linked to food security. It also fosters the development of cultural food practices and socialization among neighbors. Adult and elderly women are typically responsible for the daily tasks of maintaining and harvesting the garden, which is characterized by its diversity, including polycultures, seasonality, and the use of traditional knowledge for fertilization and pest control. Greenhouses have also been incorporated into production techniques. These systems enable bioavailability because they are considered healthy, chemical-free foods, particularly in terms of fertilizers and pesticides for vegetables and hormones for animals.

4.2. Food Safety Barriers

Regarding barriers to food security, the following codes or categories were identified: pathological old age, which refers to the perception of the elderly as sick, dependent on care, and unable to perform productive tasks. This perception is both social and cultural, based on the biomedical approach, and extends beyond self-perception and the family environment. It originates in the institutional sphere, influencing policies that focus solely on providing assistance to the elderly. This perception disrupts the cultural role traditionally assigned to the elderly, which includes being carriers of cultural wisdom and bearing the responsibility of passing down diverse knowledge, such as that related to food security, which ensures cultural survival for the community and future generations (multiple interview 1, in Table 2).

Living alone is a barrier, given the perception just indicated. The migration of young people and labor dynamics influence the elderly to be alone (interview 2, in Table 2). Water scarcity is caused by the deteriorated environment due to the loss of biodiversity and soil erosion. One of the fundamental causes referred to is the deforestation of native species and substitution with exotic species. In the case of the territory, there is also the contamination of water courses by the percolates from the Boyeco landfill. Families receive water, which is insufficient for their domestic needs and consequently does not allow the maintenance of vegetable gardens, animals, and poultry, which would contribute to the food security of the rural elderly, their family group, and the community (citation focus group 2, in Table 2).

The restrictive economy code refers to people's perception of how institutions value the needs of rural families and the lack of knowledge about these needs, particularly those related to the elderly. This can be seen in the low budget of the programs aimed at them, which do not achieve results that have an impact on the quality of life of families (citation interview 4, in Table 2). The labor dynamics category refers to the impacts on the lives of farming families who have been forced to work outside the fields, mostly in the city of Temuco. The impacts are cultural, social, and economic. The dynamics of the people who are active in the labor force imply being away from home and the farm all day, which does not leave them time to carry out productive and collaborative tasks and allow food production by the elderly. It is also cultural and social because this dynamic prevents the continuation of collective tasks and productive support in the community, which ultimately breaks family, intergenerational, neighborhood, and community relationships (quote interview 3, in Table 2).

Regarding inadequate public policies, it is linked to the references in which the participants state that these are not adapted to the needs of the rural Mapuche elderly due to a profound lack of knowledge of the culture and the territory, in addition to a lack of intersectoral coordination of the public system, which translates into a lack of public policies with a productive/economic approach aimed at this age group (quote from community leader 2, in Table 2).

It is important to highlight the situation that, according to the interviewees, refers to the conservation and reproduction of the food heritage, which is part of the role assigned to women. Specifically, this role is observed in the activities of raising poultry and small animals, as well as in the production of healthy food in a family garden. Men can collaborate in this situation when they are older if their health situation allows it.

Table 2. Food safety barriers.

Participants	Testimonials
Multiple interviews 1	"The health of the old person has nothing to do with now, that is why there are many old people who have already reached eighty-four years old, ninety-two years old, even one hundred and five years old, because that is what they were fed with another type of food, with the food from before, natural. Nowadays no, the same food brings illness, it depends on how you eat, it depends on what you are eating, it produces illnesses, sipo (reaffirms) because if one for example, is eating fatty things every day, I don't know, every day you add something fatty to the bread, in the end what does it all produce, gall bladder, you have to have a gall bladder operation, and in the old days the old people that one knew, when did they know about having a gall bladder operation?".
Interview 2	"It's not easy for them to ask for help, it's not easy to say you know that I need this or suddenly they feel that they are abusing someone who is going to help them, and they prefer not to tell him anymore, because they feel it has been too much".
Focus group 2	"But these streams do not respect [waters contaminated by a landfill], the streams follow their course, when the time of winter comes they overflow to all sides, and the water flows out, so they cannot say that there is no contamination. That estuary is called Cusaco, that is, there are two estuaries, in this case the one on this side, which is not very big, but the other one is bigger, so they come together and that estuary was analyzed and came out contaminated".
Interview 4	"the Mapuche in this case, which is us, it cost us, it costs us because the Mapuche are always used to having a lot of things, but nevertheless, it has been decreasing more and more, today the greatest food security is within the subsidies that the old people receive, that we receive (because I am part of it too), in which we have to buy things and we cannot reproduce anything, because due to the lack of water and animals, we are practically just [starting] some families again".
Interview 3	"In 1983 they begin to subdivide the lands, in which the families are left with a minimum extension of land that in this case Pinochet launches the law 2.568 where you have to subdivide the land and all the rest and many families of course agreed to this, even though there was some opposition to this law, but most of the communities in this place were subdivided and then the people began to fence their space and of course there was less space for animals and from there they began to subdivide, the people because they no longer, because in the past everything was collective there were spaces where they could install the animals and most of us had cows and oxen".
Community leader 2	"Public policies from INDAP [Institute for Agricultural Development], from agriculture, insist on programs such as PDTI [Indigenous Territorial Development Program], PRODESAL [Local Action Development Program] and PRODER [Rural Development Program], where the only thing they explain to the people is that they have to produce and hopefully a lot (emphasis), and that a lot versus quality, in my opinion, does not make sense, but for the people, according to the economic aspect, what the economic income implies, when selling those products, it makes them reach these institutions and try to maintain the link with the institutions to produce better, in parenthesis, to produce better, that is what they call it (emphasis, raises his voice). Because that is how the trained technicians come, what do I know, the engineers, right, to tell him how the farmer has to produce today, mainly because in the past production was from here upwards, and today they come from there, from the academy, perhaps to teach how to produce already, and that is where this issue is mixed, they bring you contaminants versus what used to be produced in the past, which was healthy".

The barriers are basically identified with a brake on the cultural action that allows food security through the production of healthy food, to which environmental problems, cultural changes that destabilize group identity, and inadequate public policies due to ignorance and lack of commitment to the worldview of the inhabitants of the territory contribute, in addition to poor intersectoral coordination.

4.3. Socio-Cultural and Environmental Elements Associated with Food Security

The facilitating elements are the ancestral knowledge safeguarded by rural Mapuche elders and respect for cultural traditions regarding the production of food that allows and sustains their food security.

The impossibility of having food security in a culturally diverse territory is limited by the failure to establish horizontal intercultural relations that would imply knowledge and respect on the part of the dominant social structure towards the ethnic minority with which it relates. In this case, the dominant social structure is represented by the institutions mandated by the state to fulfill this function; however, by not knowing and valuing in depth the worldview of the vulnerable group, it is not possible to strengthen or promote food security in these territorial spaces, especially due to the added social prejudice towards the elderly.

Socio-cultural and environmental elements associated with food security are present in the discourse of the study participants, with which the following associated conceptual categories are constructed.

Among the socio-cultural and environmental elements associated with food security, the following codes or categories stand out, constructed on the basis of the discourse of the participants: In this conceptual network, an important element emerges which, being an environmental element, takes on great symbolic relevance in the socio-cultural sphere for the food security of Mapuche elders; this is community water of collective service and management. The code of loss of community life refers to the denial of cultural expression to which the Mapuche people have been subjected, translated into the cessation or reduction in family, productive, and community practices as a result of the assimilation to dominant culture (quote from focus group 2, in Table 3).

The food heritage category is understood as knowledge and practices related to the production, collection, and consumption of food based on the Mapuche cosmovision that support the concept of food security specific to this culture (quote from focus group 1, in Table 3).

Finally, the labor migration code for young people, which is linked to the references in which the participants indicate that the absence of young people who contribute to the work of agricultural production for the family and community generates food insecurity in the elderly due to the scarcity and replacement of food that is culturally recognized as healthy. This absence is caused by the economic needs of the family group since there are no economic and labor solutions in the rural sector. The main impact of this phenomenon is a weakening of community ties since this age group is excluded from community participation and, therefore, their families, particularly the elderly, as they are not part of the support for the productive tasks of their families or neighbors and, consequently, they cannot be subject to such support, which weakens community ties and food security.

Among the environmental elements that influence food security from the perspective of the interviewees are drought, feral dogs, environmental aggressors, and the availability of water (quote from community leader 1, in Table 3). The code drought alludes to an environmental factor that negatively influences food security since it is not possible to grow crops or have a good and healthy diet (quote from multiple interview 2, in Table 3).

Feral dogs arrived in the territory, especially after the opening of the landfill that operated from 1992 to 2016. Families coming from the urban area of Temuco are accustomed to abandoning their dogs in the rural sector, and the Boyeco territory has become one of these preferential spaces, which has had unfortunate impacts on the family economy and the food security of the elderly (quote from community leader 1, in Table 3).

The previous element is connected to what we refer to as environmental aggressors, which, according to the research participants, are a constraint on food security. These include factors such as the presence of a landfill in the territory, which has had a profound impact on the environment and agrifood production. Participants also mentioned the use of agrochemicals, which has led to soil degradation, and the intensive use of water. All of these factors have significantly contributed to the loss of biodiversity, thereby reducing food security (citation focus group 1, in Table 3).

The use of agrochemicals is highlighted by the participants because, according to their perspective, they deteriorate the quality of the soil, causing the loss of biodiversity, soil erosion, and a lack of water (citation focus group 1, in Table 3).

The code "Intensive use of water" is associated with the use of this element by productive projects external to the communities, which produces water scarcity within the communities and does not allow for vital and productive domestic reproduction. This is related to what is defined as the problem of "water availability", which is linked to the references in which it is stated that not having good access to water is an important environmental factor that generates threats to food security (quotes from interview 2 and interview 1, in Table 3).

Table 3. Sociocultural and environmental elements associated with food security.

Participants	Testimonials
Focus group 2	"A neighbor needs help and that's it, he goes out to ask for help, but at the same time it's hard for them to return the hand, which used to be normal. The one who was going to sow was made a mingaco all together, and then he had to give his hand back. And now, what happens now, is that we suddenly work with a tractor, we run out of time and what happened, that in the long run this has also made us to be more individual".
Focus group 1	"I would separate them into two major food safety issues. One is the issue of healthy food, which is what we have talked about here, cultivating without agrochemicals, that if the tomato comes out deformed, it doesn't matter because it will have a real flavor. Of course, if it has bugs, or apply as the ancients did the ash for pests, the apple cider vinegar water, how to apply all these techniques avoiding the same thing and preserving the seed. That is liberation, sovereignty. And on the other hand, to have economic autonomy, not, as Renato said, no, to have the need to have enough money to be able to obtain food, so that gives you economic autonomy, not having to go shopping, as little as possible". Focus Group Jeronimo Melillan Community".
Community leader 1	"The drought is something that has had a great influence, people still continue to make their farms, vegetable gardens, for self-consumption, as something that everyone tries to maintain as much as possible, because there are people who are already old and have some kind of illness and do not have good access to water".
Multiple interviews 2	"Long time ago, when there were not so many eucalyptus trees, we had a water dam, we used to irrigate with a water motor where I was telling you, and we used to irrigate with a water motor, and now, even if you have a motor, you have nowhere to get water, that is the problem".
Community leader 1	"There was a big issue here a while ago with the landfill and the arrival of many dogs, but even so, they still continue to arrive, and suddenly they will kill their chickens and other poultry that they have in the house. They still continue to arrive and suddenly they are going to kill their chickens and other poultry that they have in the house, as well as sheep. Little by little, people have been raising poultry and smaller animals again".
Focus group 1	"Yes, we had a landfill for many years here, very close by, it contaminated the water table and the animals got sick, the children, who were used to bathing and drinking water from the river, also got sick, yes, we were there. The trees are no longer the same...before autumn arrives they turn yellow, but as well as with scale, many native trees began to burn, because of the focus of the landfill, for some reason it was also closed because it was there for many years, how long was it there for 18 years? 25 years! So there was a lot of pollution and that affected everything because we are right with the north wind and it took everything to this sector".
Interview 2	"The foods that were eaten before were of frequent use and valuable for us, the bloodroot they called it, also the watercress of the swamps were taken and consumed and were exquisite and that was eliminated and ended product of the chemicals".
Interview 1	"There are people who are already old and have some kind of disease and do not have good access to water, so for them it is very complex and they try to take advantage of this rainy weather to have something and try to maintain this type of food".

In this analysis, it is important to highlight that there is more than one sociological subject among the participants; that is, the group does not present characteristics of absolute homogeneity. Among them stand out those who promote and maintain their Mapuche cultural practices and the subjects that are constituted by people linked to the evangelical religion, who discontinue their cultural practices, but nevertheless, among their principles, maintain the cultural definition of the Mapuche cosmovision with the environment, which contributes to have related definitions of food security. However, this subject reinforces their cultural ties based on their religious ties, self-defined as brothers in the faith, differentiating themselves from other members of non-evangelical communities.

4.4. Conceptualization and Components of Food Security

The following codes or categories were identified in relation to the participants' perception of the conceptualization and components of food security and its implementation in rural areas.

A central element in this conceptual framework is what is referred to as the conservation of food heritage, which in symbolic and cultural terms forms the foundation of human development, as food not only nourishes but also heals. This is reinforced by what participants refer to as good food, which comes from their own traditional crops, including animal husbandry. Therefore, the concept of food security is understood as the consumption of nutritious and healthy food produced by the family, which is also meaningful within their own cultural context (quote from community leader 2, in Table 4).

The concept of food security within the culture investigated contains the components of land quality and water availability, in addition to the abundance of traditional foods known as healthy foods. Packaged foods are negatively valued because they are processed and contain unhealthy substances. These are opposed to healthy food from family and local production and a way of life that interviewees call küme mogen, a good way of living, which not only defines individual behavior but also contemplates respectful interaction and conservation of the environment and non-human species. In this way, we protect, not damage, that which allows us to survive as a species, all of which, according to the participants, contributes to and safeguards food security (quotes from interview 3 and interview 1, in Table 4).

Finally, community solidarity is highlighted, which reinforces knowledge and heritage production practices, which constitute the basis of food security for a culture (quote from focus group 1, in Table 4).

The knowledge of the heritage of food security is safeguarded by the older people of the territory; however, the current socio-cultural situation, in which young people and adults work outside the territory, prevents this knowledge from being shared and reproduced within the culture (quote from focus group 1, in Table 4). In this area, it is worth highlighting the importance of the role of women in the conservation of the food heritage and, consequently, in the strengthening of the food security of families, communities and the Mapuche people; the vegetable garden, under women's control, is an icon of family food security (quote from community leader 3, in Table 4).

In relation to the implementation of the concept of food security relevant to the territory and culture, from the perspective of the interviewed subjects, we mainly observed the need for family support for the performance in the daily life of the elderly so that they maintain and apply their knowledge in the practice of the production of food considered culturally healthy. This would be possible in the current socio-cultural and economic context through the support of state institutions for the generation of productive infrastructure necessary for food production, such as the recovery of the quality and health of the land and water management technologies, among others. A relevant and fundamental element, according to the cultural support referred to, is the existence of a vegetable garden for self-consumption, which is the element that provides permanent food security to rural Mapuche elders (interview 2, in Table 4).

To this end, it is considered essential to support participatory public policies that are based on listening to the people and their practical and cultural needs in order to solve local problems. According to those interviewed in this territory, it is important to develop the following initiatives aimed at the reforestation of natives to recover the fertility of the soil and maintain the water supply: multiculture projects, labor contracts to support infrastructure for the cultivation of vegetable gardens of the elderly, the improvement and rest of the land, community water harvesting to solve water shortages, and the use of organic fertilizers that allow the cultivation of healthy food and recover the health of the land (in Table 4).

Finally, the participants state that it is necessary to carry out actions aimed at recovering food heritage and reproducing knowledge both in Mapuche elders and in new generations. In this regard, they mentioned that currently, public institutions do not contribute to promoting its reproduction. Fundamental concepts for the definition of food security are food cultural heritage and what they call küme mogen, which are associated with good living among human beings, other species, and the environment.

Table 4. Conceptualization and components of food security and its implementation in rural areas.

Participants	Testimonials
Community leader 2	"[FEEDING] is part of the way of life, it is part of the lawen, it is part of good living, it is part of human relations, of the inter-species relation, that is to say, feeding is not only throwing food in the mouth. It is the relationship of this body, which is not only material, but also spiritual, the relationship, the interaction with nature, the interaction with the world, with the other species, basically, it is the good living associated to harmony, not to overeat, not to undereat, not to overeat, not to undereat".
Interview 3	"Security means that nothing is lacking and that hopefully in rural areas we can have a permanent surplus [of] food, which is what we see today is not happening because generally families look for resources outside the community to be able to feed themselves and bring in food from outside. And especially in young families because there is no longer a productive issue, especially in the Boyeco territory, due to water scarcity, water contamination and also because people have left aside (the Mapuche in this case) the issue of natural production because the animals that produce guano are no longer present".
Interview 1	"Food safety we could even say to protect what we grow and what we have by not adding chemicals to it, so that it can make a moderately safe food for us".
Focus group 1	"A neighbor told me that in the past, I don't know, people used to get together to fix the roads, it was because people lived here, they had the time and were the owners of their time, for example when we sowed wheat, they had to, they had to prepare the land at a certain time of the year, in a certain week of the month, then sow, then nothing is done until the harvest, and so, in between, they were doing other activities, for example picking peas, others were dedicated to breeding, but the people lived and worked here".
Focus group 1	"I tell him a lot, for example, a child was learning as he was watching the adult, and as the adult is now working in the city, the children do not learn".
Community leader 3	"That is what makes them feel good and they feel proud because I don't know, for example, the old ladies visit each other and what they see first is the vegetable garden, the gardens are shown and they invite each other, for example, the first new parents come out and visit each other and take them to their relatives or neighbors and they invite each other, the other brings back something else, for example, new beans or peas. And so on and so forth, that is the way of life that is slowly coming back, because there was a time that had definitely been lost".
Interview 2	"The PACAM [Programa de Alimentación Complementaria del Adulto Mayor] that is given to the elderly is a tremendous contribution, it is a contribution for those who have nothing, but it cannot be the solution, it is a patch. But what they should do is try to promote appropriate vegetable gardens for the elderly, that the family gets together, I don't know, other things, networks for the communities, facilitate everything that is necessary".
Interview 2	"The government should be more involved in the implementation of these projects to the communities and it should not be so bureaucratic to have to do a lot of paperwork to be able to apply for a small pool of water".

5. Discussion

Different factors that influence the food security of rural Mapuche elders are observed. One of the elements that stands out is the role of cultural heritage in food production and consumption, since older people continue to promote the practice of traditional knowledge about crops and animal husbandry, which favors their food self-sufficiency. However, the migration of young people to the cities and the lack of structural support have weakened the communities' capacity to maintain these practices.

One of the main barriers faced by these people is the limited availability of natural resources, especially water. Drought and pollution caused by human activities, such as the existence of the Boyeco landfill, negatively affect agricultural production and animal husbandry, restricting access to healthy and culturally appropriate food. This problem is aggravated by the lack of public policies consistent with the specific needs of these communities, which reflects a profound ignorance of the Mapuche cosmovision. The above evidences the scarce support of the public sector to the peasant and Indigenous sector, consistent with the analyses of the Observatory of the Right to Food of the University of Oviedo, 2019 [10].

On the other hand, a strong sense of cultural and community identity is identified as a key facilitator for food security. Older people value the use of traditional agricultural techniques and the transmission of intergenerational knowledge, although they recognize that these practices are at risk due to social and economic changes.

The impossibility of achieving food security in a territory with cultural diversity is limited by the inability to establish horizontal intercultural relations, which involve knowledge and respect from the dominant social structure toward the Indigenous people with whom it interacts. In this case, this structure is represented by institutions mandated by the State to fulfill this function through relevant public policies. However, since there is no deep understanding and appreciation of the worldview of the minoritized group, it is not possible to strengthen and promote food security in these territorial spaces, especially due to the added social prejudice and ageism against older adults.

This is how conventional agricultural production methods, which use agrochemicals in the implementation of prevailing public policies, negatively affect the perception of food security in elderly rural Mapuche people, as they contradict their concept of health in the human–nature relationship. Additionally, these practices violate the role of the rural elderly woman in traditional agriculture, who provides sustenance for the family, as is consistent with [11].

As a consequence, the State, in its interventions in Indigenous communities, has introduced a productivist paradigm based on chemical products and overexploitation of natural resources. In this context, the concern not only has to do with preserving the types of food and ways of cultivating, which for the elderly has an ancestral cultural value but also with the vulnerability in food security that these actions cause, with the lack of cultural relevance, since they are forced to consume food that they perceive as unhealthy. Likewise, in order to strengthen the food security of the rural Mapuche people, it is necessary to strengthen public policies in the use of technologies that allow for achieving the proposed objectives [31].

At the political level, it is essential to develop public policies that consider the Mapuche worldview and promote sustainable agricultural production in the rural context, as well as to overcome the ageism that these public policies entail when dealing with older people by implementing not only care-oriented actions for this age group but also productive and developmental actions, with age and cultural appropriateness. Initiatives aimed at improving access to water, rehabilitating land, and strengthening family production are also essential steps to ensure sustainable food security. Likewise, it is important to promote the active participation of communities in the creation of these policies to ensure that they are adapted to their realities and needs.

Limitations of the Study

This study presents limitations that should be considered when discussing its results. An important aspect is that being a qualitative study with an ethnographic approach, despite being conducted over a large territory and representing nine Mapuche communities, the construction of generalizing theory requires comparison with results from studies in the area with other Indigenous peoples. According to [8], regarding the topic in Latin America and the Caribbean (LAC), there are only six related studies, with the greatest productivity found in North America, with 29 studies (United States and Canada), which could present comparative difficulties for theory construction, based on the inductive qualitative method used in this study. This limitation can be overcome by carrying out other comparative ethnographic studies, both nationally and in Latin America and the Caribbean, which would allow the construction of valid generalizations through the analytical use of the comparative inductive method.

The study was conducted during the period of 2022–2023, which may have influenced the results due to the specific circumstances of the previous years due to the pandemic. This may have exacerbated some problems related to food security, such as youth migration and access to basic resources, which does not necessarily reflect a long-term situation. Another limitation is the lack of quantitative data to support the results obtained; however, the qualitative approach allowed for an exploration of the perceptions and experiences of the participants. It could be said that the absence of numerical data limits the ability to measure the scope of the problems identified and to make numerical comparisons with other populations or periods, so a mixed study could perhaps have a greater scope.

It would be interesting and innovative to approach the same topic from an intergenerational perspective because it would contribute to the construction of knowledge with a greater number of analytical dimensions.

6. Conclusions

This study provides an analysis of the factors that influence food security among Mapuche, older people in rural areas of Temuco, Chile. The results reveal the importance of cultural heritage and ancestral knowledge in food production and consumption. Older people, particularly women, play a crucial role in preserving traditional agricultural practices, which are fundamental to their food self-sufficiency and well-being.

The components of the definition of food security are closely related to the food heritage of the culture in question. The food heritage of a culture is a central element in the symbolic interpretation of the concept of food security and is the foundation for distinguishing those foods that are considered healthy, nutritious, and contributing to general health. According to older people, these foods should not be missing from a diet in order to have a long and good quality of life.

Food security in these communities faces several barriers. Key among them are environmental degradation, a lack of adequate access to water, and the decline in the youth workforce due to migration to cities. These factors have reduced the ability of older people to maintain sustainable agricultural practices and ensure a nutritious and culturally appropriate diet. Furthermore, current public policies do not effectively respond to the specific needs of rural Mapuche communities, which increases their vulnerability.

The sociological subject to which these public policies for the Mapuche people or other Indigenous peoples could be directed is not homogeneous, nor unique, that is, the group in question does not present characteristics of absolute homogeneity, so universal actions, without territorial distinction, are not very pertinent, their differentiation is based on the cultural heritage of each people, and a common aspect is that their worldview has as its axis the link of respect and horizontality with the environment. Despite these challenges, cultural heritage remains a key enabler of food security. Traditional farming and animal husbandry practices, as well as the use of ancestral knowledge about biodiversity, continue to be valuable resources. However, to ensure the survival of these practices and improve food security in these communities, it is imperative that public policies are tailored to their cultural and territorial realities.

The findings suggest that while rural Mapuche elders retain valuable practices for their food security, inadequate policies, migration, and environmental degradation present significant challenges. Comprehensive political and social intervention is required to strengthen local resources and ensure the continuity of food traditions that are crucial to the health and well-being of this population.

Author Contributions: Methodology, A.H.-M. and O.V.-P.; Formal analysis, O.V.-P. and A.H.-M.; Investigation, A.H.-M., O.V.-P. and A.G.-J.; Data curation, J.E.-R., M.G.-G. and L.C.-C.; Writing—original draft, A.H.-M., J.H.-D. and J.E.-R.; Writing—review and editing, A.H.-M., O.V.-P., M.G.-G., J.H.-D., M.C.-S., A.G.-J. and C.D.-S.; Visualization, M.C.-S.; Supervision, O.V.-P. and C.D.-S.; Project administration, L.C.-C. All authors have read and agreed to the published version of the manuscript.

Funding: The research project received financial support for field work and transcriptions from the Department of Public Health of the Universidad de La Frontera.

Institutional Review Board Statement: The study was conducted in accordance with the Declaration of Helsinki, and approved by Scientific Ethics Committee of the University of La Frontera N 075/22; 3 August 2022.

Informed Consent Statement: Informed consent was obtained from all subjects who participated in the study.

Data Availability Statement: The original contributions presented in the study are included in the article, further inquiries can be directed to the corresponding author.

Acknowledgments: We thank the Right to Food Observatory of Latin America and the Caribbean (ODA-LAC) for the approval of this project in the 10th Call for Research on the Right to Food in Latin America and the Caribbean. We also thank those who made this study possible, the Mesa Territorial de Boyeco, who supported the link with the territory, and the participants for sharing their knowledge and experience.

Conflicts of Interest: The authors declare no conflicts of interest.

References

1. Vivas, E. Los porqués del hambre. *Rev. Vinculando* **2011**. Available online: https://vinculando.org/sociedadcivil/los_porques_del_hambre.html (accessed on 15 October 2024).
2. FAO; FIDA; OMS; PMA; UNICEF. *El Estado de la Seguridad Alimentaria y la Nutrición en el Mundo 2022*; UNICEF: Roma, Italy, 2022.
3. Ramírez, R.F.; Vargas, P.L.; Cárdenas, O. La seguridad alimentaria: Una revisión sistemática con análisis no convencional. *Espacios* **2020**, *41*, 319–328. [CrossRef]
4. Jones, C.M. The moral problem of health disparities. *Am. J. Public Health* **2010**, *100*, S47–S51. [CrossRef] [PubMed]
5. Organización de las Naciones Unidas para la Alimentación y la Agricultura; Fondo Internacional de Desarrollo Agrícola; Fondo de las Naciones Unidas para la Infancia; Programa Mundial de Alimentos; Organización Panamericana de la Salud. *Panorama Regional de la Seguridad Alimentaria y Nutricional-América Latina y el Caribe 2022: Hacia una Mejor Asequibilidad de las Dietas Saludables*; Technical report; OPS: Washington, DC, USA, 2023.
6. Arriaga-Ayala, E.X.; Shamah-Levy, T.; Humarán, I.M.G.; del Carmen Morales-Ruán, M. Association of food insecurity and poor nutrition in rural women of Mexico, 2018 and 2020. *Salud Pública México* **2023**, *65*, 353–360. [CrossRef] [PubMed]
7. SENAMA. *Envejecimiento en Chile: Diagnóstico y Consulta Ciudadana*; SENAMA: Santiago, Chile, 2022.
8. Hernández-Moreno, A.; Vásquez-Palma, O.; Gutiérrez-Gutiérrez, F.; Cordero-Ahiman, O.; Celedón-Celis, N.; Hochstetter-Diez, J. Analysis of Food Security of Older Rural Indigenous People in Latin America and the Caribbean. *Foods* **2024**, *13*, 1772. [CrossRef] [PubMed]
9. Mora Biere, T.; Herrera Muñoz, F. Convención Interamericana Sobre la Protección de los Derechos Humanos de las Personas Mayores. 2018. Available online: https://www.oas.org/es/sla/ddi/docs/tratados_multilaterales_interamericanos_a-70_derechos_humanos_personas_mayores.pdf (accessed on 15 October 2024).
10. a la Alimentación, O.d.D. *Agricultura Familiar y Derecho a la Alimentación*; Universidad de Oviedo: Oviedo, Spain, 2019.
11. Guzmán Jiménez, A. Conocimientos tradicionales de mujeres mapuches en la agricultura tradicional, territorio Naqche de La Araucanía, Chile. In *Biodiversidad y Conocimientos Tradicionales. Perspectivas Históricas, Socioculturales y Jurídicas*; Universidad de la Frontera: Temuco, Chile, 2018; pp. 97–110.
12. de Salud Pública, S. Encuesta Nacional de Salud 2016–2017 Primeros Resultados. Santiago. 2017. Available online: https://www.saludmagallanes.cl/wp-content/uploads/2017/11/ENS-2016-17_PRIMEROS-RESULTADOS.pdf (accessed on 10 October 2024).
13. López Ríos, J.M.; Mejía Merino, C.M.; Frías Epinayú, C.E.; Marulanda, S.C. Estrategias comunitarias para la seguridad alimentaria en indígenas wayuu, La Guajira, Colombia. *Rev. Española Nutrición Comunitaria* **2021**, *27*, 28–34.
14. Mundo-Rosas, V.; Shamah-Levy, T.; Rivera-Dommarco, J.A. Epidemiología de la inseguridad alimentaria en México. *Salud Pública México* **2013**, *55*, S206–S213. [CrossRef]
15. OMS; PMA; UNICEF. El Estado de la Seguridad Alimentaria y la Nutrición en el Mundo 2021. 2021. Available online: https://data.unicef.org/wp-content/uploads/2021/07/SOFI2021_InBrief_SP_web.pdf (accessed on 10 October 2024).
16. Medina Rey, J.M.; Ortega Carpio, M.; Martínez Cousinou, G. Seguridad alimentaria, soberanía alimentaria o derecho a la alimentación? Estado de la cuestión. *Cuad. Desarro. Rural* **2021**, *18*, 1–19.

17. Organizacioón Mundial de la Salud. Hipertensión Arterial. Informe Técnico-OMS-1978. Available online: https://iris.who.int/bitstream/handle/10665/37027/WHO_TRS_628_?sequence=1 (accessed on 1 October 2024).
18. Gutiérrez, B. La evolución del concepto de envejecimiento y vejez¿ Por fin hablaremos de salud en vejez en el sigloXXI? *Salut. Sci. Spirit.* **2022**, *8*, 14–22.
19. Apablaza, M.; Vega, F. Perfil de Ingresos de los Adultos Mayores en Chile. 2019. Available online: https://cipem.cl/estudios/reportes/2.12.pdf (accessed on 1 October 2024).
20. Sojo, A. *Protección Social en América Latina: La Desigualdad en el Banquillo*; CEPAL: Santiago, Chile, 2017.
21. Amigo, J.A.C. El actual sistema de pensiones como mecanismo reproductor de la inequidad de género en la vejez. *Pensam. Acción Interdiscip.* **2020**, *6*, 36–70.
22. Observatorio Social. Ministerio de Desarrollo Social y Familia. Principales Resultados Segunda Ronda: Inseguridad Alimentaria. 2020. Available online: https://observatorio.ministeriodesarrollosocial.gob.cl/storage/docs/covid19/Resultados_Inseguridad_Alimentaria_Covid_II.pdf (accessed on 24 October 2024).
23. Peralta Peña, P.A. Estudio de Factibilidad Estratégica, Técnica y Económica para Establecimiento de Larga Estadía para Adultos Mayores Ubicado en la Región de Coquimbo, Chile. Master's Thesis, Universidad de Chile, Santiago, Chile, 2023.
24. Thumala, D.; Kennedy, B.; Calvo, E.; Gonzalez-Billault, C.; Zitki, P.; Lillo, P.; Villagra, P.; Ibáñez, A.; Aassar, R.; Andrade, M.; et al. Envejecimiento y políticas de salud en Chile: Nuevas agendas para la investigación. *Health Syst. Reform* **2017**, *3*, 253–260. [CrossRef] [PubMed]
25. Geertz, C. Descripción Densa: Hacia una Teoría Interpretativa de la Cultura. Available online: http://www.iunma.edu.ar/doc/MB/lic_ts_mat_bibliografico/ANTROPOLOG%C3%8DA%20PLAN%20UNSAM/t1.%20Geertz,%20la%20interpretacion%20(1).pdf (accessed on 24 October 2024).
26. Morin, E. Introducción al Pensamiento Complejo (M. Pakman, Trad.). Gedisa. (Obra Original Publicada en 1990). 1994. Available online: https://cursoenlineasincostoedgarmorin.org/images/descargables/Morin_Introduccion_al_pensamiento_complejo.pdf (accessed on 1 October 2024).
27. Strauss, A.; Corbin, J. *Bases de la Investigación Cualitativa: Técnicas y Procedimientos para Desarrollar la Teoría Fundamentada*; Universidad de Antioquia: Antoquia, Colombia, 2016.
28. Bertaux, D. El enfoque biográfico: Su validez metodológica, sus potencialidades. *Proposiciones* **1999**, *29*, 1–23. [CrossRef]
29. Cerón, M.C.; Cerâon, M.C. *Metodologías de la Investigación Social*; LOM Ediciones Santiago: Santiago, Chile, 2006.
30. Serrano, G.P. *Investigación Cualitativa: Retos e Interrogantes*; La Muralla Madrid: Madrid, Spain, 1994.
31. Deluchi Mondschein, M.; Morales, D. La horticultura mapuche: Contribuciones a la seguridad alimentaria en una comunidad rural de la estepa Patagónica. *Boletín Soc. Argent. Botánica* **2022**, *57*, 1–10. [CrossRef]

Disclaimer/Publisher's Note: The statements, opinions and data contained in all publications are solely those of the individual author(s) and contributor(s) and not of MDPI and/or the editor(s). MDPI and/or the editor(s) disclaim responsibility for any injury to people or property resulting from any ideas, methods, instructions or products referred to in the content.

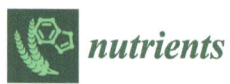 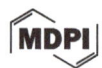

Article

Nutritional Risks of Heavy Metals in the Human Diet—Multi-Elemental Analysis of Energy Drinks

Katarzyna Czarnek [1,*], Małgorzata Tatarczak-Michalewska [2], Grzegorz Wójcik [3], Agnieszka Szopa [4], Dariusz Majerek [5], Karolina Fila [6], Muhammed Hamitoglu [7], Marek Gogacz [8] and Eliza Blicharska [2,*]

[1] Department of Basic Medical Sciences, Faculty of Medical, The John Paul II Catholic University of Lublin, Konstantynów 1 H St., 20-708 Lublin, Poland

[2] Department of Pathobiochemistry and Interdisciplinary Applications of Ion Chromatography, Medical University of Lublin, 1 Chodźki St., 20-093 Lublin, Poland; malgorzatatatarczakmichalewska@umlub.pl

[3] Department of Inorganic Chemistry, Institute of Chemical Sciences, Faculty of Chemistry, Maria Curie-Skłodowska University, Maria Curie-Skłodowska Sq. 2, 20-031 Lublin, Poland; grzegorz.wojcik2@mail.umcs.pl

[4] Department of Medicinal Plant and Mushroom Biotechnology, Faculty of Pharmacy, Jagiellonian University, 9 Medyczna St., 30-688 Kraków, Poland; a.szopa@uj.edu.pl

[5] Department of Applied Mathematics, Faculty of Mathematics and Information Technology, Lublin University of Technology, Nadbystrzycka 38 St., 20-618 Lublin, Poland; d.majerek@pollub.pl

[6] Department of Chemistry, Faculty of Food Science and Biotechnology, University of Life Sciences, 15 Akademicka St., 20-950 Lublin, Poland; karolina.fila@up.lublin.pl

[7] Department of Pharmaceutical Toxicology, Faculty of Pharmacy, Yeditepe University, 34755 Istanbul, Turkey; mohammad.saz@yeditepe.edu.tr

[8] 2nd Chair and Department of Gynecology, Medical University of Lublin, 20-090 Lublin, Poland; marek.gogacz@umlub.pl

* Correspondence: katarzyna.czarnek@kul.pl (K.C.); eliza.blicharska@umlub.pl (E.B.)

Citation: Czarnek, K.; Tatarczak-Michalewska, M.; Wójcik, G.; Szopa, A.; Majerek, D.; Fila, K.; Hamitoglu, M.; Gogacz, M.; Blicharska, E. Nutritional Risks of Heavy Metals in the Human Diet—Multi-Elemental Analysis of Energy Drinks. *Nutrients* **2024**, *16*, 4306. https://doi.org/10.3390/nu16244306

Academic Editors: Ariana Saraiva and António Raposo

Received: 15 November 2024
Revised: 5 December 2024
Accepted: 8 December 2024
Published: 13 December 2024

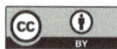

Copyright: © 2024 by the authors. Licensee MDPI, Basel, Switzerland. This article is an open access article distributed under the terms and conditions of the Creative Commons Attribution (CC BY) license (https://creativecommons.org/licenses/by/4.0/).

Abstract: Background: In recent years, the consumption of energy drinks (EDs) by adolescents and young adults has increased significantly, so concerns have been raised about the potential health risks associated with excessive ED consumption. Most analyses on EDs focus on the caffeine content. Research on the content of minerals (essential and toxic) in energy drinks can be considered scarce. Therefore, there is a need for research stating the actual status of heavy metal content in commercially available energy drinks. **Methods:** This research presents the determination of the total concentrations of macro-elements and trace elements (TEs), such as Na, K, Mg, Ca, Al, Cr, Co, Cu, Fe, Mn, Ni, B, Zn, V, Sr, Ba, Pb, Cd, and As in nine samples of energy drinks using inductively coupled plasma optical emission spectrometry (ICP-OES) and inductively coupled plasma mass spectrometry (ICP-MS) techniques. **Results:** The order in the content of macro-minerals in the EDs was as follows: Na > K > Mg > Ca. The results showed that ED 1, ED 3, and ED 7 samples had the highest micro-mineral concentrations. All the samples had a hazard quotient and hazard index < 1, indicating no non-carcinogenic risk from exposure to single or multiple heavy metals in both the adolescent and adult age groups. Some samples exceeded the threshold limit of acceptable cancer risk for As, Ni, and Cr in both adolescents and adults. **Conclusions:** This assessment showed that in addition to health implications based on the caffeine content of EDs, there might be a carcinogenic risk associated with the toxic element content of these beverages. This research also highlights notable differences in the TE levels among various ED brands, which may have important implications for consumer well-being and health.

Keywords: food safety; public health; health risks; food security; trace elements; heavy metals; energy drinks; mineral composition; ICP-OES; ICP-MS

1. Introduction

In recent years, the consumption of energy drinks (EDs) by adolescents and young adults has risen significantly, but concerns have been raised about the potential health risks associated with excessive consumption. Such drinks are aggressively advertised, and are easily accessible in local stores, supermarkets, and gas station stores in almost all European countries [1–5]. EDs are marketed as enhancers of mental acuity and physical performance. Adolescents gravitate towards these beverages to swiftly boost energy levels, and increase scholastic or athletic performance [1]. EDs have a high caffeine content which is normally combined with large amounts of vitamins, minerals, taurine, amino acids, and herbal extracts [6–8]. Most EDs contain from 50 to 505 mg of caffeine per can or bottle. Research under controlled conditions determined that 200 mg of caffeine induces atrial flutter and atrial fibrillation [1,9,10]. A growing number of case reports identifying various adverse effects following the acute ingestion of EDs, namely acute hemodynamic perturbations, disturbances in vascular function, and other cardiovascular abnormalities, have been reported [7,11–14]. Moreover, there have been reports of regular energy drink consumption being associated with anxiety and sleep disturbances [15,16].

Most analyses on EDs focus on the caffeine content. Besides caffeine, EDs generally contain high sugar and other components such as B-complex vitamins, taurine, ginseng, guarana seed extract, yerba mate, acai, and Ginkgo biloba. Some of these components (e.g., plant extracts) may lead to contamination problems in final products, including pesticide and heavy metal (HM) residues [17]. Energy drinks could also be contaminated during processing and packaging. According to some studies, most of the HMs present in alcoholic beverages can originate from agricultural pesticides or contamination from processing equipment (pipelines, containers, tanks, filtration systems, aluminum cans, etc.) [18–20].

The term "heavy metal" is based on categorization by density or molar mass. HMs are naturally occurring elements that have high atomic numbers and densities that are five times higher than water [21]. It is often used as a group name for metals (i.e., transition metals from vanadium to zinc) that are associated with contamination and potential toxicity. All so-called "heavy metals" and their compounds may have relatively high toxicity (e.g., lead or cadmium). Lead (Pb) is a toxic metal affecting nearly all organs, mimicking essential elements like calcium, iron, and zinc, and disrupting enzyme systems critical for heme synthesis, cell development, and bone growth. Arsenic (As), a widely distributed toxic metalloid, is found in water, air, food, and soil. It inactivates up to 200 enzymes involved in energy production, DNA synthesis, and repair, disrupting ATP production. Chronic exposure to As causes multisystem dysfunction and is a known carcinogen. Cadmium (Cd), a toxic element with no biological role, accumulates in plants and animal tissues, particularly the liver and kidneys. Prolonged exposure through air, water, and food can lead to cancer and damage to skeletal, urinary, cardiovascular, and nervous systems. Contamination during raw material processing may introduce Cd into beverages [22]. Aluminum (Al), abundant in the earth's crust, primarily enters the body through food. It disrupts the absorption of fluoride, calcium, and iron, and its phosphorus-binding properties may lead to phosphate depletion and osteomalacia. Al's main toxic effect is neurotoxicity [23]. Chromium occurs in various forms. Hexavalent chromium (Cr VI) is a Group 1 human carcinogen, while trivalent chromium (Cr III) is essential for carbohydrate, lipid, and protein metabolism and supports normal glucose regulation, with no classified carcinogenicity [24].

Nonetheless, metals are not always toxic and some are in fact essential and, depending on the dose and exposure levels and the receiving organism/population, the balance between essential or toxic may tip (e.g., iron or zinc) [25,26]. Trace elements (TEs) are classified as major minerals (macro-minerals) and trace minerals (micro-minerals). Major minerals include several elements such as Ca, Na, Mg, and K; while trace minerals include Zn, Cu, Fe, Mn, Co, B, and Cr. About 20 of the known elements are qualified today as essential [27]. Many TEs are essential to numerous biological, chemical, and molecular processes, regulating cellular homeostasis, humoral, and cellular immune responses, and being cofactors of many enzymes and antioxidant molecules [28,29]. Some metals, such as Fe, Zn, Cu, Co, and Mn, are required for various physiological functions in humans at low concentrations, but they become toxic at higher concentrations. Other HMs, such as cadmium and lead, are not known to have any beneficial effects on human health and their accumulation in the human body is deleterious to health [30].

The available research on the mineral content (both essential and toxic) in energy drinks remains limited. This study aimed to quantify the concentrations of Na, K, Mg, Ca, Al, Cr, Co, Cu, Fe, Mn, Ni, B, Zn, V, Sr, Ba, Pb, Cd, and As in nine commercially available energy drinks sold in Poland, packaged in aluminum cans. Inductively coupled plasma optical emission spectroscopy (ICP-OES) and inductively coupled plasma mass spectrometry (ICP-MS) were employed for the elemental analysis. Additionally, a toxicological risk assessment was conducted to evaluate the potential health risks associated with exposure to these elements through energy drink consumption in adolescents and adults. To our knowledge, this is the only study that estimated the carcinogenic risk for toxic elements from the consumption of EDs.

2. Materials and Methods

2.1. Samples and Sample Preparation

Nine different brands of energy drink samples were obtained from markets in Lublin, Poland. The energy drinks selected for research represent the most popular and most widely consumed brands in Poland based on market data. All of the packaging materials of the energy drink samples analyzed in the study were aluminum cans. The composition of each ED is shown below in Table 1.

Table 1. Composition of energy drink samples investigated in our study.

Energy Drink	Composition
ED 1	water, sugar, citric acid, carbon dioxide, taurine (400 mg/100 mL), acidity regulator (sodium citrates), glucose–fructose syrup, caffeine (30 mg/100 mL), flavors, colors (ammonia caramel and riboflavin), sweeteners (acesulfame K and sucralose), inositol (20 mg/100 mL), and vitamins (niacin, pantothenic acid, vitamin B6, and vitamin B12)
ED 2	water, sugar, carbon dioxide, acids (citric acid and tartaric acid), acidity regulator (sodium citrates), flavors, taurine (100 mg/100 mL), preservatives (potassium sorbate and sodium benzoate), caffeine (30 mg/100 mL), vitamins (niacin and vitamin B6), sweetener (sucralose), inositol, and colors (E102, E129, and E133)
ED 3	water, sucrose, glucose, acid (citric acid), carbon dioxide, taurine (400 mg/100 mL), acidity regulator (sodium carbonates and magnesium carbonate), caffeine (30 mg/100 mL), vitamins (niacin, pantothenic acid, B6, and B12), flavors, and colors (caramel and riboflavin)
ED 4	water, sugar, acidity regulators (citric acid and sodium citrates), carbon dioxide, taurine (350 mg/100 mL), flavor, caffeine (30 mg/100 mL), dyes (E 150d), riboflavin, and vitamins (niacin, pantothenic acid, vitamin B6, and vitamin B12)
ED 5	water, apple juice from concentrated apple juice, sugar, carbon dioxide, acid (citric acid), taurine (400 mg/100 mL), flavor, caffeine (30 mg/100 mL), sweeteners (acesulfame K and aspartame), color (E 150d), and vitamins (niacin, vitamin B6, and vitamin B12)
ED 6	water, sugar, acid (citric acid), carbon dioxide, taurine (300 mg/100 mL), acidity regulator (sodium citrates), flavor, caffeine (30 mg/100 mL), safflower color concentrate, inositol, and vitamins (niacin, pantothenic acid, vitamin B6, and vitamin B12)
ED 7	water, acid (citric acid), carbon dioxide, taurine (400 mg/100 mL), acidity regulator (sodium citrate), flavors, ginseng extract (0.08%), sweeteners (sucralose and acesulfame K), caffeine (30 mg/100 mL), preservatives (sorbic acid and benzoic acid), L-carnitine tartrate (0.04%), vitamins (niacin, pantothenic acid, vitamin B6, and vitamin B12), sodium chloride, D-glucuronolactone, guarana seed extract (0.002%), and inositol
ED 8	water, apple juice from concentrated juice (10%), grape juice from concentrated juice (10%), acidity regulators (citric acid, sodium citrates), carbon dioxide, sweeteners (sucralose and acesulfame K), caffeine (30 mg/100 mL), inositol, colors (ammonia caramel, sulfite caramel, and riboflavin), flavors, flavor enhancer (erythritol), and vitamins (niacin, B6, B12, and pantothenic acid)
ED 9	water, sugar, carbon dioxide, magnesium citrate, citric acid, flavorings, rhubarb gum, glycerol and vegetable resin esters, caffeine (30 mg/100 mL), and vitamins (niacin, vitamin B6, vitamin B12, and biotin)

To eliminate any dissolved CO_2, the samples were sonicated using an ultrasonic bath for 70 min. In the next step, 9 mL of the degassed sample was transferred to a Teflon cuvette and 3 mL of 65% (v/v) HNO_3 (Suprapur, Merck, Darmstadt, Germany) was added. The components were thoroughly mixed. The reaction vessel was closed and placed in a microwave mineralizer Multiwave 5000 (Anton Paar, Graz, Austria). The program used was based on temperature control with the dynamic selection of microwave power: temperature was increased from ambient temperature to 180 °C in 20 min., held at a temperature of 180 °C for 10 min., and cooled to 70 °C.

After the cooling to ambient temperature, the digested samples were diluted to 25 mL with ultrapure water, i.e., deionized water of resistance 18.3 MΩ cm^{-1} (EASYpure™ system, Barnstead, Thermolyne Corporation, Ramsey, MN, USA). The standard solution of elements was prepared by the dilution of ICP multi-element standard solution XXV for MS (Merck, Darmstadt, Germany). All the analyses were performed in triplicate. The analysis of blank samples confirmed the high purity of the used chemicals and containers.

2.2. ICP-OES Conditions

The ICP-OES analysis was performed by using a Varian 720-ES spectrometer (Varian, Melbourne, Australia). The content of four macro-minerals Na, K, Mg, and Ca was determined by this method (Table 2).

Table 2. ICP-OES instrument operating conditions.

RF power [W]	1000
Plasma flow [L min^{-1}]	15
Auxiliary flow [L min^{-1}]	1.5
Nebulizer flow [L min^{-1}]	0.75
Replicate read time [s]	1
Instrument stabilization delay [s]	15
Sample uptake delay [s]	15
Pump rate [rpm]	15
Rinse time [s]	10
Wavelength [nm]	Ca 396.847, K 766.491, Mg 279.533, Na 589.592

2.3. ICP-MS Conditions

The ICP-MS analysis was performed by using an Agilent Technologies 7700x series spectrometer (Agilent, Tokyo, Japan). The content of the fifteen elements B, Al, V, Cr, Mn, Fe, Co, Ni, Cu, Zn, As, Sr, Cd, Ba, and Pb was determined by this method (Table 3).

Table 3. ICP-MS instrument operating conditions.

RF power [W]	1600
Plasma flow [L min^{-1}]	15
Carrier gas flow rate [L min^{-1}]	0.34
Dilution gas flow rate [L min^{-1}]	0.57
Nebulizer	MicroMist
Ion Lenses	x-Lens
Replicates	3
Stabilization time [s]	30
Acquisition Mode	Spectrum
Nebulizer pump speed [rpm]	0.1
Energy discrimination [V]	5
Isotopes acquired	^{11}B, ^{27}Al, ^{51}V, ^{52}Cr, ^{55}Mn, ^{56}Fe, ^{59}Co, ^{60}Ni, ^{63}Cu, ^{66}Zn, ^{75}As, ^{88}Sr, ^{111}Cd, ^{137}Ba, ^{208}Pb

2.4. Toxicological Risk Assessment

The toxicological risk assessment for the investigated elements in the ED samples was conducted using the established equations to estimate the estimated daily intake (EDI) and non-carcinogenic risks (HQ) [22,31,32].

The EDI was calculated using the following equation:

$$EDI = (C \times IR \times EF \times EXD)/(BW \times AT)$$

The hazard quotient (HQ) for each element was calculated as follows:

$$HQ = EDI/RfD$$

where EDI is the estimated daily intake (mg/kg/day); C is the metal concentration in samples (mg/L); IR is the daily intake rate of EDs at 0.23 L/day for adolescents and 0.16 L/day for adults; EF is exposure frequency, in this study, 240 day/year; EXD is the exposure duration, in this study, 8 years (10–18 years old) for adolescents and 47 years (18–65 years old) for adults [33]; BW is the body weight at 45 kg for adolescents and 70 kg for adults; AT = EXD × 365 days is the averaging time for non-carcinogensis; HQ is the hazard quotient; and RfD is the reference oral dose in mg/kg/day (0.2 for B, 1 for Al, 0.009 for V, 0.003 for Cr, 0.14 for Mn, 0.7 for Fe, 0.0003 for Co, 0.02 for Ni, 0.04 for Cu, 0.3 for Zn, 0.0003 for As, 0.6 for Sr, 0.0005 for Cd, 0.07 for Ba and 0.0035 for Pb).

The average daily intake in our study, based on the EFSA report, was approximately 0.23 and 0.16 L/day for adolescents and adults, respectively. Adolescents (10–18 years) consumed the most, averaging 7 L per month, at least 4–5 times a week. Adults (18–65 years) averaged 4.5 L monthly, with at least 4–5 times a week [33].

To account for the additive effects of exposure to multiple elements, the total hazard index (HI) was calculated as the arithmetic sum of individual HQ values:

$$HI = \sum HQ$$

The incremental lifetime cancer risk (ILCR) was estimated to determine the probability of developing cancer over a lifetime due to exposure to potential carcinogenic elements. The formula used was as follows:

$$ILCR = EDI \times CSF$$

where CSF is the cancer slope factor (mg/kg/day). The oral values used were 0.5 for Cr, 1.7 for Ni, 1.5 for inorganic As, 0.38 for Cd, and 0.0085 for Pb. The CSF is a toxicity value that quantitatively defines the relationship between dose and response. An ILCR value greater than 10^{-4} indicates high cancer risk, while an ILCR value smaller than 10^{-6} is acceptable and safe, and a value in the range of 10^{-6} to 10^{-4} indicates a moderate risk [22,34].

2.5. Statistical Analysis

To analyze element concentrations in various energy drink products, the Kruskal–Wallis H test was used, which is a non-parametric method suitable for non-normally distributed data often seen in environmental studies. Each product was sampled three times ($n = 3$), and the test compared multiple independent groups to detect significant differences in element levels [35,36]. To control the family-wise error rate, Bonferroni adjustments were applied to the p-values, reducing the risk of Type I errors and ensuring robust significance levels despite the small sample size [37].

One-sample Student's t-tests were conducted to determine if element concentrations in individual drinks exceeded the normative values set by bodies like WHO (World Health Organization), EU (European Union), and US EPA (United States Environmental Protection Agency). Mean concentrations from three samples per product were compared to these norms. Despite the limited sample size ($n = 3$), the one-sample t-test was deemed appropriate for detecting significant exceedances. Bonferroni adjustments were also applied to control for multiple hypothesis testing, ensuring the results' reliability [38].

All the analyses were performed in R (version 4.4.1) using the tidyverse suite for data manipulation and visualization, and the rstatix package for statistical tests and Bonferroni corrections [39–41]. This approach ensured rigor, reproducibility, and adherence to statistical best practices.

3. Results

Nine energy drinks of different brands were analyzed using the techniques ICP-OES and ICP-MS, and the results are presented in Tables 4 and 5. The total concentrations of 19 elements (Na, K, Mg, Ca, B, Al, V, Cr, Mn, Fe, Co, Ni, Cu, Zn, As, Sr, Cd, Ba, and Pb), both essential and toxic, were determined in the ED samples.

Table 4. Content of the macro-minerals [mg L^{-1}] in the analyzed energy drinks (n = 27).

Elements	Min	Max	Mean	SD	p.adj *
Sodium (Na)	8.62	619.85	377.16	223.25	0.00524
Potassium (K)	5.51	189.57	65.28	72.90	0.00552
Magnesium (Mg)	0.013	543.97	83.96	184.14	0.00476
Calcium (Ca)	2.54	116.1	23.15	35.66	0.00692

* p.adj —p-values after Bonferroni correction

Table 5. Content of micro-minerals in the analyzed energy drinks (n = 27) and the WHO, EU, and US EPA regulations of maximum permissible metal levels in drinking water [µg L^{-1}].

Elements	Min	Max	Mean	SD	p.adj *	WHO [42]	EU [43]	US EPA [44–46]
Boron (B)	194.01	796.82	432.28	186.54	1.00000	2400	1500	1400
Aluminum (Al)	227.54	456.97	297.32	67.18	0.43800	N/A	200	200
Vanadium (V)	0.29	10.44	3.60	3.04	0.02640	N/A	N/A	N/A **
Chromium (Cr)	13.49	67.53	39.70	18.26	0.02520	50	50	100
Manganese (Mn)	6.69	107.27	27.38	35.27	0.05415	N/A	50	50
Iron (Fe)	121.86	308.31	205.34	66.00	0.22950	300	200	300
Cobalt (Co)	0.19	4.13	1.20	1.18	0.01830	N/A	N/A	100
Nickel (Ni)	2.04	6.57	3.36	1.57	0.14745	70	20	100
Copper (Cu)	2.94	16.76	8.02	4.31	0.02985	2000	2000	1300
Zinc (Zn)	10.34	64.56	23.98	17.27	0.03960	N/A	N/A	5000
Arsenic (As)	1.57	23.05	7.33	7.00	0.02625	10	10	10
Strontium (Sr)	2.99	3878.21	452.74	1284.72	0.02400	N/A	N/A	1500
Cadmium (Cd)	0.19	0.78	0.34	0.18	1.00000	3	5	5
Barium (Ba)	4.81	19.98	11.54	5.18	0.04095	1300	N/A	2000
Lead (Pb)	5.00	32.79	10.37	8.53	1.00000	10	10	15

* p.adj —p-values after Bonferroni correction; N/A—not available; ** a proposed notification level for vanadium at 15 µg L^{-1} in drinking water established by the OEHHA [47].

3.1. Macro-Mineral Composition Analysis of Energy Drinks

Using the ICP-OES method, the content of four macro-minerals (Na, K, Mg, and Ca) was determined, the concentrations of which, summarized in Table 4, are given in mg L^{-1}.

Among the measured elements, sodium was the element present in the investigated products at the highest concentration. The content of this macro-mineral ranged from 8.62 mg L^{-1} (ED 9) to 619.85 mg L^{-1} (ED 4). Potassium concentrations in the products tested were generally lower than Na concentrations, ranging from 5.51 mg L^{-1} (ED 3) to 189.57 mg L^{-1} (ED 5).

The determined calcium concentrations ranged from 2.54 mg L^{-1} (ED 2) to 116.1 mg L^{-1} (ED 3). The magnesium content ranged from 0.013 mg L^{-1} (ED 2) to 196 mg L^{-1} (ED 3), and was significantly higher (543.97 mg L^{-1}–ED 9) for only one ED enriched with this element at the production stage.

The Kruskal–Wallis test showed significant differences in the concentrations of all the analyzed macro-minerals—Ca, K, Mg, and Na—between the different brands of energy drinks. For each of these elements, the p-values after Bonferroni correction (p.adj) were significantly less than 0.05 (Ca: 0.00692, K: 0.00552, Mg: 0.00476, and Na: 0.00524), which indicates that there are significant differences in their concentrations between the products tested. The number of samples for each element was 27, and the test statistics exceeded the critical values for degrees of freedom of 8, which confirms the significance of the observed differences.

3.2. Micro-Mineral Composition Analysis of Energy Drinks

The results of quantitative determinations of fifteen micro-minerals (B, Al, V, Cr, Mn, Fe, Co, Ni, Cu, Zn, As, Sr, Cd, Ba, and Pb), obtained using the ICP-MS technique, are given in $\mu g\ L^{-1}$ of the initial drink solution in Table 5 and in Figures 1–6.

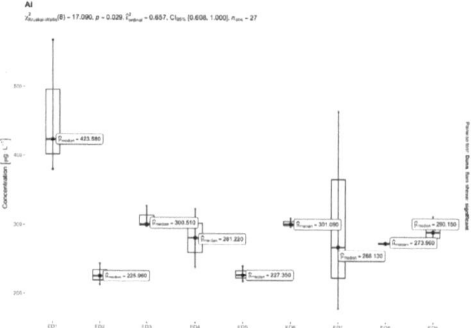

Figure 1. Content of aluminum (Al) [mg L^{-1}] in the analyzed energy drinks (n = 3).

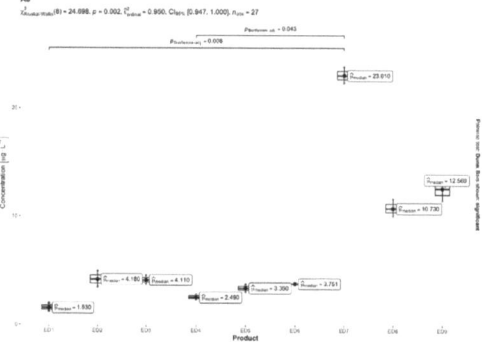

Figure 2. Content of arsenic (As) [mg L^{-1}] in the analyzed energy drinks (n = 3).

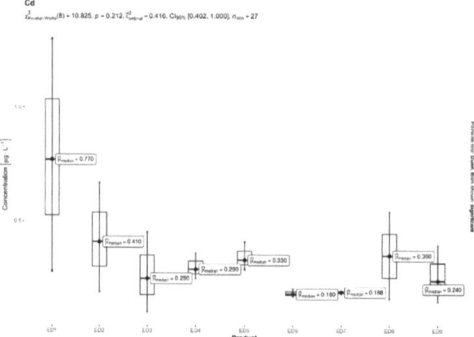

Figure 3. Content of cadmium (Cd) [mg L^{-1}] in the analyzed energy drinks (n = 3).

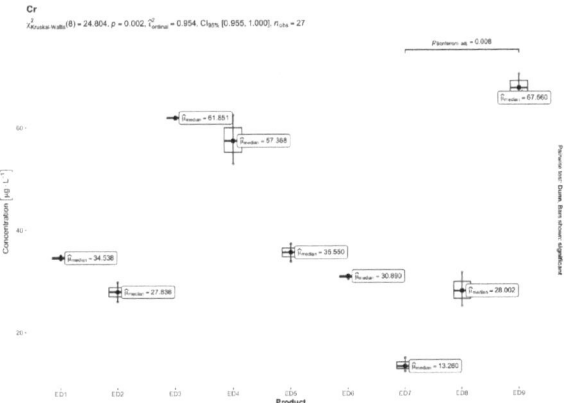

Figure 4. Content of chromium (Cr) [mg L^{-1}] in the analyzed energy drinks (n = 3).

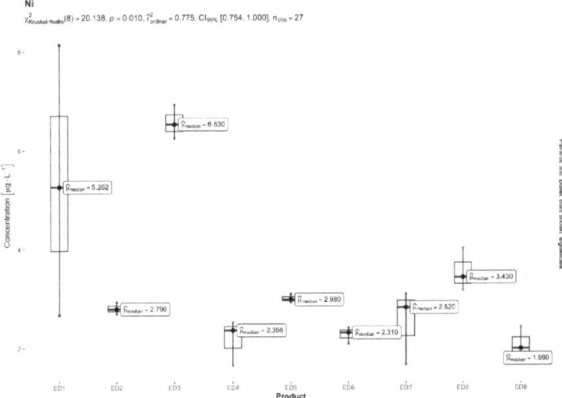

Figure 5. Content of nickel (Ni) [mg L^{-1}] in the analyzed energy drinks (n = 3).

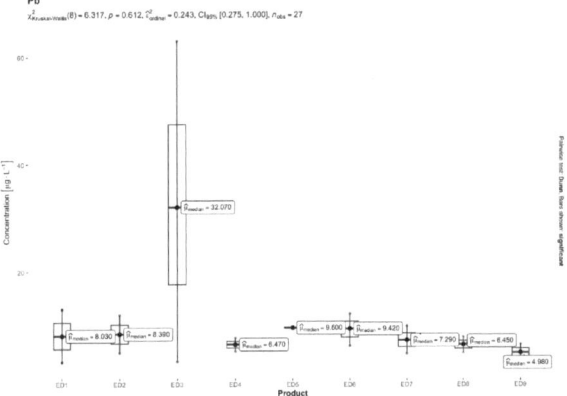

Figure 6. Content of lead (Pb) [mg L^{-1}] in the analyzed energy drinks (n = 3).

Of the elements listed above, the essential TEs include Fe, B, Cu, Cr, Mn, Zn, and Co, with Fe, Cu, Cr, and Zn also classified as heavy metals. Conversely, Ni, As, Cd, and Pb are examples of HMs that do not have any biological role. Some trace elements like Al, V, Sr, and Ba have not been demonstrated to be essential in humans.

Among the essential TEs analyzed, B and Fe exhibited the greatest levels in the examined EDs. The B concentration varied between 194.01 µg L^{-1} in ED 3 and 796.82 µg L^{-1} in ED 7, with the Fe levels ranging from 121.86 µg L^{-1} in ED 2 to 308.31 µg L^{-1} in ED 7. Concentrations for the other essential TEs varied within the following ranges: Mn (6.69–107.27 µg L^{-1}), Cr (13.49–67.53 µg L^{-1}), Zn (10.34–64.56 µg L^{-1}), Cu (2.94–16.76 µg L^{-1}), and Co (0.19–4.13 µg L^{-1}).

Among the most hazardous toxic elements, Pb and As exhibited the highest concentration in th EDs. The average Pb levels in the energy drinks tested were consistent (ranging from 5.00 to 9.61 µg L^{-1}), except for one ED 3 sample, which contained 32.79 µg L^{-1} of Pb. The highest concentrations of Ni and As were found in ED 3 and ED 7, with concentration ranges of 2.04–6.57 µg L^{-1} and 1.57–23.05 µg L^{-1}, respectively. Cd was found in very small amounts in the EDs tested, ranging from 0.19 µg L^{-1} in ED 7 and ED 6 to 0.78 µg L^{-1} in the ED 1 sample.

It was noticed that Al was present in the highest concentrations among the non-essential TEs, with a range from 227.54 µg L^{-1} (ED 2) to 456.97 µg L^{-1} (ED 1). Toxic Ba was also found in the ED samples (the lowest concentration of 4.81 µg L^{-1} was recorded for ED 7, and the highest 19.98 µg L^{-1} for ED 3). Interestingly, of the EDs tested, the highest Sr concentration was reported for the ED 3 sample, which was 3878.21 µg L^{-1}. Unlike the sample of ED 3, the other EDs had low Sr concentrations (between 2.99 and 72.36 µg L^{-1}). Additional non-essential TEs, like V, were found in the EDs analyzed at levels between 0.29 (ED 9) and 10.44 µg L^{-1} (ED 1).

The result of the Kruskal–Wallis test for micro-minerals indicates that for some elements, there are significant differences in concentrations between product groups, while for others, these differences are not statistically significant after taking into account the Bonferroni correction. Trace elements such as As, Ba, Co, Cr, Cu, Sr, V, and Zn showed significant differences in concentrations between products. The values of the adjusted p ($p.adj$) for these trace elements were lower than the accepted level of significance (e.g., 0.05), which suggests that their concentrations differ depending on the type of product. On the other hand, trace elements such as Al, B, Cd, Fe, Mn, Ni, and Pb did not show significant differences after applying the Bonferroni correction. This means that the differences in their concentrations between the tested product groups are not statistically significant, so it cannot be stated that these products differ significantly in terms of their content. In summary, the Kruskal–Wallis test showed significant differences in the concentrations of some micro-minerals, which indicates that some of them may be more dependent on the type of product. The Bonferroni correction provided control for the first-type error in the multiple comparison analysis, allowing a more conservative assessment of statistical significance.

The EDI for fifteen micro-minerals via the consumption of the EDs is summarized in Tables 6 and 7. The HQ was calculated to evaluate the risk of chronic systemic toxicity posed by exposure to each toxic and essential element. The HQ represents the ratio of EDI to the RfD, which is the maximum acceptable dose assumed to be without adverse health effects in humans. When the HQ value for an element exceeds 1 (HQ > 1), it indicates a potential health risk, meaning the exposure surpasses the maximum permissible RfD. Conversely, if HQ $\leq$ 1, adverse health effects are unlikely, and the exposed population is presumed to be safe.

The HQ values for the investigated elements through the consumption of the EDs are presented in Tables 6 and 7. For the nine analyzed ED samples, all the HQ values for both adolescent and adult age groups were below the risk threshold (HQ < 1), indicating no significant non-carcinogenic risks to consumers.

The potential cumulative hazard from exposure to the fifteen micro-minerals was also assessed, with the results presented in Tables 6 and 7. The HI ranged from 0.10 to 0.32 for the nine ED samples in adolescents and from 0.04 to 0.13 in adults. All the HI values were below the critical threshold of one, confirming that the cumulative exposure to these micro-minerals does not pose a significant non-carcinogenic risk for consumers.

Table 6. Estimated daily intake and health risks associated with micro-mineral exposure in adolescents from energy drink consumption.

Sample	B	Al	V	Cr	Mn	Fe	Co	Ni	Cu	Zn	As	Sr	Cd	Ba	Pb	HI
								EDI THQ								
ED 1	1.6×10^{-3} 8.1×10^{-3}	1.5×10^{-4} 1.5×10^{-3}	3.4×10^{-5} 3.7×10^{-3}	1.2×10^{-4} 3.9×10^{-2}	4.0×10^{-5} 2.9×10^{-4}	5.8×10^{-4} 8.3×10^{-4}	4.4×10^{-6} 1.5×10^{-2}	1.8×10^{-5} 9.0×10^{-4}	5.6×10^{-5} 1.4×10^{-3}	2.2×10^{-4} 7.2×10^{-4}	5.3×10^{-6} 1.8×10^{-2}	1.3×10^{-4} 2.1×10^{-4}	2.6×10^{-6} 5.2×10^{-3}	4.8×10^{-5} 6.8×10^{-4}	2.7×10^{-5} 7.7×10^{-3}	0.10
ED 2	6.7×10^{-4} 3.4×10^{-3}	7.7×10^{-4} 7.7×10^{-3}	6.7×10^{-6} 7.5×10^{-4}	9.4×10^{-5} 3.1×10^{-2}	2.4×10^{-5} 1.7×10^{-4}	4.1×10^{-4} 5.9×10^{-4}	6.4×10^{-7} 2.1×10^{-3}	9.4×10^{-6} 4.7×10^{-4}	2.4×10^{-5} 6.1×10^{-4}	6.7×10^{-5} 2.2×10^{-4}	1.4×10^{-5} 4.7×10^{-2}	1.1×10^{-5} 1.8×10^{-5}	1.4×10^{-6} 2.8×10^{-3}	2.2×10^{-5} 3.1×10^{-4}	2.8×10^{-5} 8.1×10^{-3}	0.10
ED 3	6.4×10^{-4} 3.2×10^{-3}	1.0×10^{-3} 1.0×10^{-2}	1.7×10^{-5} 1.9×10^{-3}	2.1×10^{-4} 6.9×10^{-2}	2.4×10^{-5} 1.7×10^{-4}	5.1×10^{-4} 7.3×10^{-4}	1.4×10^{-5} 4.6×10^{-2}	2.2×10^{-5} 1.1×10^{-3}	3.6×10^{-5} 8.9×10^{-4}	3.5×10^{-5} 1.2×10^{-4}	1.4×10^{-5} 4.6×10^{-2}	1.3×10^{-5} 2.2×10^{-5}	9.1×10^{-7} 1.8×10^{-3}	6.7×10^{-5} 9.6×10^{-4}	1.1×10^{-4} 3.1×10^{-2}	0.23
ED 4	1.9×10^{-3} 9.7×10^{-3}	9.4×10^{-4} 9.4×10^{-4}	1.0×10^{-5} 1.1×10^{-3}	1.9×10^{-4} 6.5×10^{-2}	2.4×10^{-5} 1.7×10^{-4}	6.7×10^{-4} 9.6×10^{-4}	1.6×10^{-6} 5.5×10^{-3}	7.3×10^{-6} 3.6×10^{-4}	2.2×10^{-5} 5.5×10^{-4}	5.1×10^{-5} 1.7×10^{-4}	8.5×10^{-6} 2.8×10^{-2}	8.0×10^{-5} 1.3×10^{-4}	1.0×10^{-6} 2.0×10^{-3}	2.6×10^{-5} 3.8×10^{-4}	2.2×10^{-5} 6.2×10^{-3}	0.12
ED 5	1.6×10^{-3} 8.1×10^{-3}	7.7×10^{-4} 7.7×10^{-3}	1.7×10^{-5} 1.9×10^{-3}	1.2×10^{-4} 4.0×10^{-2}	2.2×10^{-5} 1.6×10^{-4}	7.2×10^{-4} 1.0×10^{-3}	3.5×10^{-6} 1.2×10^{-2}	1.0×10^{-5} 5.0×10^{-4}	1.8×10^{-5} 4.4×10^{-4}	9.7×10^{-5} 3.2×10^{-4}	1.1×10^{-5} 3.8×10^{-2}	7.7×10^{-5} 1.3×10^{-4}	1.1×10^{-6} 2.3×10^{-3}	5.1×10^{-5} 7.3×10^{-4}	3.2×10^{-5} 9.2×10^{-3}	0.12
ED 6	1.4×10^{-3} 6.9×10^{-3}	1.0×10^{-3} 1.0×10^{-3}	1.0×10^{-5} 1.1×10^{-3}	1.0×10^{-4} 3.5×10^{-2}	8.1×10^{-5} 5.8×10^{-4}	8.7×10^{-4} 1.2×10^{-3}	1.3×10^{-6} 4.3×10^{-3}	7.6×10^{-6} 3.8×10^{-4}	2.4×10^{-5} 6.1×10^{-4}	6.6×10^{-5} 2.2×10^{-4}	1.3×10^{-5} 4.2×10^{-2}	6.1×10^{-5} 1.0×10^{-4}	6.4×10^{-7} 1.3×10^{-3}	4.2×10^{-5} 6.0×10^{-4}	3.1×10^{-5} 8.9×10^{-3}	0.10
ED 7	2.7×10^{-3} 1.3×10^{-2}	1.0×10^{-3} 1.0×10^{-3}	1.0×10^{-5} 1.1×10^{-3}	4.7×10^{-5} 1.6×10^{-2}	4.0×10^{-5} 2.9×10^{-4}	1.0×10^{-3} 1.5×10^{-3}	4.7×10^{-6} 1.6×10^{-2}	8.5×10^{-6} 4.3×10^{-4}	1.3×10^{-5} 3.4×10^{-4}	3.8×10^{-5} 1.3×10^{-4}	7.7×10^{-5} 2.6×10^{-1}	1.0×10^{-5} 1.7×10^{-5}	6.4×10^{-7} 1.3×10^{-3}	1.6×10^{-5} 2.3×10^{-4}	2.5×10^{-5} 7.0×10^{-3}	0.32
ED 8	1.3×10^{-3} 6.7×10^{-3}	9.1×10^{-4} 9.1×10^{-3}	1.7×10^{-5} 1.9×10^{-3}	9.4×10^{-5} 3.1×10^{-2}	3.7×10^{-5} 2.6×10^{-4}	9.5×10^{-4} 1.4×10^{-3}	3.9×10^{-6} 1.3×10^{-2}	1.2×10^{-5} 5.9×10^{-4}	3.9×10^{-5} 9.7×10^{-4}	1.2×10^{-4} 3.8×10^{-4}	3.6×10^{-5} 1.2×10^{-1}	2.4×10^{-4} 4.1×10^{-4}	1.2×10^{-6} 2.4×10^{-3}	5.3×10^{-5} 7.5×10^{-4}	2.2×10^{-5} 6.2×10^{-3}	0.19
ED 9	1.2×10^{-3} 5.9×10^{-3}	9.7×10^{-4} 9.7×10^{-4}	1.0×10^{-5} 1.1×10^{-3}	2.3×10^{-4} 7.6×10^{-2}	2.4×10^{-5} 1.7×10^{-4}	4.6×10^{-4} 6.6×10^{-4}	2.5×10^{-6} 8.4×10^{-3}	6.9×10^{-6} 3.4×10^{-4}	9.9×10^{-6} 2.5×10^{-4}	3.9×10^{-5} 1.3×10^{-4}	4.2×10^{-5} 1.4×10^{-1}	5.1×10^{-5} 8.5×10^{-5}	8.7×10^{-7} 1.7×10^{-3}	2.4×10^{-5} 3.4×10^{-4}	1.7×10^{-5} 4.8×10^{-3}	0.24

Table 7. Estimated daily intake and health risks associated with micro-mineral exposure in adults from energy drink consumption.

Sample	B	Al	V	Cr	Mn	Fe	Co	Ni	Cu	Zn	As	Sr	Cd	Ba	Pb	HI
								EDI THQ								
ED 1	6.8×10^{-4} 3.4×10^{-3}	6.5×10^{-4} 6.5×10^{-4}	1.4×10^{-5} 1.6×10^{-3}	4.9×10^{-5} 1.6×10^{-2}	1.7×10^{-5} 1.2×10^{-4}	2.4×10^{-4} 3.5×10^{-4}	1.8×10^{-6} 6.1×10^{-3}	7.6×10^{-6} 3.8×10^{-4}	2.4×10^{-5} 5.9×10^{-4}	9.1×10^{-5} 3.0×10^{-4}	2.2×10^{-6} 7.4×10^{-3}	5.3×10^{-5} 8.9×10^{-5}	1.1×10^{-6} 2.2×10^{-3}	2.0×10^{-5} 2.9×10^{-4}	1.1×10^{-5} 3.2×10^{-3}	0.04
ED 2	2.8×10^{-4} 1.4×10^{-3}	3.2×10^{-4} 3.2×10^{-4}	2.8×10^{-6} 3.1×10^{-4}	3.9×10^{-5} 1.3×10^{-2}	9.9×10^{-6} 7.0×10^{-5}	1.7×10^{-4} 2.5×10^{-4}	2.7×10^{-7} 8.9×10^{-4}	3.9×10^{-6} 2.0×10^{-4}	1.0×10^{-5} 2.6×10^{-4}	2.8×10^{-5} 9.4×10^{-5}	5.9×10^{-6} 2.0×10^{-2}	4.4×10^{-6} 7.4×10^{-6}	5.9×10^{-7} 1.2×10^{-3}	9.1×10^{-6} 1.3×10^{-4}	1.2×10^{-5} 3.4×10^{-3}	0.04
ED 3	2.7×10^{-4} 1.3×10^{-3}	4.4×10^{-4} 4.4×10^{-4}	7.0×10^{-6} 7.8×10^{-4}	8.7×10^{-5} 2.9×10^{-2}	9.9×10^{-6} 7.0×10^{-5}	2.1×10^{-4} 3.1×10^{-4}	5.8×10^{-6} 1.9×10^{-2}	9.3×10^{-6} 4.6×10^{-4}	1.5×10^{-5} 3.7×10^{-4}	1.5×10^{-5} 4.9×10^{-5}	5.8×10^{-6} 1.9×10^{-2}	5.5×10^{-5} 9.1×10^{-5}	3.8×10^{-7} 7.6×10^{-4}	2.8×10^{-5} 4.0×10^{-4}	4.6×10^{-5} 1.3×10^{-2}	0.10
ED 4	8.2×10^{-4} 4.1×10^{-3}	3.9×10^{-4} 3.9×10^{-4}	4.2×10^{-6} 4.7×10^{-4}	8.2×10^{-5} 2.7×10^{-2}	9.9×10^{-6} 7.0×10^{-5}	2.8×10^{-4} 4.0×10^{-4}	6.9×10^{-7} 2.3×10^{-3}	3.1×10^{-6} 1.5×10^{-4}	9.2×10^{-6} 2.3×10^{-4}	2.1×10^{-5} 7.1×10^{-5}	3.6×10^{-6} 1.2×10^{-2}	3.4×10^{-5} 5.6×10^{-5}	4.2×10^{-7} 8.5×10^{-4}	1.1×10^{-5} 1.6×10^{-4}	9.1×10^{-6} 2.6×10^{-3}	0.05
ED 5	6.8×10^{-4} 3.4×10^{-3}	3.2×10^{-4} 3.2×10^{-4}	7.0×10^{-6} 7.8×10^{-4}	5.1×10^{-5} 1.7×10^{-2}	9.2×10^{-6} 6.5×10^{-5}	3.0×10^{-4} 4.3×10^{-4}	1.5×10^{-6} 4.9×10^{-3}	4.2×10^{-6} 2.1×10^{-4}	7.4×10^{-6} 1.8×10^{-4}	4.1×10^{-5} 1.4×10^{-4}	4.7×10^{-6} 1.6×10^{-2}	3.2×10^{-5} 5.4×10^{-5}	4.8×10^{-7} 9.6×10^{-4}	2.1×10^{-5} 3.0×10^{-4}	1.4×10^{-5} 3.9×10^{-3}	0.05

Table 7. Cont.

Sample	B	Al	V	Cr	Mn	Fe	Co	EDI THQ Ni	Cu	Zn	As	Sr	Cd	Ba	Pb	HI
ED 6	5.8×10^{-4} 2.9×10^{-3}	4.2×10^{-4} 4.2×10^{-4}	4.2×10^{-6} 4.7×10^{-4}	4.4×10^{-5} 1.5×10^{-2}	3.4×10^{-5} 2.4×10^{-4}	3.6×10^{-4} 5.2×10^{-4}	5.4×10^{-7} 1.8×10^{-3}	3.2×10^{-6} 1.6×10^{-4}	1.0×10^{-5} 2.6×10^{-4}	2.8×10^{-5} 9.2×10^{-5}	5.3×10^{-6} 1.8×10^{-2}	2.6×10^{-5} 4.3×10^{-5}	2.7×10^{-7} 5.4×10^{-4}	1.8×10^{-5} 2.5×10^{-4}	1.3×10^{-5} 3.7×10^{-3}	0.04
ED 7	1.1×10^{-3} 5.6×10^{-3}	4.2×10^{-4} 4.2×10^{-4}	4.2×10^{-6} 4.7×10^{-4}	2.0×10^{-5} 6.6×10^{-3}	1.7×10^{-5} 1.2×10^{-4}	4.3×10^{-4} 6.2×10^{-4}	2.0×10^{-6} 6.6×10^{-3}	3.6×10^{-6} 1.8×10^{-4}	5.7×10^{-6} 1.4×10^{-4}	1.6×10^{-5} 5.4×10^{-5}	3.2×10^{-5} 1.1×10^{-1}	4.2×10^{-6} 7.0×10^{-6}	2.7×10^{-7} 5.4×10^{-4}	6.8×10^{-6} 9.7×10^{-5}	1.0×10^{-5} 3.0×10^{-3}	0.13
ED 8	5.6×10^{-4} 2.8×10^{-3}	3.8×10^{-4} 3.8×10^{-4}	7.0×10^{-7} 7.8×10^{-5}	3.9×10^{-5} 1.3×10^{-2}	1.5×10^{-4} 1.1×10^{-3}	4.0×10^{-4} 5.7×10^{-4}	1.6×10^{-6} 5.4×10^{-3}	5.0×10^{-6} 2.5×10^{-4}	1.6×10^{-5} 4.1×10^{-4}	4.8×10^{-5} 1.6×10^{-4}	1.5×10^{-5} 5.1×10^{-2}	1.0×10^{-4} 1.7×10^{-4}	4.9×10^{-7} 9.9×10^{-4}	2.2×10^{-5} 3.2×10^{-4}	9.0×10^{-6} 2.6×10^{-3}	0.08
ED 9	4.9×10^{-4} 2.5×10^{-3}	4.1×10^{-4} 4.1×10^{-4}	4.2×10^{-7} 4.7×10^{-5}	9.6×10^{-5} 3.2×10^{-2}	9.9×10^{-6} 7.0×10^{-5}	1.9×10^{-4} 2.8×10^{-4}	1.1×10^{-6} 3.5×10^{-3}	2.9×10^{-6} 1.4×10^{-4}	4.1×10^{-6} 1.0×10^{-4}	1.6×10^{-5} 5.4×10^{-5}	1.8×10^{-5} 5.9×10^{-2}	2.1×10^{-5} 3.6×10^{-5}	3.7×10^{-7} 7.3×10^{-4}	9.9×10^{-6} 1.4×10^{-4}	7.0×10^{-6} 2.0×10^{-3}	0.10

The carcinogenic risk for Cr, Ni, As, Cd, and Pb via the consumption of the EDs for both adolescents and adults was determined and is presented in Table 8. To our knowledge, this is the only study that estimated the carcinogenic risk for toxic elements from the consumption of EDs. For Pb and Cd, the ILCR values were consistently below the safe limit of 10^{-6} for both adolescents and adults, indicating no carcinogenic concern for these metals.

Table 8. Incremental lifetime cancer risk (ILCR) for adolescents and adults due to Cr, Ni, As, Cd, and Pb exposure from the analyzed energy drinks.

Sample	ILCR *				
	Cr	Ni	As	Cd	Pb
Adolescents					
ED 1	5.9×10^{-5}	3.1×10^{-5}	7.9×10^{-6}	1.0×10^{-6}	2.3×10^{-7}
ED 2	4.7×10^{-5}	1.6×10^{-5}	2.1×10^{-5}	5.4×10^{-7}	2.4×10^{-7}
ED 3	1.0×10^{-4}	3.8×10^{-5}	2.1×10^{-5}	3.4×10^{-7}	9.4×10^{-7}
ED 4	9.7×10^{-5}	1.2×10^{-5}	1.3×10^{-5}	3.8×10^{-7}	1.8×10^{-7}
ED 5	6.0×10^{-5}	1.7×10^{-5}	1.7×10^{-5}	4.3×10^{-7}	2.7×10^{-7}
ED 6	5.2×10^{-5}	1.3×10^{-5}	1.9×10^{-5}	2.4×10^{-7}	2.6×10^{-7}
ED 7	2.4×10^{-5}	1.4×10^{-5}	1.2×10^{-4}	2.4×10^{-7}	2.1×10^{-7}
ED 8	4.7×10^{-5}	2.0×10^{-5}	5.4×10^{-5}	4.5×10^{-7}	1.8×10^{-7}
ED 9	1.1×10^{-4}	1.2×10^{-5}	6.3×10^{-5}	3.3×10^{-7}	1.4×10^{-7}
Adults					
ED 1	2.5×10^{-5}	1.3×10^{-5}	3.3×10^{-6}	4.2×10^{-7}	9.7×10^{-8}
ED 2	2.0×10^{-5}	6.7×10^{-6}	8.9×10^{-6}	2.2×10^{-7}	1.0×10^{-7}
ED 3	4.4×10^{-5}	1.6×10^{-5}	8.7×10^{-6}	1.4×10^{-7}	3.9×10^{-7}
ED 4	4.1×10^{-5}	5.2×10^{-6}	5.3×10^{-6}	1.6×10^{-7}	7.7×10^{-8}
ED 5	2.5×10^{-5}	7.2×10^{-6}	7.1×10^{-6}	1.8×10^{-7}	1.2×10^{-7}
ED 6	2.2×10^{-5}	5.4×10^{-6}	7.9×10^{-6}	1.0×10^{-7}	1.1×10^{-7}
ED 7	9.9×10^{-6}	6.1×10^{-6}	4.9×10^{-5}	1.0×10^{-7}	8.8×10^{-8}
ED 8	2.0×10^{-5}	8.5×10^{-6}	2.3×10^{-5}	1.9×10^{-7}	7.7×10^{-8}
ED 9	4.8×10^{-5}	4.9×10^{-6}	2.7×10^{-5}	1.4×10^{-7}	6.0×10^{-8}

* ILCR was calculated by multiplying the EDI by the cancer slope factor (CSF). Oral CSF for Cr, Ni, inorganic As, Cd, and Pb is 0.5, 1.7, 1.5, 0.38, and 0.0085 mg/kg/day, respectively [48].

For As, in adolescents, the ILCR values for most samples (except ED 1 and ED 7) ranged between 10^{-6} and 10^{-4}, signifying a moderate cancer risk. ED 1 was within the safe limit, while ED 7 exceeded the 10^{-4} threshold, indicating a high cancer risk for this age group. Among adults, the ILCR values for As ranged from 3.3×10^{-6} (ED 1) to 4.9×10^{-5} (ED 7). While most samples were below the safe limit, ED 7, ED 8, and ED 9 indicated a moderate risk (10^{-6} to 10^{-4}).

For Ni, the ILCR values in adolescents ranged from 1.2×10^{-5} (ED 9) to 4.7×10^{-5} (ED 8), all within the moderate risk range of 10^{-6} to 10^{-4}. For adults, most samples fell within the safe limit ($<10^{-6}$), except ED 1 (1.3×10^{-5}) and ED 3 (1.6×10^{-5}), which presented a moderate carcinogenic risk.

For Cr, the ILCR values in adolescents ranged from 2.4×10^{-5} (ED 7) to 1.1×10^{-4} (ED 9). Two samples (ED 3 and ED 9) approached or slightly exceeded the 10^{-4} threshold, indicating a high cancer risk, while the others fell within the moderate risk range. In adults, the ILCR values for Cr ranged from 9.9×10^{-6} (ED 7) to 4.8×10^{-5} (ED 9), with all the samples falling within the moderate risk range.

4. Discussion

4.1. Energy Drink Macro-Mineral Composition

The results of the energy drinks showed a high content of Na, followed by K, Mg, and Ca. In a previous study, Leśniewicz et al. [4] reported that the concentration of Na in energy drinks consumed in Poland varied from 174 mg L^{-1} to 943 mg L^{-1}. In the study by Martins et al. [49], the Na concentrations in the seventeen energy drinks were very different depending on the type of packaging; they ranged from 31.5 to 1216.7 mg L^{-1} in PET bottles and 8.73 to 630.4 mg L^{-1} in aluminum cans. The results obtained in our study (8.62 mg L^{-1}–619.85 mg L^{-1}) are similar to them. The potassium concentrations determined by Martins' research team ranged from 2.4 to 210 mg L^{-1} [49]. The results of our experiments are consistent with this range. The relationship between sodium and potassium at the cellular level is responsible for many essential functions, including maintaining fluid balance. Na and K play important roles in various bodily functions, and an imbalance in their intake can have significant health implications, particularly concerning cardiovascular diseases and hypertension. Reducing the amount of Na intake in foods remains an essential concern for the food processing industry. The WHO recommends a Na–K molar ratio of <1 to help lower blood pressure. Therefore, it is very important to monitor the content of these elements in energy drinks, which are becoming an important part of the diet of young people [50–54].

The Mg and Ca levels in our study ranged from 0.013 mg L^{-1} to 196 mg L^{-1} and 2.54 mg L^{-1} to 116.1 mg L^{-1}, respectively. Of all the macro-minerals tested, the largest differences between the minimum and maximum concentrations were obtained for Mg, as have other researchers. Calcium concentrations determined by the ICP-OES technique by other researchers ranged from 12.9 mg L^{-1} to 106 mg L^{-1} [49], and from 2.39 mg L^{-1} to 120 mg L^{-1} [55], so they were consistent with our results. In contrast, the Ca levels determined by Leśniewicz et al. [4] and Mohammed et al. [56] were lower, not exceeding 41.2 mg L^{-1} and 66 mg L^{-1}, respectively.

4.2. Energy Drink Micro-Mineral Composition

The concentrations of V, B, and Co in EDs were examined only in the study conducted by Leśniewicz et al. [4], with the levels ranging from 0.19 to 4.25 μg L^{-1}, 36.3 to 92.8 μg L^{-1}, and 0.41 to 1.63 μg L^{-1}, respectively. These findings showed a considerable decrease in comparison to our research, where the highest average levels of these substances were 10.44 μg L^{-1} (for V), 796.82 μg L^{-1} (for B), and 4.13 μg L^{-1} (for Co). The WHO guidelines for drinking water quality do not establish a specific limit for Co, V, and Sr, among others [42]. We found that the concentrations of V and Co in our study were within the ranges recommended by the California Office of Environmental Health Hazard Assessment (OEHHA) and US EPA [44,47], respectively (Table 5). B's outcome was significantly lower than the standard suggested by the WHO. Leśniewicz et al. [4] reported Sr concentrations ranging from 12.8 to 117 μg L^{-1}, while Szymczycha-Madeja et al. [55] found concentrations ranging from 1.8 to 608 μg L^{-1}. However, our study showed a significant increase in the Sr levels for the ED 3 sample to a value equal to 3878.21 μg L^{-1} (statistic = 918.030) with an adjusted p-value of 0.000, indicating that the Sr concentration in this product significantly exceeds the US EPA standards. This supports the hypothesis that the Sr levels in ED 3 are higher than the normative values. The researchers also found Ba levels ranging from 4.28 to 23.7 μg L^{-1} [4] and from 19 to 82 μg L^{-1} [55]. In our research, the levels of Ba found fell within the lowest range reported in their study (4.81–19.98 μg L^{-1}).

The findings revealed that in the several ED samples in our research, the Al concentrations showed significant deviations from the EU and US EPA norms (Table 5). Specifically, ED 6 (statistic = 28.372, $p.adj$ = 0.006), ED 3 (statistic = 11.656, $p.adj$ = 0.033), and ED 8 (statistic = 96.162, $p.adj$ = 0.000) all exhibited Al levels that significantly exceed the standards mentioned. The elevated Al levels in the tested EDs are linked to the specific packaging material used. Martins and colleagues [49] found higher levels of aluminum (150–7150 μg L^{-1}) in EDs within aluminum cans compared to the levels in PET bottles (10–120 μg L^{-1}). Leśniewicz et al. [4] and Bunu et al. [57] found that the highest levels in EDs were 1260 μg L^{-1} and 2049 μg L^{-1}, respectively. It is well known that aluminum cans are covered with a thin polymer layer, which may impact the Al content in EDs [49]. Francisco et al. [58] stated that if cans are mishandled, it may result in the beverage coming into contact with the metal can material. Even though the highest average concentration of Al in our study was significantly lower (456.97 μg L^{-1}) compared to previous studies by Leśniewicz et al. [4], Martins et al. [49], and

Bunu et al. [57], the levels of this metal found still exceed the permissible limits in drinking water as per the specified standards (Table 5). Furthermore, as stated by Kilic et al. [17], Cr, Ni, and Fe are among the other metals that have the ability to move from the metal container into the ED sample. The Al levels in non-carbonated samples ranged from 26.12 µg L^{-1} to 48.16 µg L^{-1}, with a mean of 37.74 µg L^{-1}, according to Ahmed et al. [59]. The aforementioned study also discovered that orange juice samples had an average Al content of 36.98 µg L^{-1}. Fruit juices and non-alcoholic beverage samples were the subject of another study conducted in the USA; the results showed a broad range of concentrations, ranging from 0.017 to 2.6 mg L^{-1}, with an average of 0.36 mg L^{-1} [60]. Across different brands in Egypt, the Al content of soft drink samples, whether in glass, plastic, or can bottles, varied from 20 µg L^{-1} to 507.35 µg L^{-1} [61].

Despite these elevated Al levels, the calculated HQs for aluminum in all the tested EDs for adolescents and adults were below the threshold of 1 (HQ $\leq$ 1), indicating no significant non-carcinogenic risk to consumers. This finding aligns with evidence suggesting that while aluminum is present in various foods, beverages, and water, orally ingested Al at typical levels is not immediately harmful to humans. However, potential long-term exposure risks, including its speculated role in neurodegenerative conditions such as Alzheimer's disease, remain a topic of ongoing scientific investigation [62]. The results underscore the need for the careful monitoring of Al concentrations in EDs, particularly those packaged in aluminum cans, to ensure compliance with regulatory standards and minimize potential health risks.

As, Cd, and Pb are frequently found in the environment as pollutants. These metals have adverse effects on the human body and there is no known mechanism of homeostasis for them [63]. HMs are potentially toxic in high amounts or after long-term exposure. These metals manifest the ability to move and concentrate in different organs, leading to various health issues [19]. Therefore, monitoring their concentrations in various foods, including EDs, is warranted.

Comparing the concentrations of harmful HMs in the EDs to the available literature data, the following conclusions can be drawn: The studies by Kilic et al. [17], Adepoju and Ojo [64], and Bunu et al. [57] reported As levels ranging from 0.76 to 6.73 µg L^{-1}, 2.1 to 7.1 µg L^{-1}, and 0.5 to 60.3 µg L^{-1}, respectively. The As levels in our study were significantly elevated in ED 7, with a statistic of 30.466 and an adjusted p-value of 0.005, which is below the 0.05 threshold for significance. This indicates that the As concentration in ED 7 surpasses the WHO, EU, and US EPA norms (Table 5), supporting the hypothesis that the As levels in this particular energy drink are higher than recommended. In addition, slightly increased levels of As were found in ED 8 and ED 9. Early symptoms of low As exposure in drinking water include melanosis (abnormal black-brown skin pigmentation) and keratosis (the hardening of the palms and soles). Ongoing exposure, on the other hand, leads to leukomelanosis (skin depigmentation with white patches), hyperkeratosis, and potentially skin cancer [65].

In previous research, Ni levels were reported to range between 0.93 and 22.7 µg L^{-1} [4], 12 and 59 µg L^{-1} [55], and 35.98 and 303.97 µg L^{-1} [17], significantly higher than our findings, which revealed Ni concentrations to be 3–46 times lower. Despite the relatively lower levels detected, the results of our risk assessment indicated that Ni posed no carcinogenic risk in adults, with the ILCR values falling below the safe threshold of 10^{-6} for most samples, except for ED 1 and ED 3, which presented a moderate risk. In adolescents, however, an intermediate cancer risk was identified across all the samples. Nickel exposure, depending on its concentration and duration, is associated with various adverse health effects, including contact dermatitis, cardiovascular diseases, asthma, lung fibrosis, and respiratory tract cancer [66].

In our investigation, the levels of Cd and Pb ranged from 0.19 to 0.78 µg L^{-1} and 5.00 to 32.79 µg L^{-1}, respectively. It is important to mention that the levels of Pb in ED 3 exceeded the permitted levels for this metal in drinking water as stated in Table 5. Among the studies that were conducted, only the research by Adepoju and Ojo [64] reported significantly reduced levels of Cd (0.1–0.2 µg L^{-1}) and Pb (1.6–4.8 µg L^{-1}). In research conducted in Poland, Szymczycha-Madeja et al. [55] observed elevated levels of Cd (1.2–2.5 µg L^{-1}) and Pb (19–53 µg L^{-1}) compared to the findings of Leśniewicz et al. [4], who reported lower concentrations of Cd and Pb at 0.21–0.88 µg L^{-1} and 5.91–17.2 µg L^{-1}, respectively. Our findings on the levels of these HMs were most similar to those of Leśniewicz et al. [4]. Kilic et al. [17] also reported comparable results for Cd and Pb. Moreover, Bunu et al. [57] found maximum Pb concentrations of 23.4 µg L^{-1} for Pb in their study. In the case of HM content in carbonated and non-carbonated beverages [59], the lowest mean concentration of Cd (7.4–18.6 µg L^{-1}) followed by Pb (4.1–4.5 µg L^{-1}) was observed in both types of beverage samples. A Pb range of 0.0014–6.0 µg L^{-1} was found in a prior investigation of fruit juices and non-alcoholic beverage samples from the USA [60]. Pb levels in a variety of soft drink samples packaged in glass bottles, plastic, and cans ranged from 0.5 to 6.44 µg L^{-1} [67]. According to earlier Egyptian research on soft drink samples, several soft drink brands had Cd concentrations ranging from 0.5 µg L^{-1} to 1.96 µg L^{-1} [61].

Researchers from Nigeria and Iraq observed particularly high levels of Cd and Pb concentrations [56,57,68–70] that were above the acceptable limits of these HMs in drinking water (Table 5). In the study conducted by Yahaya et al. [69], Cd levels ranged from 769 to 779 µg L^{-1} while Pb levels fell between 12 and 323 µg L^{-1}. Mohammed and his colleagues [56] found Cd levels between 140 and 340 µg L^{-1} and Pb levels ranging from 100 to 140 µg L^{-1}. Pb concentrations determined in the studies by Bunu et al. [68] and Gimba et al. [70] ranged from 18 to 332 µg L^{-1} and 28 to 139 µg L^{-1}, respectively. Contamination with Pb is a significant issue in Nigeria. According to Momodu and Anyakora [71], 36.7% of the drinking water wells in Nigeria had Pb levels exceeding the WHO guideline value. Over a long period of intake, Cd can build up in the kidneys and liver, potentially causing kidney damage due to its extended biological half-life [72]. Excessive exposure to Pb can result in bone weakness, metallic taste, insomnia, seizures, microcytic anemia, glucosuria, cognitive issues, anorexia, reticulocytosis, and more. The organs affected are the brain, bone, blood, kidney, and thyroid [73].

The concentration levels of Cr found in this research (13.49–67.53 µg L^{-1}), and also documented by Kilic et al. [17] (13.25–100.96 µg L^{-1}) and Adepoju and Ojo [64] (534.3–608.9 µg L^{-1}) are significantly greater than those reported in the ED samples in the Leśniewicz et al. [4] (2.56–19.7 µg L^{-1}) and Szymczycha-Madeja et al. [55] (3.5–14 µg L^{-1}) studies. The Cr concentrations exhibited significant deviations from the WHO and EU norms in two energy drinks: ED 9 and ED 3. ED 9 showed a moderate increase in the Cr levels (statistic = 10.746) with an adjusted p-value of 0.038, which is below the significance threshold of 0.05. ED 3 presented a substantial increase in the Cr concentration (statistic = 308.273) with an adjusted p-value of 0.000 indicating a highly significant departure from the norm. It is essential to maintain regular glucose metabolism in human nutrition by ensuring that Cr levels in drinking water are within the recommended range. However, excessive intake of Cr can result in stomach issues, ulcers, seizures, and damage to the kidneys and liver, possibly leading to death [74].

Our risk assessment revealed that the THQs for As, Pb, Cd, and Cr were below the threshold value of one, indicating no non-carcinogenic concerns for long-term exposure. However, the ILCR values in the adolescent age group highlighted notable carcinogenic risks for both As and Cr. Specifically, the ILCR values for As exceeded the safe threshold of 10^{-6} in seven samples, indicating intermediate cancer risk, while one sample surpassed the 10^{-4} level, signifying a high cancer risk. For Cr, the ILCR values exceeded 10^{-6} in seven samples, with two samples surpassing the 10^{-4} threshold, pointing to a high cancer risk. Importantly, our study measured the total Cr levels, encompassing both Cr^{6+} and Cr^{3+}. While Cr^{6+} is recognized as a genotoxic and carcinogenic compound, Cr^{3+} is an essential trace element for human nutrition. This underscores the necessity for further speciation analysis to accurately assess the health risks associated with Cr exposure.

Our study found elevated levels of Mn, similar to the findings in the studies conducted by Kilic et al. [17] (5.45–489.93 µg L^{-1}), Szymczycha-Madeja et al. [55] (9.4–586 µg L^{-1}), and Mohammed et al. [56] (100–210 µg L^{-1}). Leśniewicz et al. [4] discovered noticeably lower amounts of this element in ED samples (15.1–40.9 µg L^{-1}). The Mn concentrations exceeded the EU and US EPA norms in two energy drinks: ED 5 and ED 8. ED 5 showed a significant increase in the Mn levels (statistic = 57.898) with an adjusted p-value of 0.001, while ED 8 also demonstrated elevated Mn concentrations (statistic = 37.589) with an adjusted p-value of 0.003. The carbonated and non-carbonated beverage samples examined by Ahmed et al. [59] showed mean Mn concentrations in the range 119.0–146.4 µg L^{-1}, which was higher compared to our results. A previous report from Brazil also demonstrated the elevated mean content of Mn 150.4 µg L^{-1} in orange juices [75]. As widely recognized, Mn is a powerful neurotoxic in addition to being an essential element. Numerous enzymes involved in energy metabolism, the generation of neurotransmitters, the regulation of reproductive hormones, and endogenous antioxidant enzyme systems use it as a cofactor. On the other hand, excessive Mn exposure is hazardous, particularly to the central nervous system (CNS), since it gradually destroys nerve cells [76].

Except for Yahaya et al.'s research [69] reporting the highest Cu concentration of 14,041 µg L^{-1}, other studies found Cu levels in EDs below drinking water standards (Table 5). The Cu concentrations in our study and in Martins et al. [49] did not exceed 20 µg L^{-1}. However, Kilic et al. [17] observed Cu levels ranging from 23.67 to 60.48 µg L^{-1}, Leśniewicz et al. [4] found concentrations between 0.87 and 109 µg L^{-1}, and Szymczycha-Madeja et al. [55] recorded levels between 11 and 79 µg L^{-1}. Juices and soft beverages' Cu content was also examined in the literature. A comparison with our results showed that there are significantly lower Cu levels in EDs than in the aforementioned drinks. For example, in Brazil, orange fruit juices have been shown to contain Cu at concentrations between 21.6 and 293 µg L^{-1}. According to Godebo et al. [60], orange juices have a Cu concentration of 75.15 to 141.66 µg L^{-1}, which is higher than the concentration in another study [59]. Remarkably, a recent study on non-alcoholic juice found that two varieties had significantly higher mean concentrations of copper: 280.0 µg L^{-1} in fresh mango juice and 240.0 µg L^{-1} in cappy mango juice [61]. According to reports, the Cu concentration in samples of different soft drink brands in Egypt ranges from 10.0 to 66.64 µg L^{-1} [67]. Conversely, Abdel-Rahman et al. [61] found that the Cu concentrations in canned and plastic-bottled Pepsi drinks were 210.0 µg L^{-1} and 160.0 µg L^{-1}, respectively. Cu acts as a cofactor for various enzymes (referred to as cuproenzymes) that play a role in energy production, iron metabolism, neuropeptide activation, connective tissue production, and neurotransmitter creation [70]. But, prolonged exposure to elevated copper levels can lead to liver damage and symptoms in the gastrointestinal tract such as abdominal pain, cramps, nausea, diarrhea, and vomiting [77].

Kilic et al. [17], Leśniewicz et al. [4], Bunu et al. [68], Yahaya et al. [69], and Mohammed et al. [56] all reported significantly high concentrations of Fe in their respective studies (334.77–937.12, 139–1380, 26–1850, 1083–1157, and 120–1030 µg L^{-1}). In our research, the Fe levels varied between 121.86 and 308.31 µg L^{-1}. All ED samples, with the exception of the EDs in the studies by Szymczycha-Madeja et al. [55] (35–78 µg L^{-1}) and Martins et al. [49] (70–190 µg L^{-1}), had higher Fe concentrations compared to the permitted levels (Table 5). Fe concentrations were generally within the EU and US EPA norms across most EDs. However, ED 8 exhibited a significant increase in Fe levels (statistic = 71.735) with an adjusted p-value of 0.001, indicating a substantial deviation from the norm. Fe is an important element in many biological processes, as on the one hand, it serves as an excellent oxygen carrier, and on the other, it can act as a protein-bound redox element [78]. Iron deficiency is common worldwide and in infants can cause severe neurological deficit. However, excessive iron intake is generally connected with an increased risk of colorectal cancer [79].

The analysis of Zn concentrations in our study, as well as in studies conducted by other researchers [4,49,55,57,68,69], revealed that Zn was present in different brands of EDs within acceptable limits (Table 5). The maximum Zn concentrations of 1005 µg L^{-1} and 2907 µg L^{-1} were observed by Yahaya et al. [69] and Bunu et al. [57], respectively. In turn, the Zn concentration in soft drinks packaged in cans, glass, and plastic bottles collected from

Giza's Egyptian market places was found to be in the range of 10 μg L^{-1} and 197.63 μg L^{-1} [67], which is less than the ranges obtained in both carbonated (265.15–315.78 μg L^{-1}) and non-carbonated (168.81–301.81 μg L^{-1}) beverage samples in the research study presented by Ahmed et al. [59]. Zinc plays a significant role in the metabolism of proteins, lipids, nucleic acids, and gene transcription [80]. Its function in the human body is wide-ranging in terms of reproduction, immune function, and wound healing. Zinc deficiency may manifest as growth issues, sexual problems, inflammation, digestive symptoms, or skin problems [81].

The present study and other available scientific reports have shown that EDs are not inert to human health. Nevertheless, there is no document in the EU legal system that specifies what an "energy drink" is. Regulation (EU) No 1169/2011 on the provision of food information to consumers mainly refers to a non-alcoholic caffeine-rich soft drink. From 2014 onwards, drinks containing more than 15 mg caffeine/100 mL had to be labeled with the warning: 'High caffeine content. Not recommended for serving to children, pregnant and breastfeeding women' and information on the caffeine content in mg/100 mL [82]. In Denmark, it is illegal to produce or distribute soft drinks and to add more than 15 mg of caffeine per 100 milliliters to food. EDs are only allowed to be sold to people above 16 in the UK and Germany, but only to people above 18 in Lithuania and Latvia [83]. Energy drinks are categorized as dietary supplements or ordinary foods in the US. The Dietary Supplement Health and Education Act of 1994 (DSHEA) states that substances used in normal foods, including caffeine, cannot be used in dietary supplements without previous FDA approval. Despite caffeine's classification as a medication, the DSHEA does not mandate that components in herbal supplements be disclosed [84]. Since 1 January 2024, Poland has prohibited the sale of energy drinks to anyone younger than 18. With the exception of natural sources, it covers items that contain more than 150 mg of taurine or caffeine per liter. This rule attempts to shield youth from health consequences that can impair everyday functioning and education, such as sleeplessness, anxiety, or difficulty focusing. These rules were put in place with the goal of encouraging a healthy lifestyle and helping children develop good eating habits at a young age.

5. Conclusions

The analysis of nine ED samples revealed the presence of Na, K, Mg, and Ca, with Na being the most abundant. These macro-elements are crucial for the overall health of the body. Overall, the majority of the elements analyzed in the EDs adhered to the WHO, EU, and US EPA norms, with no significant deviations observed. However, notable exceptions included elevated levels of Cr (in ED 3 and ED 9), Mn (in ED 5 and ED 8), Fe (in ED 8), As (in ED 7), Sr (in ED 3), and Al (in ED 6, ED 3 and ED 8). The observed differences in heavy metal content may be due to their heterogeneity, raw material sources, origin, production, and packaging processes. Consequently, caution is advised when consuming EDs, as excessive drinking can lead to increased build-up of both essential and non-essential TEs and/or HMs in the human body. In general, the accumulation of these metals can increase the risk of non-communicable diseases such as cardiovascular diseases and various types of cancer. These findings raise specific concerns regarding the safety of certain EDs concerning the Cr, Mn, Fe, As, Sr, and Al content, warranting further investigation and potential regulatory scrutiny to ensure consumer safety.

The analysis of nine ED samples revealed the presence of Na, K, Mg, and Ca, with Na being the most abundant. These macro-elements are essential for maintaining overall health. Most of the elements analyzed adhered to the WHO, EU, and US EPA norms, with no significant deviations observed for non-carcinogenic risks, as indicated by the THQ values below one for all the elements, including Cr, Mn, Fe, As, Sr, and Al. This confirms that in terms of long-term non-carcinogenic exposure, the investigated EDs are generally safe for consumption.

However, carcinogenic risk assessments highlighted concerns, particularly for certain elements like As and Cr in some ED samples, especially in the adolescent age group. The ILCR values for these elements exceeded the thresholds for moderate to high carcinogenic risk in specific cases, necessitating caution. The variability in heavy metal content among the ED samples may be attributed to differences in raw material sources, production processes, and packaging.

While no immediate non-carcinogenic risks were identified, excessive and prolonged consumption of EDs could contribute to the accumulation of both essential and non-essential trace elements and/or heavy metals in the human body, posing potential long-term health risks, including carcinogenic risks. These findings underscore the importance of regulatory oversight and further studies, including longitudinal and clinical research, to ensure the safety of energy drink consumption and protect consumer health.

Author Contributions: Conceptualization, E.B., K.C., M.T.-M. and A.S.; methodology, E.B., K.C., M.T.-M. and G.W.; software, D.M.; validation, K.C., M.T.-M. and E.B.; formal analysis, E.B., K.C., G.W. and M.T.-M.; investigation, K.C., E.B. and M.T.-M.; resources, K.C. and E.B.; writing—original draft preparation, E.B., K.C., K.F. and M.T.-M.; writing—review and editing, E.B., A.S., K.C., M.H., M.G. and M.T.-M.; supervision, E.B. and K.C.; project administration, E.B. and K.C.; funding acquisition, K.C. and E.B. All authors have read and agreed to the published version of the manuscript.

Funding: The research work was carried out as part of the commissioned project entitled *'The study on the impact of energy drink consumption and selected plant adaptogens on the health and mental state of young adults–a research project'*, funded by the Minister of Science and Higher Education and conducted at the John Paul II Catholic University of Lublin.

Institutional Review Board Statement: Not applicable.

Informed Consent Statement: Not applicable.

Data Availability Statement: Data are contained within the article.

Conflicts of Interest: The authors declare no conflicts of interest.

References

1. Costantino, A.; Maiese, A.; Lazzari, J.; Casula, C.; Turillazzi, E.; Frati, P.; Fineschi, V. The Dark Side of Energy Drinks: A Comprehensive Review of Their Impact on the Human Body. *Nutrients* **2023**, *15*, 3922. [CrossRef] [PubMed]
2. Erdmann, J.; Wiciński, M.; Wódkiewicz, E.; Nowaczewska, M.; Słupski, M.; Otto, S.W.; Kubiak, K.; Huk-Wieliczuk, E.; Malinowski, B. Effects of Energy Drink Consumption on Physical Performance and Potential Danger of Inordinate Usage. *Nutrients* **2021**, *13*, 2506. [CrossRef] [PubMed]
3. Hladun, O.; Papaseit, E.; Martín, S.; Barriocanal, A.M.; Poyatos, L.; Farré, M.; Pérez-Mañá, C. Interaction of Energy Drinks with Prescription Medication and Drugs of Abuse. *Pharmaceutics* **2021**, *13*, 1532. [CrossRef] [PubMed]
4. Leśniewicz, A.; Grzesiak, M.; Żyrnicki, W.; Borkowska-Burnecka, J. Mineral Composition and Nutritive Value of Isotonic and Energy Drinks. *Biol. Trace Elem. Res.* **2016**, *170*, 485–495. [CrossRef] [PubMed]
5. Nowak, D.; Jasionowski, A. Analysis of the Consumption of Caffeinated Energy Drinks among Polish Adolescents. *Int. J. Environ. Res. Public Health* **2015**, *12*, 7910–7921. [CrossRef]
6. Gutiérrez-Hellín, J.; Varillas-Delgado, D. Energy Drinks and Sports Performance, Cardiovascular Risk, and Genetic Associations; Future Prospects. *Nutrients* **2021**, *13*, 715. [CrossRef]
7. Jagim, A.R.; Harty, P.S.; Barakat, A.R.; Erickson, J.L.; Carvalho, V.; Khurelbaatar, C.; Camic, C.L.; Kerksick, C.M. Prevalence and Amounts of Common Ingredients Found in Energy Drinks and Shots. *Nutrients* **2022**, *14*, 314. [CrossRef]
8. Kumar, G.; Park, S.; Onufrak, S. Perceptions about Energy Drinks Are Associated with Energy Drink Intake among U.S. Youth. *Am. J. Health Promot.* **2015**, *29*, 238–244. [CrossRef]
9. Dobmeyer, D.J.; Stine, R.A.; Leier, C.V.; Greenberg, R.; Schaal, S.F. The Arrhythmogenic Effects of Caffeine in Human Beings. *N. Engl. J. Med.* **1983**, *308*, 814–816. [CrossRef]
10. Tomanic, M.; Paunovic, K.; Lackovic, M.; Djurdjevic, K.; Nestorovic, M.; Jakovljevic, A.; Markovic, M. Energy Drinks and Sleep among Adolescents. *Nutrients* **2022**, *14*, 3813. [CrossRef]
11. Ehlers, A.; Marakis, G.; Lampen, A.; Hirsch-Ernst, K.I. Risk Assessment of Energy Drinks with Focus on Cardiovascular Parameters and Energy Drink Consumption in Europe. *Food Chem. Toxicol.* **2019**, *130*, 109–121. [CrossRef] [PubMed]
12. Fletcher, E.A.; Lacey, C.S.; Aaron, M.; Kolasa, M.; Occiano, A.; Shah, S.A. Randomized Controlled Trial of High-volume Energy Drink versus Caffeine Consumption on ECG and Hemodynamic Parameters. *J. Am. Heart Assoc.* **2017**, *6*, e004448. [CrossRef] [PubMed]
13. Higgins, J.P.; Liras, G.N.; Liras, I.N.; Jacob, R.; Husain, F.; Pabba, K.C.; Schultea, M. Energy Drink Effects on Hemodynamics and Endothelial Function in Young Adults. *Cardiology* **2021**, *146*, 258–262. [CrossRef] [PubMed]

14. Shah, S.A.; Szeto, A.H.; Farewell, R.; Shek, A.; Fan, D.; Quach, K.N.; Bhattacharyya, M.; Elmiari, J.; Chan, W.; O'Dell, K.; et al. Impact of High Volume Energy Drink Consumption on Electrocardiographic and Blood Pressure Parameters: A Randomized Trial. *J. Am. Heart Assoc.* **2019**, *8*, e011318. [CrossRef] [PubMed]
15. Trapp, G.S.; Hurworth, M.; Jacoby, P.; Maddison, K.; Allen, K.; Martin, K.; Christian, H.; Ambrosini, G.L.; Oddy, W.; Eastwood, P.R. Energy Drink Intake Is Associated with Insomnia and Decreased Daytime Functioning in Young Adult Females. *Public Health Nutr.* **2021**, *24*, 1328–1337. [CrossRef]
16. Trapp, G.S.A.; Allen, K.; O'Sullivan, T.A.; Robinson, M.; Jacoby, P.; Oddy, W.H. Energy Drink Consumption Is Associated with Anxiety in Australian Young Adult Males. *Depress. Anxiety* **2014**, *31*, 420–428. [CrossRef]
17. Kilic, S.; Cengiz, M.F.; Kilic, M. Monitoring of Metallic Contaminants in Energy Drinks Using ICP-MS. *Environ. Monit. Assess.* **2018**, *190*, 202. [CrossRef]
18. Eticha, T.; Hymete, A. Health Risk Assessment of Heavy Metals in Locally Produced Beer to the Population in Ethiopia. *J. Bioanal. Biomed.* **2014**, *6*, 65–68. [CrossRef]
19. Scutarașu, E.C.; Trincă, L.C. Heavy Metals in Foods and Beverages: Global Situation, Health Risks and Reduction Methods. *Foods* **2023**, *12*, 3340. [CrossRef]
20. Shaheen, N.; Irfan, N.M.; Khan, I.N.; Islam, S.; Islam, M.S.; Ahmed, M.K. Presence of Heavy Metals in Fruits and Vegetables: Health Risk Implications in Bangladesh. *Chemosphere* **2016**, *152*, 431–438. [CrossRef]
21. Izah, S.C.; Inyang, I.R.; Angaye, T.C.N.; Okowa, I.P. A Review of Heavy Metal Concentration and Potential Health Implications of Beverages Consumed in Nigeria. *Toxics* **2016**, *5*, 1. [CrossRef] [PubMed]
22. Charehsaz, M.; Helvacıoğlu, S.; Çetinkaya, S.; Demir, R.; Erdem, O.; Aydin, A. Heavy Metal and Essential Elements in Beers from Turkey Market: A Risk Assessment Study. *Hum. Exp. Toxicol.* **2021**, *40*, 1241–1249. [CrossRef] [PubMed]
23. Helvacıoğlu, S.; Charehsaz, M.; Gulhane, O.E.; Aydın, A. Assessment of Toxic Element Content of Some Grape Molasses Produced by Conventional and Industrial Techniques: Insights into Human Safety. *Toxin Rev.* **2021**, *40*, 1198–1205. [CrossRef]
24. DesMarais, T.L.; Costa, M. Mechanisms of Chromium-Induced Toxicity. *Curr. Opin. Toxicol.* **2019**, *14*, 1–7. [CrossRef]
25. Pourret, O.; Hursthouse, A. It's Time to Replace the Term "Heavy Metals" with "Potentially Toxic Elements" When Reporting Environmental Research. *Int. J. Environ. Res. Public Health* **2019**, *16*, 4446. [CrossRef]
26. Witkowska, D.; Słowik, J.; Chilicka, K. Heavy Metals and Human Health: Possible Exposure Pathways and the Competition for Protein Binding Sites. *Molecules* **2021**, *26*, 6060. [CrossRef]
27. El Hosry, L.; Sok, N.; Richa, R.; Al Mashtoub, L.; Cayot, P.; Bou-Maroun, E. Sample Preparation and Analytical Techniques in the Determination of Trace Elements in Food: A Review. *Foods* **2023**, *12*, 895. [CrossRef]
28. Ali, H.; Khan, E.; Ilahi, I. Environmental Chemistry and Ecotoxicology of Hazardous Heavy Metals: Environmental Persistence, Toxicity, and Bioaccumulation. *J. Chem.* **2019**, *2019*, 6730305. [CrossRef]
29. Cannas, D.; Loi, E.; Serra, M.; Firinu, D.; Valera, P.; Zavattari, P. Relevance of Essential Trace Elements in Nutrition and Drinking Water for Human Health and Autoimmune Disease Risk. *Nutrients* **2020**, *12*, 2074. [CrossRef]
30. Czarnek, K.; Tatarczak-Michalewska, M.; Szopa, A.; Klimek-Szczykutowicz, M.; Jafernik, K.; Majerek, D.; Blicharska, E. Bioaccumulation Capacity of Onion (*Allium cepa* L.) Tested with Heavy Metals in Biofortification. *Molecules* **2024**, *29*, 101. [CrossRef]
31. Nduka, J.K.; Kelle, H.I.; Amuka, J.O. Health Risk Assessment of Cadmium, Chromium and Nickel from Car Paint Dust from Used Automobiles at Auto-Panel Workshops in Nigeria. *Toxicol. Rep.* **2019**, *6*, 449–456. [CrossRef] [PubMed]
32. Eze, V.; Ndife, C.; Muogbo, M. Carcinogenic and Non-Carcinogenic Health Risk Assessment of Heavy Metals in Njaba River, Imo State, Nigeria. *Braz. J. Anal. Chem.* **2021**, *8*, 57–70. [CrossRef]
33. EFSA. Gathering Consumption Data on Specific Consumer Groups of Energy Drinks. Available online: https://www.efsa.europa.eu/en/supporting/pub/en-394 (accessed on 29 November 2024).
34. US. EPA Human Health Risk Assessment. Available online: https://semspub.epa.gov/work/03/2339323.pdf (accessed on 29 November 2024).
35. Montgomery, D.C. The Kruskal-Wallis Test. In *Design and Analysis of Experiments*; John Wiley & Sons: Hoboken, NJ, USA, 2017.
36. Liu, H. Comparing Welch's ANOVA, a Kruskal-Wallis Test and Traditional ANOVA in Case of Heterogeneity of Variance. Master Thesis, Virginia Commonwealth University, Richmond, VA, USA, 2015.
37. Hochberg, Y. A Sharper Bonferroni Procedure for Multiple Tests of Significance. *Biometrika* **1988**, *75*, 800–802. [CrossRef]
38. Fay, M.P.; Proschan, M.A. Wilcoxon-Mann-Whitney or t-Test? on Assumptions for Hypothesis Tests and Multiple Interpretations of Decision Rules. *Stat. Surv.* **2010**, *4*, 1–39. [CrossRef]
39. R Core Team. *R: A Language and Environment for Statistical Computing*; R Foundation for Statistical Computing: Vienna, Austria, 2024.
40. Wickham, H.; Averick, M.; Bryan, J.; Chang, W.; McGowan, L.; François, R.; Grolemund, G.; Hayes, A.; Henry, L.; Hester, J.; et al. Welcome to the Tidyverse. *J. Open Source Softw.* **2019**, *4*, 1686. [CrossRef]
41. Kassambara, A. Rstatix: Pipe-Friendly Framework for Basic Statistical Tests 2023. Available online: https://cran.r-project.org/web/packages/rstatix/index.html (accessed on 29 October 2024).
42. World Health Organization. *Guidelines for Drinking-Water Quality—Fourth Edition Incorporating the First Addendum*; World Health Organization: Geneva, Switzerland, 2017; ISBN 978-92-4-154995-0.

43. European Commission Directive (EU) 2020/2184 of the European Parliament and of the Council of 16 December 2020 on the Quality of Water Intended for Human Consumption (Recast) (Text with EEA Relevance) 2020. Available online: https://eur-lex.europa.eu/eli/dir/2020/2184/oj (accessed on 21 October 2024).
44. US. EPA Announcement of Preliminary Regulatory Determinations for Contaminants on the Third Drinking Water Contaminant Candidate List. U.S. Environmental Protection Agency Web. Available online: https://www.federalregister.gov/documents/2014/10/20/2014-24582/announcement-of-preliminary-regulatory-determinations-forcontaminants-on-the-third-drinking-water (accessed on 23 July 2024).
45. US EPA National Primary Drinking Water Regulations 2008. Available online: https://www.epa.gov/ground-water-and-drinking-water/national-primary-drinking-water-regulations (accessed on 3 October 2024).
46. US EPA Secondary Drinking Water Regulations: Guidance for Nuisance Chemicals 2013. Available online: https://www.epa.gov/sdwa/secondary-drinking-water-standards-guidance-nuisance-chemicals (accessed on 3 October 2024).
47. OEHHA Proposed Notification Level for Vanadium. California Office of Environmental Health Hazard Assessment (OEHHA). Available online: https://oehha.ca.gov/water/notification-level/proposed-notification-level-vanadium (accessed on 24 July 2024).
48. US EPA. Risk Assessment Guidance for Superfund Volume I: Human Health Evaluation Manual (Part E, Supplemental Guidance for Dermal Risk Assessment). 2004, EPA/540/R/99/005. Available online: https://www.epa.gov/sites/default/files/2015-09/documents/part_e_final_revision_10-03-07.pdf (accessed on 7 December 2024).
49. Martins, A.S.; Junior, J.B.P.; De Araújo Gomes, A.; Carvalho, F.I.M.; Filho, H.A.D.; Das Graças Fernandes Dantas, K. Mineral Composition Evaluation in Energy Drinks Using ICP OES and Chemometric Tools. *Biol. Trace Elem. Res.* **2020**, *194*, 284–294. [CrossRef]
50. Calliope, S.R.; Samman, N.C. Sodium Content in Commonly Consumed Foods and Its Contribution to the Daily Intake. *Nutrients* **2020**, *12*, 34. [CrossRef]
51. Nurmilah, S.; Cahyana, Y.; Utama, G.L.; Aït-Kaddour, A. Strategies to Reduce Salt Content and Its Effect on Food Characteristics and Acceptance: A Review. *Foods* **2022**, *11*, 3120. [CrossRef]
52. Salman, E.; Kadota, A.; Miura, K. Global Guidelines Recommendations for Dietary Sodium and Potassium Intake. *Hypertens. Res.* **2024**, *47*, 1620–1626. [CrossRef]
53. *World Health Organization Guideline: Sodium Intake for Adults and Children*; World Health Organization: Geneva, Switzerland, 2012; ISBN 978-92-4-150483-6.
54. World Health Organization Tackling NCDs: "best Buys" and Other Recommended Interventions for the Prevention and Control of Noncommunicable Diseases 2017. Available online: https://iris.who.int/bitstream/handle/10665/259232/WHO-NMH-NVI-17.9-eng.pdf?sequence=1 (accessed on 9 October 2024).
55. Szymczycha-Madeja, A.; Welna, M.; Pohl, P. Determination of Elements in Energy Drinks by ICP OES with Minimal Sample Preparation. *J. Braz. Chem. Soc.* **2013**, *24*, 1606–1612. [CrossRef]
56. Mohammed, S.G.; Al-Hashimi, A.G.; Al-Hussainy, K.S. Determination of Caffeine and Trace Minerals Contents in Soft and Energy Drinks Available in Basrah Markets. *Pak. J. Nutr.* **2012**, *11*, 845–848. [CrossRef]
57. Bunu, S.J.; Ebeshi, B.U.; Kpun, H.F.; Kashimawo, A.J.; Vaikosen, E.N.; Itodo, C.B. Atomic Absorption Spectroscopic (AAS) Analysis of Heavy Metals and Health Risks Assessment of Some Common Energy Drinks. *Pharmacol. Toxicol. Nat. Med.* **2023**, *1*, 1–10. [CrossRef]
58. Francisco, B.B.A.; Brum, D.M.; Cassella, R.J. Determination of Metals in Soft Drinks Packed in Different Materials by ETAAS. *Food Chem.* **2015**, *185*, 488–494. [CrossRef] [PubMed]
59. Ahmed, M.; Yousaf, A.; Khaleeq, A.; Saddiqa, A.; Sanaullah, M.; Ahmad, W.; Ali, I.; Khalid, K.; Wani, T.A.; Zargar, S. Chemometric Analysis and Human Health Implications of Trace and Heavy/Non-Essential Metals through Ingestion of Carbonated and Non-Carbonated Beverages. *Biol. Trace Elem. Res.* **2024**, *202*, 5828–5849. [CrossRef]
60. Godebo, T.R.; Stoner, H.; Pechilis, M.; Taylor-Arnold, H.; Ashmead, J.; Claman, L.; Guest, L.; Consolati, W.; DiMatteo, O.; Johnson, M.; et al. Toxic Metals and Essential Elements Contents in Commercially Available Fruit Juices and Other Non-Alcoholic Beverages from the United States. *J. Food Compos. Anal.* **2023**, *119*, 105230. [CrossRef]
61. Abdel-Rahman, G.N.; Ahmed, M.B.M.; Sabry, B.A.; Ali, S.S.M. Heavy Metals Content in Some Non-Alcoholic Beverages (Carbonated Drinks, Flavored Yogurt Drinks, and Juice Drinks) of the Egyptian Markets. *Toxicol. Rep.* **2019**, *6*, 210–214. [CrossRef]
62. WHO Aluminium in Drinking-Water. Background Document for Preparation of WHO Guidelines for Drinking-Water Quality 2010. Available online: https://cdn.who.int/media/docs/default-source/wash-documents/wash-chemicals/aluminium.pdf?sfvrsn=e54f4db9_4 (accessed on 15 October 2024).
63. Llobet, J.M.; Falcó, G.; Casas, C.; Teixidó, A.; Domingo, J.L. Concentrations of Arsenic, Cadmium, Mercury, and Lead in Common Foods and Estimated Daily Intake by Children, Adolescents, Adults, and Seniors of Catalonia, Spain. *J. Agric. Food Chem.* **2003**, *51*, 838–842. [CrossRef]
64. Adepoju, O.T.; Ojo, V.O. Consumption Pattern of Energy Drinks by University of Ibadan Students and Associated Health Risks Factors. *FNS* **2014**, *05*, 2209–2216. [CrossRef]
65. Dastgiri, S.; Mosaferi, M.; Fizi, M.A.H.; Olfati, N.; Zolali, S.; Pouladi, N.; Azarfam, P. Arsenic Exposure, Dermatological Lesions, Hypertension, and Chromosomal Abnormalities among People in a Rural Community of Northwest Iran. *J. Health Popul. Nutr.* **2010**, *28*, 14–22.

66. Genchi, G.; Carocci, A.; Lauria, G.; Sinicropi, M.S.; Catalano, A. Nickel: Human Health and Environmental Toxicology. *Int. J. Environ. Res. Public. Health* **2020**, *17*, 679. [CrossRef]
67. Ghuniem, M.M.; Khorshed, M.A.; El-Safty, S.M.; Souaya, E.R.; Khalil, M.M. Potential Human Health Risk Assessment of Potentially Toxicelements Intake via Consumption of Soft Drinks Purchasedfrom Different Egyptian Markets. *Int. J. Environ. Anal. Chem.* **2022**, *102*, 3485–3507. [CrossRef]
68. Bunu, S.J.; George, D.; Alfred-Ugbenbo, D.; Ebeshi, B.U. Heavy Metals Quantification and Correlative Carcinogenic Risks Evaluation in Selected Energy Drinks Sold in Bayelsa State Using Atomic Absorption Spectroscopic Technique. *Int. J. Chem. Res.* **2023**, *7*, 1–4. [CrossRef]
69. Yahaya, T.O.; Gulumbe, B.H.; Umar, A.K.; Yusuf, A.; Mohammed, A.Z.; Izuafa, A.; Abubakar, A. Heavy Metal Content and Associated Health Risks in Selected Energy Drinks Sold in Birnin Kebbi, Nigeria. *AJHSE* **2022**, *3*, 26–34. [CrossRef]
70. Gimba, C.E.; Abechi, S.E.; Abbas, N.S. Studies on Physicochemical Properties, Trace Mineral and Heavy Metal Contents of Common Energy Drinks. *Int. J. Adv. Res.* **2014**, *2*, 131–138.
71. Momodu, M.A.; Anyakora, C.A. Heavy Metal Contamination of Ground Water: The Surulere Case Study. *Res. J. Environ. Earth Sci.* **2010**, *2*, 39–43.
72. Rafati Rahimzadeh, M.; Rafati Rahimzadeh, M.; Kazemi, S.; Moghadamnia, A. Cadmium Toxicity and Treatment: An Update. *Casp. J. Intern. Med.* **2017**, *8*, 135–145. [CrossRef]
73. Sachdeva, C.; Thakur, K.; Sharma, A.; Sharma, K.K. Lead: Tiny but Mighty Poison. *Indian. J. Clin. Biochem.* **2018**, *33*, 132–146. [CrossRef]
74. Khan, S.A.; Uddin, Z.; Zubair, A. Levels of Selected Heavy Metals in Drinking Water of Peshawar City. *Int. J. Sci. Nat.* **2011**, *2*, 648–652.
75. De Souza, M.J.; Barciela-Alonso, M.C.; Aboal-Somoza, M.; Bermejo-Barrera, P. Determination of the Trace Element Contents of Fruit Juice Samples by ICP OES and ICP-MS. *Braz. J. Anal. Chem.* **2021**, *9*, 49–61. [CrossRef]
76. Gunter, T.E.; Miller, L.M.; Gavin, C.E.; Eliseev, R.; Salter, J.; Buntinas, L.; Alexandrov, A.; Hammond, S.; Gunter, K.K. Determination of the Oxidation States of Manganese in Brain, Liver, and Heart Mitochondria. *J. Neurochem.* **2004**, *88*, 266–280. [CrossRef]
77. National Research Council (US). *Copper in Drinking Water. Committee on Copper in Drinking Water*; National Academies Press: Washington, DC, USA, 2000; ISBN 0-309-59406-5.
78. Huang, X. Iron Overload and Its Association with Cancer Risk in Humans: Evidence for Iron as a Carcinogenic Metal. *Mutat. Res.* **2003**, *533*, 153–171. [CrossRef]
79. Ashmore, J.H.; Rogers, C.J.; Kelleher, S.L.; Lesko, S.M.; Hartman, T.J. Dietary Iron and Colorectal Cancer Risk: A Review of Human Population Studies. *Crit. Rev. Food Sci. Nutr.* **2016**, *56*, 1012–1020. [CrossRef]
80. McClung, J.P. Iron, Zinc, and Physical Performance. *Biol. Trace Elem. Res.* **2019**, *188*, 135–139. [CrossRef]
81. Sanna, A.; Firinu, D.; Zavattari, P.; Valera, P. Zinc Status and Autoimmunity: A Systematic Review and Meta-Analysis. *Nutrients* **2018**, *10*, 68. [CrossRef]
82. Binder, J.-H.; Gortsos, C.V. *The European Banking Union: A Compendium*; Nomos Verlagsgesellschaft: Baden-Baden, Germany, 2015.
83. Schroeder, W. Age Restrictions on the Sale of Energy Drinks from an EU Law Perspective. *Eur. Food Feed. Law Rev. (EFFL)* **2016**, *11*, 400.
84. Generali, J.A. Energy Drinks: Food, Dietary Supplement, or Drug? *Hosp. Pharm.* **2013**, *48*, 5–9. [CrossRef]

Disclaimer/Publisher's Note: The statements, opinions and data contained in all publications are solely those of the individual author(s) and contributor(s) and not of MDPI and/or the editor(s). MDPI and/or the editor(s) disclaim responsibility for any injury to people or property resulting from any ideas, methods, instructions or products referred to in the content.

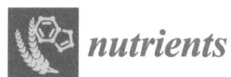

Article

Comparative Analysis of Dietary Behavior in Children and Parents During COVID-19 Lockdowns in Greece: Insights from a Non-Representative Sample

Odysseas Androutsos [1,*], George Saltaouras [1,2], Michail Kipouros [1], Maria Koutsaki [1], Athanasios Migdanis [1], Christos Georgiou [1], Maria Perperidi [1], Sousana K. Papadopoulou [3], Rena I. Kosti [1], Constantinos Giaginis [4] and Theodora Mouratidou [5]

[1] Laboratory of Clinical Nutrition and Dietetics (CND-lab), Department of Nutrition and Dietetics, University of Thessaly, 42132 Trikala, Thessaly, Greece; gsalt@hua.gr (G.S.); mihalis.kip@gmail.com (M.K.); mkoutsaki@uth.gr (M.K.); amigdanis@uth.gr (A.M.); cri.georgiou@gmail.com (C.G.); mperperidi@uth.gr (M.P.); renakosti@uth.gr (R.I.K.)
[2] Department of Nutrition and Dietetics, School of Health Sciences and Education, Harokopio University of Athens, 17671 Athens, Greece
[3] Department of Nutritional Sciences and Dietetics, Faculty of Health Sciences, International Hellenic University, 57400 Thessaloniki, Greece; souzpapa@gmail.com
[4] Department of Food Science and Nutrition, School of the Environment, University of the Aegean, 81400 Lemnos, Greece; cgiaginis@aegean.gr
[5] Department of Nutrition and Dietetic Sciences, School of Health Sciences, Hellenic Mediterranean University, 72300 Sitia, Greece; tmouratidou@hmu.gr
* Correspondence: oandroutsos@uth.gr; Tel.: +30-2431047108

Academic Editors: António Raposo and Ariana Saraiva

Received: 3 December 2024
Revised: 27 December 2024
Accepted: 28 December 2024
Published: 30 December 2024

Citation: Androutsos, O.; Saltaouras, G.; Kipouros, M.; Koutsaki, M.; Migdanis, A.; Georgiou, C.; Perperidi, M.; Papadopoulou, S.K.; Kosti, R.I.; Giaginis, C.; et al. Comparative Analysis of Dietary Behavior in Children and Parents During COVID-19 Lockdowns in Greece: Insights from a Non-Representative Sample. *Nutrients* **2025**, *17*, 112. https://doi.org/10.3390/nu17010112

Copyright: © 2024 by the authors. Licensee MDPI, Basel, Switzerland. This article is an open access article distributed under the terms and conditions of the Creative Commons Attribution (CC BY) license (https://creativecommons.org/licenses/by/4.0/).

Abstract: Background/Objectives: Home isolation measures during the COVID-19 lockdown periods may have influenced individuals' lifestyles. The COVEAT study aimed to identify differences in children's and their parents' dietary behavior, children's body weight and parental body mass index (BMI) between two lockdown periods implemented in Greece. Methods: In total, 61 participants (children 2–18 years and their parents) completed questionnaires about their lifestyle, body weight and height, and family socio-demographic data, during both lockdown periods (LDs) implemented in Greece (LD1 in March–May 2020; LD2 in December 2020–January 2021). Results: No significant differences in parents' BMI and fluctuations in children's/adolescents' body weight and BMI were observed in LD2 compared to LD1. Regarding dietary behavior, in LD2 fewer parents were found to have dinner and prepared home meals and more families reported to order fast food. Furthermore, a significant decrease in the consumption of fresh and prepacked juices and an increase in fast-food consumption were observed for children/adolescents in LD2 compared to LD1. Conclusions: The findings of the COVEAT study indicate that each lockdown period had a different impact on children's/adolescents' and their parents' dietary behavior, with less favorable changes observed in LD2, suggesting that the implementation of additional lockdowns may have had a negative impact on individuals' lifestyles.

Keywords: COVID-19; lockdown; nutrition; diet; COVEAT

1. Introduction

At the end of 2019, the city of Wuhan, China was confronted with virus of Sars-CoV2 for the first time. The spread of the virus was rapid at a global basis. As a result, on 11 March 2020, the World Health Organization declared that the coronavirus disease 2019 (COVID-19) was a pandemic. In Greece, the first confirmed case of COVID-19 was recorded on 26 February 2020 and in March 2020 the Greek government implemented a nationwide closure of educational institutions of all levels and all public areas, such as cafes, restaurants, shopping centers, and churches. On 23 March 2020, the first national lockdown was implemented and only certain commuting activities (e.g., walking, cycling) and work were allowed upon individuals' request and the approval of the national authorities. On 5 November 2020, the government announced the second national lockdown and the relevant regulations for community activities and work were reactivated. The lockdown period in Greece ended in early 2021 with the reopening of the preschools and primary schools on 11 January 2021 and secondary schools on February 1st and the termination of the restrictions for all age groups.

The implementation of lockdowns led to changes in individuals' lifestyles, previously described [1–3]. Specifically, during the first lockdown, where the fear of this unknown disease prevailed, citizens tended to have higher compliance with the home isolation measures [4]. Previous studies have shown that this home isolation led to significant changes in eating behavior [3,4]. Two studies reported that children, adolescents, and young adults increased their consumption of healthy foods such as fruits, vegetables, and juices with simultaneous reduction in fast-food consumption. In addition, an increase in sedentary time and a decrease in physical activity level were recorded, even though citizens had the opportunity to perform outdoor physical activities [5–7]. Similar findings were observed in the second lockdown. Some studies reported that during the second lockdown, individuals increased healthy foods, mostly fresh fruits and vegetables, and decreased processed foods and added sugar, compared to the first lockdown [8]. However, other studies revealed contradictory findings, indicating that certain lifestyle indices, including diet quality, worsened during the second lockdown [9].

Therefore, this study aims to explore the variations in dietary behavior and body mass index (BMI) between the first and second lockdowns in children, adolescents, and their parents in Greece, addressing a critical gap in the existing literature.

2. Materials and Methods

2.1. Study Design and Participants

The COVEAT study had a cross-sectional design. Its detailed protocol has been previously presented elsewhere [10]. In brief, families (parents and their children aged 2–18 years) from 63 municipalities in Greece were recruited from networks of dietitians-nutritionists, personal networks, and social media and provided data in two time-points: in March–May 2020 (1st lockdown) and in December 2020–January 2021 (2nd lockdown).

This study adhered to the Declaration of Helsinki and the conventions of the Council of Europe on Human Rights and Biomedicine; received ethical clearance from the Ethical Committee of the Department of Physical Education and Sport Science, University of Thessaly; and was registered at clinicaltrials.org (NCT04437121). Prior to their enrollment in this study, participants signed an online informed consent form.

2.2. Questionnaires

The questionnaires, based on a Food Frequency Questionnaire (FFQ), were completed online at both lockdowns, using Google-forms. These questionnaires collected data on family sociodemographic characteristics (e.g., age, family composition, region of residence, parental occupation, and educational level), anthropometric indices (e.g., parental and children's/adolescents' weight and height) and parents' and children's/adolescents' lifestyle behaviors (e.g., main meals, snacks and fast-food consumption, and consumption of various foods). More specifically, the frequency of each main meal (breakfast, lunch, dinner) was self-reported by the participants and variables were then dichotomized to "Yes" (for those consuming each meal every day) and "No" (for the rest of participants). Furthermore, the frequencies and servings of each food (fruit, fresh juices, prepacked juices, vegetables, dairy, red meat, poultry, fish, pasta, legumes, homemade sweets, ready-made sweets, salty snacks, fast food, and soda beverages) was also self-reported by the participants and servings per week of each food were calculated. All dietary intake data were collected retrospectively for the lockdown periods, with no prospective meal recordings. Parents (one partner: husband or wife) provided data on behalf of their children, reporting both dietary intake and anthropometric measurements. Each family contributed data for one child only. Body mass index (BMI) was calculated according to the following equation: Weight (kg)/ Height (m^2).

2.3. Statistical Analysis

Continuous data are presented as mean ± standard deviation (SD). Categorical variables are presented as absolute (n) and relative (%) frequencies. The variables "preparing meal at home" and "ordering fast food" were transformed from ordinal to continuous. For paired comparisons of continuous data that were normally distributed (Shapiro–Wilk test for evaluation of data distribution), Student's test for paired data was applied. For paired comparisons of continuous data that were not normally distributed and for categorical data, the Wilcoxon matched-pairs signed-rank test was applied. The level of statistical significance was set to $p < 0.05$ for analyses. All analyses were performed with SPSS V26 software package (IBM, Armonk, NY, USA).

3. Results

In total, 61 participants completed the survey during both the 1st and the 2nd lockdown. Table 1 summarizes the demographic and occupational characteristics of the study participants, providing critical context for interpreting the findings. Most surveys were completed by females/mothers (93.4% for both lockdowns). The table reveals educational differences among parents: 39.3% of fathers and 19.7% of mothers had completed secondary school, while 21.3% of fathers and 31.1% of mothers held postgraduate qualifications. Family status data indicate that 95.1% of participants came from families with married parents, and 4.9% were from single-parent households. Employment changes during the lockdowns varied significantly between fathers and mothers. Among fathers, 37.7% reported no change in employment status, while 29.5% experienced reduced working hours. In contrast, 49.2% of mothers experienced no employment changes, while 16.4% reported reduced hours. Additionally, fathers were more likely to work from home (8.2% compared to 4.9% for mothers) and to leave for personal or exceptional reasons (13.1% versus 8.2% for mothers).

Table 1. Parental demographic characteristics (n = 61).

Characteristics		N (%)
Father's education	Primary school	2 (3.3)
	Secondary school	24 (39.3)
	Clerical/Commercial/Professional qualification (IEK)	5 (8.2)
	University qualification	17 (27.9)
	Postgraduate qualification	13 (21.3)

Table 1. *Cont.*

Characteristics		N (%)
Mother's education	Primary school	1 (1.6)
	Secondary school	12 (19.7)
	Clerical/Commercial/Professional qualification (IEK)	4 (6.6)
	University qualification	25 (41)
	Postgraduate qualification	19 (31.1)
Family status	Married parents	58 (95.1)
	Single-parent families	3 (4.9)
Changes in father's job during lockdown	No change	23 (37.7)
	Work from home	5 (8.2)
	Increased hours at work	1 (1.6)
	Reduced hours at work	18 (29.5)
	Leave for personal or exceptional reasons	8 (13.1)
	Unemployed	3 (4.9)
	Other	3 (4.9)
Changes in mother's job during lockdown	No change	30 (49.2)
	Work from home	3 (4.9)
	Increased hours at work	1 (1.6)
	Reduced hours at work	10 (16.4)
	Leave for personal or exceptional reasons	5 (8.2)
	Unemployed	2 (3.3)
	Other	10 (16.4)

At baseline, mean (SD) age was 43.0 (6.6) years and 39.9 (5.7) years for fathers and mothers, respectively, and 7.7 (4.2) for their children. Table 2 presents the anthropometric characteristics of parents and children/adolescents during both lockdowns, and Table 1 presents the baseline demographic characteristics of the parents during the 1st lockdown. Both parents' weight (Figure 1) and body mass index (BMI) were similar during lockdowns and did not fluctuate during the period before the imposing of the 1st lockdown until the second lockdown ($p > 0.05$ for all comparisons). On the other hand, there was a significant increase in children's/adolescents' body weight and body mass index (Table 2; Figure 1). Interestingly, there was a significant decrease in children's/adolescents' body weight during the first lockdown, compared to the period before the first COVID-19 lockdown (mean difference 1.14 kg; $p < 0.001$).

Table 2. Anthropometric characteristics for parents and child/adolescent.

Characteristics	LD1 (Mean (SD))	LD2 (Mean (SD))	*p* Value
Father's weight (kg) (n = 57)	90.4 (13.5)	91.0 (14.4)	0.294
Father's body mass index (kg/m^2) (n = 57)	28.4 (4.3)	28.7 (4.2)	0.239
Mother's weight (kg) (n = 61)	69.7 (16.7)	69.5 (16.3)	0.880
Mother's body mass index (kg/m^2) (n = 57)	25.6 (5.1)	25.6 (4.8)	0.179
Child/Adolescent's weight (n = 60)	31.9 (15.4)	34.8 (15.7)	<0.001

SD: Standard Deviation; LD1: First COVID-19 lockdown; LD2: Second COVID-19 lockdown.

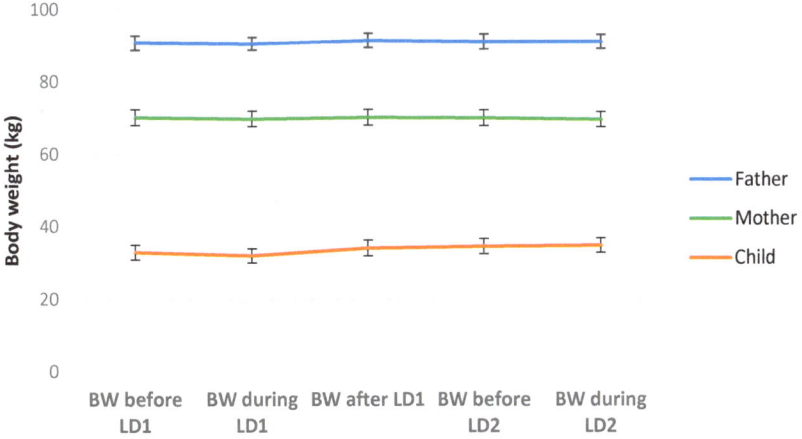

Figure 1. Changes in parents' and children's body weight at different time points (before first COVID-19 lockdown until during second COVID-19 lockdown). BW: Body weight; LD1: First COVID-19 lockdown; LD2: Second COVID-19 lockdown. Data presented as mean (SE). $p < 0.05$ for all comparisons (child/adolescent): BW before LD1 vs. BW during LD1, BW during LD1 vs. BW after LD1, BW after LD1 vs. BW before LD2, BW before LD2 vs. BW during LD2, BW during LD1 vs. BW before LD2.

In relation to changes in dietary habits and practices, there were no changes in the consumption of all three main meals (breakfast, lunch, and dinner) with the exception of a decreased percentage of parents reporting having dinner during the second COVID-19 lockdown ($p = 0.025$). Similarly, no changes were detected in the consumption of snacks for either parents or children (Table 3). There was a significant increase in ordering/consuming fast foods for both parents and children ($p < 0.001$). Parents ordered/consumed fast foods 0.64 times/week during LD1 and 1.17 times/week during LD2 ($p < 0.001$), while children consumed fast foods 0.55 and 1.08 times/week, respectively ($p < 0.001$). Parents also reported preparing home meals less often during LD2, compared to LD1 (6.09 times/week vs. 6.43 times/week; $p = 0.027$).

Table 3. Dietary practices for parents and children during the first and second COVID-19 lockdown (n = 61).

Practices		Parent			Child		
		LD1 N (%)	LD2 N (%)	*p* Value	LD1 N (%)	LD2 N (%)	*p* Value
Consumption of breakfast	Yes	58 (95.1)	54 (88.5)	0.157	60 (98.4)	58 (95.1)	0.317
Consumption of lunch	Yes	59 (96.7)	61 (100)	0.157	61 (100)	60 (98.4)	0.317
Consumption of dinner	Yes	60 (98.4)	55 (90.2)	0.025	59 (96.7)	57 (93.4)	0.414
Consumption of snacks	No snack	0 (0)	0 (0)	0.826	1 (1.6)	1 (1.6)	0.854
	1	12 (19.7)	12 (19.7)		7 (11.5)	7 (11.5)	
	2	30 (49.2)	30 (49.2)		31 (50.8)	31 (50.8)	
	3	13 (21.3)	15 (24.6)		14 (23.0)	15 (24.6)	
	>=4	6 (9.8)	4 (6.6)		8 (13.1)	7 (11.5)	
Ordering/eating fast food	Never	27 (44.3)	10 (16.4)	<0.001 *	30 (49.2)	10 (16.4)	<0.001 *
	1–3 times/month	18 (29.5)	21 (34.4)		19 (31.1)	25 (41.0)	
	1–2 times/week	13 (21.3)	22 (36.1)		9 (14.8)	20 (32.8)	
	3–4 times/week	3 (4.9)	8 (13.1)		3 (4.9)	5 (8.2)	
	5–6 times/week	0 (0)	0 (0)		0 (0)	1 (1.6)	
	Every day	0 (0)	0 (0)		0 (0)	0 (0)	

LD1: First COVID-19 lockdown; LD2: Second COVID-19 lockdown; * Paired *t*-tests for continuous variables, as mentioned in text (transformed from nominal variables).

Table 4 presents the changes in the consumption of different food groups (available only for children). There was a significant decrease in the weekly consumption of fresh and prepacked juices (−1 and −0.47 servings/week, respectively) and fish (−0.14 servings/week) and a significant increase in weekly consumption of fast foods (+0.53 servings/week).

Table 4. Children's and adolescents' eating habits * during the first and second COVID-19 lockdown (n = 60).

Food Groups	LD1	LD2	p Value
Fruits	5.11 (2.32)	4.92 (2.30)	0.591
Fresh juices	4.03 (2.48)	3.03 (2.38)	0.004
Prepacked juices	1.50 (2.01)	1.03 (1.72)	0.044
Vegetables	4.15 (2.65)	4.00 (2.56)	0.836
Dairy	6.52 (1.45)	6.34 (1.38)	0.401
Red meat	2.12 (1.27)	2.16 (1.15)	0.704
Poultry	1.65 (0.73)	1.66 (0.98)	0.902
Fish	1.21 (0.52)	1.07 (0.73)	0.035
Pasta	3.60 (2.09)	3.74 (1.97)	0.490
Legumes	1.46 (0.94)	1.43 (0.73)	0.783
Homemade sweets	2.55 (2.06)	2.39 (2.14)	0.533
Ready-made sweets	2.51 (2.31)	2.65 (2.29)	0.669
Salty snacks	1.21 (1.61)	1.29 (1.59)	0.679
Fast food	0.55 (0.85)	1.08 (1.09)	<0.001
Soda beverages	0.71 (1.63)	0.58 (1.39)	0.205

* Data presented as mean (SD) consumption (in servings/week) of each food. LD1: First lockdown; LD2: Second lockdown.

4. Discussion

The COVEAT study assessed differences in parents' and their children's BMI or body weight, respectively, and their dietary behavior between the two lockdown periods implemented in Greece. The results of this study did not identify any significant changes in fathers' and mothers' parental BMI. However, significant changes in children's/adolescents' body weight were recorded during the second lockdown (LD2) compared to the first lockdown (LD1). Regarding dietary behavior, fewer parents were found to prepare home meals in LD2, and they increased fast-food consumption. In addition, a significant decrease in fresh and prepacked juices consumption and an increase in fast-food consumption were recorded in children/adolescents in LD2 compared to LD1.

Only a few studies focused on individuals' change in dietary behavior and anthropometric indices between different lockdown periods. The vast majority of the studies are based on data obtained in LD1. The study of Parker et al. observed that over 40% of adults 18–28 years old living in the United States of America had an increase and approximately 17% a decrease in their body weight. Interestingly, a higher increase occurred among the lower income participants and in females [11]. The study by Al Zaman et al. included 439 adults 18–59 years old in the United Arab Emirates. Based on the results of this study, 51.1% of the participants gained weight, 36.2% lost weight, and 12.7% maintained their body weight [12]. Rizzo et al. presented the results of a large-scale, online study in 140 countries (n = 19.903) and showed that a large number of citizens, especially in the USA, increased their body weight during LD1 [13]. In addition, Khan et al. conducted a review of studies (n = 41) and concluded that body weight increased in LD1 in 6–8-year-old children, especially in those who were already living with overweight or obesity. On the other hand, Bahatheg conducted a study with 330 parents from three countries (Great Britain, Saudi Arabia, and Turkey) and revealed that 63% of the parents reported that their children did not gain weight in LD1 [14].

Regarding the changes in dietary behavior in LD1, the studies by Phillippe et al. and Caso et al. reported a significant increase in healthy food consumption in parents and their children and preparation of home meals [15,16]. Moreover, Phillippe et al. observed that parents preferred to prepare local recipes and to use raw materials and Caso et al. observed a decrease in adults' fast-food consumption [15,16]. During LD1, Gaa et al. recorded a significant increase in homemade foods consumption and a decrease in meal skipping in a sample of 220 students in Uganda [17]. Regarding the number of main meals, Bahatheg showed that the majority of participants consumed three main meals per day (59.7%) and prepared those meals at home, but also captured an increase in consumption of soft drinks, sweetened juices, juice blends, fruit juice, and frozen food (e.g., pizza, nuggets) in children [14]. Furthermore, the study revealed that a high number of children were eating meat and drinking milk, but fewer were consuming fish. Gomes et al. reported minor changes in fruits, vegetables, and ultra-processed foods consumption in Brazilian adolescents [18]. On the other hand, the study of Parker et al. reported an increase in fast-food consumption, especially among young adults with lower incomes, while the high-income participants had a significant increase in homemade food consumption [11].

Previous studies have also explored individuals' changes of lifestyle and BMI in LD2. According to Bell et al., there was a significant increase in self-reported body mass and BMI at LD1 compared to LD2 [9]. Additionally, there was an increase in the proportion of participants meeting the criteria for overweight between LD1 and LD2 [9]. Comparable results were reported in the study by Kriaučionienė et al., where the most significant increase in BMI was observed in participants who were already overweight. According to the changes in dietary behaviors, this study observed a significant increase in fast-food consumption among both parents and children in LD2 compared to LD1. Furthermore, a decline in the preparation of homemade meals was recorded, although no significant change was observed. A reduction in dinner consumption was accompanied by a simultaneous decrease in the intake of both fresh and prepackaged juices, as well as fish. In accordance with the findings of Kriaučionienė et al., a significant increase in the consumption of fast food, sugary beverages, along with a greater volume of food ordered for home delivery or takeaway, was strongly correlated with weight gain in more than 60% of the participants [19]. According to Pfiefer et al., during LD2 the consumption of certain unhealthy foods (e.g., processed meat products and sweets) was observed among Croatian students [20]. In accordance with the aforementioned, the study by Abdelkawy also reported that participants under 20 years old increased their consumption of carbonated beverages, commercial pastries, fried foods, and fast food, along with difficulties in finding certain foods such as honey, olive oil, broccoli, oranges, and pineapples [21].

The differences observed in individuals' dietary behaviors between LD1 and LD2 could be attributed to the limited knowledge regarding the health effects of COVID-19 during LD1, which in combination with the home isolation measures seem to have led them in adopting a healthier dietary pattern. More specifically, Di Renzo et al. [4] highlighted that the initial fear of infection during LD1 motivated individuals to focus on healthier behaviors, such as preparing meals at home and consuming fresh foods. However, the progressive normalization of the pandemic and the opening of retail and food services during LD2 facilitated the higher consumption of fast food [19,22]. Understanding the differences in dietary behavior between LD1 and LD2 provides crucial insights for public health strategies. The findings suggest that increased stress and lifestyle changes during the second lockdown were associated with less healthy dietary choices, such as a higher consumption of fast-food. These results can inform targeted interventions aimed at promoting home meal preparation and healthy food consumption, particularly during health crises. By providing educational tools and support to families, future strategies could mitigate the impact of restrictions on diet and weight, fostering long-term health and well-being.

The findings of the present study should be interpreted under the light of its strengths and limitations. The COVEAT study was the first study in Greece which investigated the differences in dietary behavior in parents and children/adolescents and the changes in their body weight and BMI during LD1 and LD2. As a result, its methodological design offers the opportunity to obtain some insights in this field, using data obtained by the same study participants in both lockdown periods. The limitations of this study focus on the small, non-representative sample size and the fact that participants were mainly females and well-educated participants; therefore, the results may not be generalizable to the general population. Furthermore, given the restrictions which were in place during the lockdown periods, the data were collected via networks of dietitians-nutritionists which might have caused selection bias. Also, data were based on self-reported questionnaires, since objective methods (e.g., anthropometric measurements such as body weight and height) could not be applied. Finally, due to the limited number of participants, it was not possible to conduct additional statistical analyses to identify differences among sub-groups of the population which may have been affected more, due to the home isolation, such as individuals with different socio-economic backgrounds, weight categories, genders, age groups, health status, etc. Future meta-analyses should aim to explore differences in citizens' lifestyle behaviors and health indices among the lockdown periods, using larger sample sizes from pre-existing cohorts to better understand the impact that home isolation had in individuals' health status.

5. Conclusions

The COVEAT study revealed that dietary behaviors varied across the different lockdown periods implemented in Greece. The findings suggest that each lockdown period had a different impact on individuals' (children's/adolescent' and parents') dietary behaviors. Notably, more unfavorable changes were observed during LD2, indicating that the potential implementation of additional lockdowns could negatively affect individuals' lifestyle choices. The changes in 61 individuals' dietary patterns during the lockdowns implemented during the COVID-era underscore the need of applying careful monitoring and lifestyle interventions to prevent long-term negative impacts on individuals' health status and well-being, particularly among vulnerable population groups. Further research with larger and more diverse populations is necessary to validate these results and ensure that they are representative of broader groups.

Author Contributions: Conceptualization, O.A. and M.P.; methodology, O.A.; statistical analysis, G.S.; data curation, O.A., M.P. and C.G. (Christos Georgiou); writing—original draft preparation, O.A.; writing—review and editing, G.S., M.K. (Michail Kipouros), A.M., M.K. (Maria Koutsaki), C.G. (Christos Georgiou), M.P., S.K.P., R.I.K., C.G. (Constantinos Giaginis) and T.M.; supervision, O.A. All authors have read and agreed to the published version of the manuscript.

Funding: This research received no external funding.

Institutional Review Board Statement: This study was conducted according to the guidelines of the Declaration of Helsinki and the conventions of the Council of Europe on Human Rights and Biomedicine. The study protocol was approved by the Ethical Committee of the Department of Physical Education and Sport Science in the School of Physical Education, Sport Science, and Dietetics,

University of Thessaly (protocol code 1655 and date of approval: 6 June 2020), and registered at clinicaltrials.org (NCT04437121).

Informed Consent Statement: Informed consent was obtained from all subjects involved in this study.

Data Availability Statement: The data presented in this study are available on request from the corresponding author. The data are not publicly available due to ethical restrictions.

Acknowledgments: The authors would like to thank the study participants.

Conflicts of Interest: The authors declare no conflicts of interest.

References

1. Naja, F.; Hamadeh, R. Nutrition amid the COVID-19 pandemic: A multi-level framework for action. *Eur. J. Clin. Nutr.* **2020**, *74*, 1117–1121. [CrossRef] [PubMed]
2. Butler, M.J.; Barrientos, R.M. The impact of nutrition on COVID-19 susceptibility and long-term consequences. *Brain Behav. Immun.* **2020**, *87*, 53–54. [CrossRef]
3. Pietrobelli, A.; Pecoraro, L.; Ferruzzi, A.; Heo, M.; Faith, M.; Zoller, T.; Antoniazzi, F.; Piacentini, G.; Fearnbach, S.N.; Heymsfield, S.B. Effects of COVID-19 Lockdown on Lifestyle Behaviors in Children with Obesity Living in Verona, Italy: A Longitudinal Study. *Obesity* **2020**, *28*, 1382–1385. [CrossRef]
4. Di Renzo, L.; Gualtieri, P.; Pivari, F.; Soldati, L.; Attinà, A.; Cinelli, G.; Leggeri, C.; Caparello, G.; Barrea, L.; Scerbo, F.; et al. Eating habits and lifestyle changes during COVID-19 lockdown: An Italian survey. *J. Transl. Med.* **2020**, *18*, 229. [CrossRef] [PubMed]
5. Robinson, T.N.; Banda, J.A.; Hale, L.; Robinson, T.N.; Banda, J.A.; Hale, L.; Lu, A.S.; Fleming-Milici, F.; Calvert, S.L.; Wartella, E. Screen Media Exposure and Obesity in Children and Adolescents. *Pediatrics* **2017**, *140* (Suppl. S2), S97–S101. [CrossRef]
6. Tambalis, K.D.; Panagiotakos, D.B.; Psarra, G.; Sidossis, L.S. Insufficient Sleep Duration Is Associated with Dietary Habits, Screen Time and Obesity in Children. *J. Clin. Sleep Med.* **2018**, *14*, 1689–1696. [CrossRef] [PubMed]
7. Avery, A.; Anderson, C.; McCullough, F. Associations between children's diet quality and watching television during meal or snack consumption: A systematic review. *Matern. Child Nutr.* **2017**, *13*, e12428. [CrossRef]
8. Woods, N.; Seabrook, J.A.; Schaafsma, H.; Burke, S.; Tucker, T.; Gilliland, J. Dietary changes of youth during the COVID-19 pandemic: A systematic review. *J. Nutr.* **2024**, *154*, 1376–1403. [CrossRef]
9. Bell, M.; Duncan, M.J.; Patte, K.A.; Roy, B.D.; Ditor, D.S.; Klentrou, P. Changes in Body Mass, Physical Activity, and Dietary Intake during the COVID-19 Pandemic Lockdowns in Canadian University Students. *Biology* **2023**, *12*, 326. [CrossRef]
10. Androutsos, O.; Perperidi, M.; Georgiou, C.; Chouliaras, G. Lifestyle Changes and Determinants of Children's and Adolescents' Body Weight Increase during the First COVID-19 Lockdown in Greece: The COV-EAT Study. *Nutrients* **2021**, *13*, 930. [CrossRef] [PubMed]
11. Parker, J.; Kaur, S.; Medalla, J.M.; Imbert-Sanchez, A.; Bautista, J. Dietary trends among young adults during the COVID-19 lockdown: Socioeconomic and gender disparities. *BMC Nutr.* **2023**, *9*, 107. [CrossRef]
12. Zaman, K.A.; Ahmed, S.; Alshamsi, A.; Alshamsi, A.; Alshdaifat, B.; Alaleeli, S.; Mussa, B.M. Impact of COVID-19 Pandemic on Weight Change Among Adults in the UAE. *Int. J. Gen. Med.* **2023**, *16*, 1661–1670. [CrossRef]
13. Rizzo, N. Quarantine Weight Gain: 35.82% Gained Weight During Pandemic [19,903 Person Study]. 2021. Available online: https://runrepeat.com/quarantine-15-weight-gain-study (accessed on 6 August 2021).
14. Bahatheg, R.O. Young Children's Nutrition During the COVID-19 Pandemic Lockdown: A Comparative Study. *Early Child. Educ. J.* **2021**, *49*, 915–923. [CrossRef] [PubMed]
15. Philippe, K.; Issanchou, S.; Monnery-Patris, S. Contrasts and ambivalences in French parents' experiences regarding changes in eating and cooking behaviours during the COVID-19 lockdown. *Food Qual. Prefer.* **2021**, *96*, 104386. [CrossRef]
16. Caso, D.; Guidetti, M.; Capasso, M.; Cavazza, N. Finally, the chance to eat healthily: Longitudinal study about food consumption during and after the first COVID-19 lockdown in Italy. *Food Qual. Prefer.* **2021**, *95*, 104275. [CrossRef] [PubMed]
17. Gaa, P.K.; Sulley, S.; Boahen, S.; Bogobiri, S.; Mogre, V. Reported dietary habits and lifestyle behaviors of students before and during COVID-19 lockdown: A cross-sectional survey among university students from Ghana. *J. Public Health Res.* **2022**, *11*, 22799036221129417.
18. Gomes, C.S.; Santi, N.M.M.; da Silva, D.R.P.; Werneck, A.O.; Szwarcwald, C.L.; de Azevedo Barros, M.B.; Malta, D.C. The COVID-19 pandemic and changes in eating habits of Brazilian adolescents. *Dialogues Health* **2022**, *1*, 100070. [CrossRef]
19. Kriaučionienė, V.; Grincaitė, M.; Raskilienė, A.; Petkevičienė, J. Changes in Nutrition, Physical Activity, and Body Weight among Lithuanian Students during and after the COVID-19 Pandemic. *Nutrients* **2023**, *15*, 4091. [CrossRef] [PubMed]
20. Pfeifer, D.; Rešetar, J.; Czlapka-Matyasik, M.; Bykowska-Derda, A.; Kolay, E.; Stelcer, B.; Gajdoš Kljusurić, J. Changes in diet quality and its association with students' mental state during two COVID-19 lockdowns in Croatia. *Nutr. Health* **2023**, *12*, 2532. [CrossRef]

21. Abdelkawy, K.; Elbarbry, F.; El-Masry, S.M.; Zakaria, A.Y.; Rodríguez-Pérez, C.; El-Khodary, N.M. Changes in dietary habits during Covid-19 lockdown in Egypt: The Egyptian COVIDiet study. *BMC Public Health* **2023**, *23*, 956. [CrossRef] [PubMed]
22. Bohlouli, J.; Moravejolahkami, A.R.; Ganjali Dashti, M.; Balouch Zehi, Z.; Hojjati Kermani, M.A.; Borzoo-Isfahani, M.; Bahreini-Esfahani, N. COVID-19 and fast foods consumption: A review. *Int. J. Food Prop.* **2021**, *24*, 203–209. [CrossRef]

Disclaimer/Publisher's Note: The statements, opinions and data contained in all publications are solely those of the individual author(s) and contributor(s) and not of MDPI and/or the editor(s). MDPI and/or the editor(s) disclaim responsibility for any injury to people or property resulting from any ideas, methods, instructions or products referred to in the content.

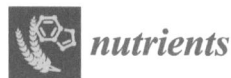

Article

Dietary Intakes Among University Students in Iceland: Insights from the FINESCOP Project

Brittany M. Repella and Greta Jakobsdottir *

Faculty of Health Promotion, Sport and Leisure Studies, School of Education, University of Iceland, 105 Reykjavik, Iceland; brittany@hi.is
* Correspondence: gretaja@hi.is

Abstract: Objectives: Using data from the Food Insecurity among European University Students during the COVID-19 Pandemic (FINESCOP) project, this study aims to investigate the dietary intakes among university students in Iceland, focusing specifically on their current diet after March 2020. Additionally, it examines correlations among different food groups to reveal associations in dietary patterns. **Methods**: The investigation uses data from the observational FINESCOP project in Iceland. Spearman's correlation coefficients were used to identify associations between different dietary intakes. p values show significance at a level of <0.05. **Results**: Icelandic university students have a low intake of vegetables and salad ("3–4 times per week", n = 159, 24.8%), fruit ("1–2 times per week", n = 164, 25.6%), and whole wheat ("3–4 times per week", n = 147, 23.2%). Lower than these was legume intake ("Never/seldom", n = 203, 32.0%). Meat and eggs were consumed more frequently ("3–4 times per week", n = 231, 36.3%) compared to fish and seafood ("1–2 times per week", n = 277, 43.5%). While the findings do indicate a significant correlation between vegetables and salad and fruit intake ($p < 0.001$) and between vegetable and salad and legume intake ($p < 0.001$), causal relationships cannot be established. Among discretionary foods, sweets and snacks were moderately and significantly correlated ($p < 0.001$). **Conclusions**: This study explores dietary intakes and correlations between dietary factors among university students in Iceland. Further research is needed to explore the potential for causal inferences and better understand these dietary behaviors of university students in Iceland.

Keywords: health promotion; nutrition; diet; food choice; dietary patterns

1. Introduction

What university students eat is important for their mental and physical health. Among university students in Iceland, 17% (n = 125) experienced some level of food insecurity and nearly 4% (n = 28) went an entire day without eating due to the lack of food or other resources to purchase food [1]. Food intake has been associated with university students' ability to function as well as their ability to concentrate and to properly study and absorb information [2,3]. Students must be able to consume enough nourishing food throughout the day regardless of their socioeconomic status. The following research looks deeper into what university students in Iceland are eating, and which foods are correlated. The first investigation in Iceland was published in October 2023 and looked at the prevalence of food insecurity and associations with academic performance, consumption patterns, and social support among university students during the COVID-19 pandemic [1].

The Nordic Nutrition Recommendations, which guide the national Icelandic recommendations, are a set of nutritional and health promoting guidelines that are evidence-based. The current guidelines also consider the environment, with an emphasis on plant-based foods [4]. Plant foods, namely vegetables and fruits, are crucial for human health and are the basis of nearly all national dietary recommendations around the world, including the recommendations put forth by the World Health Organization [5]. In addition to the right quantities of food, everyone, including university students, benefits from consuming nutritious foods. Higher intake of plants, like vegetables, fruits, and legumes, can reduce a person's risk of many noncommunicable diseases, for instance, cardiovascular disease and certain cancers [6,7], and reduce all-cause mortality [7,8].

In Iceland, the dietary recommendations advise adults from the age of two and older to consume five servings of fruits and vegetables, with three of these preferably being a vegetable, whole grains two times a day, fish two to three times a week, a reasonable amount of dairy and dairy products, about twice a day, and a moderate amount of meat, limiting red meat to around two servings a week. Legume intake is recommended at a few times a week. While there is no intake level, the recommendations promote limiting processed foods such as sugar-sweetened beverages, salty snacks, sweets, and processed meat [9]. Even with the national guidelines, Icelanders fall short to reach the intake of plant foods. In the most recent national dietary survey of Icelanders, "What are Icelanders Eating (Hvað borða Íslendingar)" [10], only about 2% of the respondents consumed the recommended five servings (500 g) of vegetables and fruit per day. Iceland falls far behind the consumption range in the European Union, which has an average five serving intake of 12%, ranging from 20% (France) to 33% (Ireland) [11,12].

Legumes are also an important part of the diet and have been linked to reduced noncommunicable diseases and reduced all-cause mortality [13]. As seen in the Icelandic national dietary survey, only 17% of respondents ate beans or lentils and 25% ate a plant-based meal as the main course once or more during the week [10]. While the Nordic Dietary Recommendations are promoting an increase in plant-based foods, especially protein-rich plant foods such as beans and lentils, consuming protein from fish and seafood is also important. Fish and seafood, especially fatty fish, have been linked to an improvement in cardiovascular health [14], mostly due to the omega fatty acids in fatty fish like salmon or cod liver oil [15]. Meat and eggs can also be part of a balanced diet. Most guidelines, including the Nordic and Icelandic, recommend meat in moderation and priority should be placed on leaner cuts of meat, such as chicken and turkey.

The Food Insecurity among European University Students during the COVID-19 Pandemic (FINESCOP) is a cross-sectional investigation of university students, with data collected throughout Europe, such as Iceland, Norway, Finland, Germany, Poland, the Netherlands, Belgium, Portugal, Spain, and Italy. The primary focus of this paper is to analyze dietary intakes of university students in Iceland. The Icelandic dietary guidelines are used for comparisons and to identify specific food groups that are over- or under-consumed relative to the recommendations. Additionally, correlations between foods and food groups are explored.

2. Materials and Methods

2.1. Study Design

The data for this research come from the FINESCOP project. The following dissemination refers to Icelandic data only, which were collected from the 11th of January until the 31st of March 2022 [1].

2.2. Participant Recruitment and Enrollment

Information on participants and enrollment can be found in more detail in the first Icelandic publication about FINESCOP [1]. Eligibility criteria included being a university student at one of the participating universities, aged 18 years or older, and having access to their university email.

2.3. Questionnaire Development

In collaboration with participating FINESCOP countries, the questionnaire was developed. Further insights and details can be seen in previously published FINESCOP papers [1,16].

2.4. Dietary Intakes Questions

The following food groups were in the FINESCOP questionnaire: vegetables and salad [(juice and potatoes are not included) (one plate, 1–2 cups or 150–200 g each time)]; fruit [(juice not included) (one large piece or two small ones, 1 cup or 120–200 g each time)]; legumes (beans and lentils) [(4 tablespoons of cooked beans, about 60–80 g)]; dairy and dairy products [(one glass or container, about 200–250 g)]; whole wheat products [bowl of cereal, 1 slice of bread, 3 tablespoons of pasta/rice (about 60–80 g each)]; fish and seafood (one portion, about 125–150 g each); meat and eggs [unprocessed products (one portion, about 100–125 g each)]; processed meat [e.g., sausages, ham, bacon (about 100–125 g each)]; salty snacks [salt sticks and flakes (one small bag, about 50–100 g each time)]; sweets [chocolate, biscuits, muffins, pastries, ice cream, and candy (one medium-sized piece, about 50–100 g each)]; sugary drinks/soda [other than energy drinks (one can, about 330 mL each time)]; sugar-free soda [other than energy drinks (one can, about 330 mL each)]; energy drinks (one can, about 330 mL each). Responses included rarely/never; less than once a week; 1–2 times a week; 3–4 times a week; 5–6 times a week; 1 time a day; 2 times a day; 3 times or more a day; don't know.

Dietary data were collected twice in the questionnaire and the following questions were included: (1) "Before the COVID-19 pandemic (March 2019-March 2020), how many times a week on average did you eat/drink..." and (2) "Since the COVID-19 epidemic started, in March 2020, how many times a week on average did you eat/drink...". For this study, we focus only on the diet after March 2020, or the current diet of the respondents, and do not include any pre-pandemic data. Dietary intake descriptives are shown as both the number of respondents and the percentage of the total and cumulative percentage.

When making statements about correct dietary intakes, the researchers use and refer to either the Icelandic dietary recommendations or the Nordic recommendations [4,9]. Since Iceland bases its recommendations on the Nordic recommendations, for the sake of brevity, all statements will be referred to as dietary recommendations.

2.5. Data Analysis

Descriptives and analysis were completed using RStudio v4.6.4 (R Core Team 2022) and jamovi (Version 2.5).

A correlation matrix was created with the dietary intake variables, and Spearman's correlation coefficients were used to assess how well the relationship is between the variables. Spearman's rank correlation was chosen due to the responses in the dietary questions, which are measured using an ordinal scale. A positive correlation suggests that both variables move in the same direction, while a negative correlation suggests that variables move in the opposite direction. The closer the correlation comes to one ($\pm$), the stronger the correlation is. The correlation ranges include Spearman's rho (ρ) = ± 1 (perfect correlation), $\pm 0.7 < \rho < \pm 1$ (strong correlation), $\pm 0.4 < \rho \leq \pm 0.7$ (moderate correlation), and $0 < \rho \leq \pm 0.4$ (weak correlation). Additionally, the correlation can be non-existent or zero, $\rho = 0$, which implies no relationship between the two variables.

2.6. Ethical Consideration

This study complied with ethical standards aimed at protecting participant confidentiality and rights. Each participant completed a digital consent form before taking part in the survey, and participation was contingent upon receiving this consent. The institutional review board of the university's Ethics Committee for Scientific Research reviewed and approved this study (SHV2021-038).

3. Results

3.1. Respondent Demographics

The university cohort's demographics can be seen in the first published paper from Repella et al. [1]. The students were mostly female (74.5%) originating in Iceland (78.5%). The average age of the respondents was 31.7 years (SD 8.4).

3.2. Dietary Intakes

Table 1 shows dietary intakes. The dietary recommended level will be in bold text if applicable and as accurately as possible. Since vegetables and salad and fruit are combined in the dietary recommendations as five per day, more than one intake level will be bold in fruit.

For the food groups that have a recommendation in Iceland, the respondent's dietary intake fell short. For vegetables and salad, just 15 respondents (2.3%) reached the "3 times or more per day" recommended intake level. Fruit was also low, with only 46 respondents (7.2%) reaching the recommended "2 times per day". Intake of whole wheat had just 50 respondents (7.9%) and dairy and dairy products had 49 respondents (7.7%) reach the recommended intake. Nearly half of the respondents consumed fish and seafood "1–2 times per week" (n = 277, 43.5%) and meat and eggs at a higher frequency ("3–4 times per week") but with slightly fewer respondents (n = 231, 36.3%).

Salty snacks were consumed "1–2 times per week" (n = 198, 30.9%) and sweets were consumed slightly more frequently at "3–4 times per week" (n = 180, 28.1%). About three-quarters of the respondents consumed processed meat less than two times per week, split nearly evenly among the three frequency groups: "1–2 times per week" (n = 164, 25.8%), "less than once a week" (n = 163, 25.7%), and "never/seldom" (n = 164, 25.8%). When looking at beverages, the highest intake group, "never/seldom", was the same for sugar-sweetened beverages, sugar-free beverages, and energy drinks, as seen in Table 1.

Table 1. Dietary intakes of university students in Iceland.

	Counts	% of Total	Cumulative %
Vegetable and Salad			
3 times or more per day	15	2.3%	2.3%
2 times per day	69	10.8%	13.1%
Once per day	112	17.5%	30.6%
5–6 times per week	101	15.8%	46.3%
3–4 times per week	159	24.8%	71.1%
1–2 times per week	111	17.3%	88.5%
Less than once a week	41	6.4%	94.9%
Never/seldom	29	4.5%	99.4%
Don't know	4	0.6%	100.0%

Table 1. *Cont.*

	Counts	% of Total	Cumulative %
Fruit			
3 times or more per day	**22**	**3.4%**	**3.4%**
2 times per day	**46**	**7.2%**	**10.6%**
Once per day	86	13.4%	24.0%
5–6 times per week	73	11.4%	35.4%
3–4 times per week	128	20.0%	55.4%
1–2 times per week	164	25.6%	81.0%
Less than once a week	90	14.0%	95.0%
Never/seldom	28	4.4%	99.4%
Don't know	4	0.6%	100.0%
Legumes			
3 times or more per day	3	0.5%	0.5%
2 times per day	3	0.5%	0.9%
Once per day	15	2.4%	3.3%
5–6 times per week	21	3.3%	6.6%
3–4 times per week	**68**	**10.7%**	**17.4%**
1–2 times per week	120	18.9%	36.3%
Less than once a week	179	28.2%	64.5%
Never/seldom	203	32.0%	96.5%
Don't know	22	3.5%	100.0%
Whole Wheat			
3 times or more per day	13	2.1%	2.1%
2 times per day	**50**	**7.9%**	**9.9%**
Once per day	132	20.8%	30.8%
5–6 times per week	110	17.4%	48.1%
3–4 times per week	147	23.2%	71.3%
1–2 times per week	95	15.0%	86.3%
Less than once a week	48	7.6%	93.8%
Never/seldom	39	6.2%	100.0%
Don't know	0	0	0
Dairy and Dairy Products			
3 times or more per day	11	1.7%	1.7%
2 times per day	**49**	**7.7%**	**9.5%**
Once per day	122	19.3%	28.8%
5–6 times per week	71	11.2%	40.0%
3–4 times per week	114	18.0%	58.0%
1–2 times per week	103	16.3%	74.2%
Less than once a week	70	11.1%	85.3%
Never/seldom	91	14.4%	99.7%
Don't know	2	0.3%	100.0%

Table 1. *Cont.*

	Counts	% of Total	Cumulative %
Fish and Seafood			
3 times or more per day	0	0	0
2 times per day	0	0	0
Once per day	3	0.5%	0.5%
5–6 times per week	4	0.6%	1.1%
3–4 times per week	**72**	**11.3%**	**12.4%**
1–2 times per week	**277**	**43.5%**	**55.9%**
Less than once a week	167	26.2%	82.1%
Never/seldom	112	17.6%	99.7%
Don't know	2	0.3%	100.0%
Meat and Eggs			
3 times or more per day	0	0	0
2 times per day	9	1.4%	1.4%
Once per day	41	6.4%	7.8%
5–6 times per week	88	13.8%	21.7%
3–4 times per week	**231**	**36.3%**	**57.9%**
1–2 times per week	**144**	**22.6%**	**80.5%**
Less than once a week	41	6.4%	87.0%
Never/seldom	80	12.6%	99.5%
Don't know	3	0.5%	100.0%
Salty Snacks			
3 times or more per day	4	0.6%	0.6%
2 times per day	6	0.9%	1.6%
Once per day	18	2.8%	4.4%
5–6 times per week	49	7.6%	12.0%
3–4 times per week	117	18.3%	30.3%
1–2 times per week	**198**	**30.9%**	**61.2%**
Less than once a week	174	27.1%	88.3%
Never/seldom	71	11.1%	99.4%
Don't know	4	0.6%	100.0%
Sweets			
3 times or more per day	12	1.9%	1.9%
2 times per day	20	3.1%	5.0%
Once per day	63	9.8%	14.8%
5–6 times per week	94	14.7%	29.5%
3–4 times per week	180	28.1%	57.7%
1–2 times per week	**139**	**21.7%**	**79.4%**
Less than once a week	100	15.6%	95.0%
Never/seldom	31	4.8%	99.8%
Don't know	1	0.2%	100.0%

Table 1. *Cont.*

	Counts	% of Total	Cumulative %
Sugar Drinks and Soda			
3 times or more per day	5	0.8%	0.8%
2 times per day	5	0.8%	1.6%
Once per day	19	3.0%	4.5%
5–6 times per week	14	2.2%	6.7%
3–4 times per week	51	8.0%	14.7%
1–2 times per week	**97**	**15.2%**	**29.9%**
Less than once a week	139	21.8%	51.6%
Never/seldom	309	48.4%	100.0%
Don't know	0	0	0
Processed Meat			
3 times or more per day	0	0	0
2 times per day	2	0.3%	0.3%
Once per day	15	2.4%	2.7%
5–6 times per week	25	3.9%	6.6%
3–4 times per week	100	15.7%	22.4%
1–2 times per week	164	25.8%	48.2%
Less than once a week	163	25.7%	73.9%
Never/seldom	164	25.8%	99.7%
Don't know	2	0.3%	100.0%
Sugar-Free Soda			
3 times or more per day	23	3.6%	3.6%
2 times per day	23	3.6%	7.2%
Once per day	41	6.4%	13.6%
5–6 times per week	40	6.3%	19.9%
3–4 times per week	85	13.3%	33.2%
1–2 times per week	84	13.2%	46.4%
Less than once a week	84	13.2%	59.6%
Never/seldom	253	39.7%	99.2%
Don't know	5	0.8%	100.0%
Energy Drinks			
3 times or more per day	7	1.1%	1.1%
2 times per day	17	2.7%	3.8%
Once per day	61	9.5%	13.3%
5–6 times per week	28	4.4%	17.7%
3–4 times per week	50	7.8%	25.5%
1–2 times per week	53	8.3%	33.8%
Less than once a week	80	12.5%	46.3%
Never/seldom	343	53.7%	100.0%
Don't know	0	0	0

3.3. Correlation and Association

A correlation matrix was created for the food recommended by the dietary recommendations: vegetables and salad, fruit, fish and seafood, meat and eggs, legumes, dairy and dairy products, and whole wheat products, as can be seen in Table 2. The strength of correlations is categorized based on Spearman's coefficient thresholds [17]. Fifteen significant correlations were found, though the strength of the correlations was weak. One strong positive correlation was found between the intake of vegetables and salad and fruit (Spearman's rho = 0.647, $p < 0.001$). Another significant correlation was found between the intake of vegetables and salad and legumes, moderately positive (Spearman's rho = 0.403, $p < 0.001$).

A correlation matrix was also created for processed foods and drinks with the assumption that all correlations would be positive: salty snacks, sweets, sugar drinks and soda, sugar-free soda, energy drinks, and processed meat, as shown in Table 3. Among these pairs, only one was ranked moderately positive, salty snacks and sweets (Spearman's rho = 0.405, $p < 0.001$), while the remaining pairs were significant, but with a weak correlation strength.

Table 2. Correlation matrix of dietary recommended foods.

Variable 1	Variable 2	Spearman's Rho	Strength	df [1]	p-Value
Vegetables and Salad					
	Fruit (n = 637)	0.647 ***	Strong (+)	635	<0.001
	Legumes (n = 612)	0.403 ***	Moderate (+)	610	<0.001
	Whole Wheat (n = 630)	0.279 ***	Weak (+)	628	<0.001
	Dairy and Dairy Products (n = 629)	0.078	Weak (+)	627	0.05
	Fish and Seafood (n = 633)	0.106 **	Weak (+)	631	<0.01
	Meat and Eggs (n = 632)	0.001	No correlation	630	0.972
Fruit					
	Legumes (n = 612)	0.208 ***	Weak (+)	610	<0.001
	Whole Wheat (n = 630)	0.271 ***	Weak (+)	628	<0.001
	Dairy and Dairy Products (n = 629)	0.104 **	Weak (+)	627	<0.01
	Fish and Seafood (n = 633)	0.152 ***	Weak (+)	631	<0.001
	Meat and Eggs (n = 632)	0.009	No correlation	630	0.822
Legumes					
	Whole Wheat (n = 611)	0.175 ***	Weak (+)	609	<0.001
	Dairy and Dairy Products (n = 611)	−0.113 **	Weak (−)	609	0.005
	Fish and Seafood (n = 612)	−0.053	Weak (−)	610	0.189
	Meat and Eggs (n = 611)	−0.280 ***	Weak (−)	609	<0.001
Whole Wheat					
	Dairy and Dairy Products (n = 630)	0.219 ***	Weak (+)	628	<0.001
	Fish and Seafood (n = 632)	−0.056	Weak (−)	630	0.160
	Meat and Eggs (n = 631)	−0.046	Weak (−)	629	0.25

Table 2. Cont.

Variable 1	Variable 2	Spearman's Rho	Strength	df [1]	p-Value
Dairy and Dairy Products					
	Fish and Seafood (n = 631)	0.235 ***	Weak (+)	629	<0.001
	Meat and Eggs (n = 630)	0.214 ***	Weak (+)	628	<0.001
Fish and Seafood					
	Meat and Eggs (n = 634)	0.294 ***	Weak (+)	632	<0.001

[1] degrees of freedom: $df = n - 2$. Note: ** $p < 0.01$, *** $p < 0.001$, one-tailed.

Table 3. Correlation matrix of processed food and drinks.

Variable 1	Variable 2	Spearman's Rho	Strength	df [1]	p-Value
Salty Snacks					
	Sweets (n = 636)	0.405 ***	Moderate (+)	634	<0.001
	Sugar Drinks and Soda (n = 635)	0.234 ***	Weak (+)	633	<0.001
	Processed Meat (n = 631)	0.131 ***	Weak (+)	629	<0.001
	Sugar-Free Soda (n = 629)	0.124 ***	Weak (+)	627	<0.001
	Energy Drinks (n = 635)	0.097 **	Weak (+)	633	<0.01
Sweets					
	Sugar Drinks and Soda (n = 637)	0.209 ***	Weak (+)	635	<0.001
	Processed Meat (n = 632)	0.143 ***	Weak (+)	630	<0.001
	Sugar-Free Soda (n = 631)	0.094 **	Weak (+)	629	<0.01
	Energy Drinks (n = 637)	0.036	No correlation	635	0.179
Sugar Drinks and Soda					
	Processed Meat (n = 633)	0.209 ***	Weak (+)	631	<0.001
	Sugar-Free Soda (n = 633)	−0.035	No correlation	631	0.812
	Energy Drinks (n = 639)	0.071 *	Weak (+)	637	<0.05
Processed Meat					
	Sugar-Free Soda (n = 627)	0.182 ***	Weak (+)	625	<0.001
	Energy Drinks (n = 633)	0.144 ***	Weak (+)	631	<0.001
Sugar-Free Soda					
	Energy Drinks (n = 633)	0.213 ***	Weak (+)	631	<0.001

[1] degrees of freedom: $df = n - 2$. Note: * $p < 0.05$, ** $p < 0.01$, *** $p < 0.001$, one-tailed.

4. Discussion

The purpose of this research was to describe the dietary intake of university students in Iceland and identify correlations among dietary intake variables from the FINESCOP questionnaire. While other variables were measured in the questionnaire, this research looks only at dietary intake and only after the COVID-19 pandemic and, therefore, the current diet of university students in Iceland. For results on other variables from the Icelandic study, see the first paper by Repella et al. [1].

The dietary guidelines in Iceland recommend five servings of vegetables and fruits per day, with the idea that more than half of them comprise vegetables. According to the most recent Icelandic national dietary survey, "What are Icelanders Eating (Hvað borða Íslendingar)" [10], only about 2% of respondents reached the recommended intake level of five servings per day of vegetables and fruit, or about 500 g. The average intake was about 213 g, just slightly under half of the recommendations [9]. The current research shows similar failings to reach the recommended amount, with 24.8% (n = 159) respondents consuming vegetables three to four times per week, far from three times per day. For fruit intake, only 7.2% (n = 46) reached the recommendation, while the greatest number of respondents consumed fruit one to two times per week, 25.6% (n = 164).

The current FINESCOP questionnaire kept vegetables and fruit separate. To make the comparison possible, the minimum intake of three vegetables and two to three fruits per day were combined to create a vegetable and fruit intake grouping. This revealed that 11.1% (n = 71) met the recommended minimum of five servings of produce per day. This low percentage, only 11%, is not ideal for the health of university students. Vegetables and fruit should be the basis of the diet, and they provide many necessary vitamins and minerals. The intake of vegetables and fruits has been linked to concentration improvements in university students [3], in addition to better mood and lower depression [18]. While the percentage calculated from the Icelandic FINESCOP cohort is much higher than that of the national survey results, it is close to the EU average of 12% [11,12]. However, both percentages still reveal a low intake of fruits and vegetables. This could be due to many reasons such as time restrictions, convenience, taste, and knowledge of the benefits of consuming these foods. The exact reason as to why both Iceland and the EU have low intake of vegetables and fruit is unknown; therefore, more research into the exact reasons is needed.

Concerning other food groups, 43.5% (n = 277) of respondents consumed fish and seafood "1–2 times per week" and 72 respondents (11.3%) consumed it "3–4 times per week". This falls in line with the recommended intake of several times per week, a vague amount that lets the person decide for themselves. The consumption of dairy and dairy products also comes close to the dietary recommendations (two times per day), with the most respondents consuming dairy and dairy products "once per day" (n = 122, 19.3%). Meat and eggs, which do not specify the type of meat, such as white or dark meat, were consumed "3–4 times per week" by the greatest number of respondents (n = 231, 36.3%). This does follow the national dietary guidelines, which recommend meat in moderation with red meat consumption not exceeding 500 g per week. Legumes and whole wheat products are the furthest from the recommendations, with 32.0% (n = 203) consuming legumes "never/seldom" and 23.2% (n = 147) consuming whole wheat "3–4 times per week", rather than a few times a week and twice per day, respectively.

For processed foods, such as processed meat, salty snacks, sweets, sugary drinks/soda, sugar-free soda, and energy drinks, the respondents follow dietary recommendations of limiting consumption to less than four times per week. Intake of processed meat showed an interesting response split, with nearly a triple tie at about 25% each over three frequencies. After combining the frequencies, just around 75% of respondents consumed processed meat no more than two times per week (77.3%, n = 491). Processed meats have been linked to many chronic diseases, such as heart disease and certain cancers [19,20] and most national dietary recommendations, including those from Iceland, recommend people consume as little as possible [9]. Salty snacks were consumed four or less times a week (76.3%, n = 489) and sweets by slightly fewer respondents (65.4%, n = 419). These two food groups were also moderately positively correlated with each other (Spearman's rho = 0.405, $p < 0.001$), suggesting that as snack consumption increases, the consumption of sweets tends to increase as well. However, it is important to note that this association is not perfectly strong, so other factors may also be influencing this relationship and further investigation is needed. These results are not similar to what other research shows on university students' processed food habits, which shows university students consume a large part of their daily diet from processed foods [21,22]. Processed foods, such as salty snacks and sweets, have been associated with increased BMI and an increased risk all-cause mortality [22,23]. Why this is different within the Icelandic population is not known; therefore, further dietary intake research can benefit this body of knowledge.

Concerning how other variables were associated, there was a strong positive correlation between vegetable and salad intake and fruit intake (Spearman's rho = 0.647, $p < 0.001$) and a moderate positive correlation between vegetable and salad intake and legumes (Spearman's rho = 0.403, $p < 0.001$), which indicates that as university students increase their consumption of vegetables and salads, they are also likely to increase their fruit intake, and vice versa; similarly, if their vegetable and salad consumption decreases, their fruit intake is likely to decrease as well. While the intake of vegetables and salad and fruit was low (frequency), it may be that those who choose healthy foods, such as vegetables, will also choose other healthy ingredients, such as fruit [21,22,24]. While further analysis is needed to show and further confirm causality, it may benefit students for the university commissaries to promote these foods together. Interestingly, there were no correlations found between meat and eggs and vegetables and salad or with fruit. There was a significant, but weak, negative correlation between meat and eggs and legumes (Spearman's rho = −0.280, $p < 0.001$); however, without knowing more about the respondent's diet, such as if they follow a vegetarian or vegan food pattern, it is not possible to infer why these correlations occur.

The reasons behind food purchases and preferences among university students have been shown to be mostly taste, value, convenience, and cost [25,26]. A Dutch study looked at the effects of a conveniently located and free farm stand in university buildings and its effects on the intake of produce. The study revealed an increase in both vegetables and fruit, especially among those who had a lower intake prior to the farm stand being set up [27]. Any approach which promotes an increased intake of recommended food groups helps to improve health and well-being [28]. By having more offerings at school, in and around campus buildings, hopefully the intake of these important food groups will increase.

The findings from this study are important for understanding the dietary habits of university students in Iceland. When comparing the dietary intakes to the recommended dietary intakes, the diet of university students in Iceland falls short. The most recent report of dietary intake among people residing in Iceland also found the diet of the general population to have trouble reaching the national dietary recommendations. First and foremost, for both university students and the public, education can be used to promote healthier diets. Food and nutrition education may increase cooking self-efficacy, the use of vegetables and fruits, and behavioral outcomes, such as increased fruit and vegetable consumption [1,29]. Therefore, it is important to promote education, specifically nutrition education, for all students.

Further research must be conducted to explain the causal relationship between vegetables and fruit. Correlation does not imply causation, but it does indicate associations, which can be useful when planning promotions for dietary intakes, as seen in the Dutch food stand study [27]. FINESCOP was not designed to collect comprehensive dietary intake data [1]. The results from Iceland (n = 924) do represent a sample of university students in Iceland, a strength of this study. The sample largely represents the student population, as seen in the ratio of male and female students at the University of Iceland, approximately 32% and 68% in 2022, respectively, which is similar to, but not exactly the same as, our respondents, 22% male and 75% female [1,30]. According to Statistics Iceland, in 2022, 45% of university students were between 18 and 25 years old and 55% were aged 26 and older. While we had fewer students aged 18–25 (29%), our study also had a high number of students aged 26 and older (71%) [31]. Ph.D. students were also included in our research, which may have brought the students' age up. The general academic spread was also comparable to our respondents, with 53% being undergraduates and 43% being either postgraduate or other compared to the universities' figures, which show 57% undergraduates and 42% postgraduate or other [1,32]. A limitation of the research includes a low response rate (4.4%), which may have been due to the need to advertise the questionnaire more. Additionally, the dietary data were self-reported; therefore, bias may have occurred, such as under- or over-reporting and recall bias. The findings are limited to university students.

5. Conclusions

The overall dietary intake of recommended foods among these university respondents is generally low in comparison to the dietary recommendations in Iceland, except for fish and seafood and meat and eggs. The significant correlations between dietary behaviors suggest a pattern of eating, which can be used to promote healthier foods to university students. Future research would be valuable in establishing whether increased vegetable and salad intake directly causes an increase in intake of fruit and legumes and how we can use this knowledge to increase healthy patterns of eating in general. Therefore, a longitudinal study design with a food frequency questionnaire is recommended.

Author Contributions: Methodology, B.M.R. and G.J.; formal analysis, B.M.R.; investigation, B.M.R. and G.J.; writing—original draft preparation, B.M.R.; writing—review and editing, B.M.R. and G.J.; visualization, B.M.R.; supervision, G.J.; funding acquisition, G.J. All authors have read and agreed to the published version of the manuscript.

Funding: This research was funded by the University of Iceland Research Fund (No. 15625), and the Icelandic Public Health Fund (No. P-2021-11-09-0001).

Institutional Review Board Statement: This study was conducted in accordance with the Declaration of Helsinki and approved by the institutional review board of the university's Ethics Committee for Scientific Research, which reviewed and approved this study (SHV2021-038, date 9 September 2021).

Informed Consent Statement: Informed consent was obtained from all subjects involved in this study.

Data Availability Statement: The original contributions presented in this study are included in the article. Further inquiries can be directed to the corresponding author.

Acknowledgments: The authors would like to express their gratitude to Marta Arroyo-Izaga (https://orcid.org/0000-0001-5592-4241, accessed on 21 January 2025) and Liv E. Torheim (https://orcid.org/0000-0002-3161-1635, accessed on 21 January 2025) for the opportunity to participate in the FINESCOP project.

Conflicts of Interest: The authors declare no conflicts of interest. The funders had no role in the design of this study; in the collection, analyses, or interpretation of data; in the writing of the manuscript; or in the decision to publish the results.

References

1. Repella, B.M.; Rice, J.G.; Arroyo-Izaga, M.; Torheim, L.E.; Birgisdottir, B.E.; Jakobsdottir, G. Prevalence of Food Insecurity and Associations with Academic Performance, Food Consumption and Social Support among University Students during the COVID-19 Pandemic: FINESCOP Project in Iceland. *Nutrients* **2024**, *16*, 764. [CrossRef] [PubMed]
2. Pilato, I.B.; Beezhold, B.; Radnitz, C. Diet and lifestyle factors associated with cognitive performance in college students. *J. Am. Coll. Health* **2020**, *70*, 2230–2236. [CrossRef] [PubMed]
3. Reuter, P.R.; Forster, B.L.; Brister, S.R. The influence of eating habits on the academic performance of university students. *J. Am. Coll. Health* **2020**, *69*, 921–927. [CrossRef]
4. Nordic Nutrition Recommendations 2023. (20 June 2023). Available online: https://www.norden.org/en/publication/nordic-nutrition-recommendations-2023 (accessed on 25 December 2024).

5. *Plant-Based Diets and Their Impact on Health, Sustainability and the Environment: A Review of the Evidence: WHO European Office for the Prevention and Control of Noncommunicable Diseases*; License: CC BY-NC-SA 3.0 IGO; WHO Regional Office for Europe: Copenhagen, Denmark, 2021.
6. Nguyen, B.; Bauman, A.; Gale, J.; Banks, E.; Kritharides, L.; Ding, D. Fruit and vegetable consumption and all-cause mortality: Evidence from a large Australian cohort study. *Int. J. Behav. Nutr. Phys. Act.* 2016, *13*, 9. [CrossRef]
7. Liu, W.; Hu, B.; Dehghan, M.; Mente, A.; Wang, C.; Yan, R.; Rangarajan, S.; Tse, L.A.; Yusuf, S.; Liu, X.; et al. Fruit, vegetable, and legume intake and the risk of all-cause, cardiovascular, and cancer mortality: A prospective study. *Clin. Nutr.* 2021, *40*, 4316–4323. [CrossRef]
8. Miller, V.; Mente, A.; Dehghan, M.; Rangarajan, S.; Zhang, X.; Swaminathan, S.; Dagenais, G.; Gupta, R.; Mohan, V.; Lear, S.; et al. Fruit, vegetable, and legume intake, and cardiovascular disease and deaths in 18 countries (PURE): A prospective cohort study. *Lancet* 2017, *390*, 2037–2049. [CrossRef] [PubMed]
9. Næring—Ráðleggingar Embættis Landlæknis. Embætti Landlæknis. 2014. Available online: https://island.is/naering-radleggingar-landlaeknis (accessed on 25 December 2024).
10. Hvað Borða Íslendingar? 2022. Available online: https://maturinnokkar.hi.is/wp-content/uploads/2022/03/Hvadbordaislendingar_vefur_endanlegt.pdf (accessed on 25 December 2024).
11. *Daily Consumption of Fruit and Vegetables by Sex, Age and Educational Attainment Level*; Europa.Eu: Brussels, Belgium, 2022. [CrossRef]
12. Eurostat. *How Much Fruit and Vegetables Do You Eat Daily?* Eurostat: Luxembourg, 2022. Available online: http://ec.europa.eu/eurostat/web/products-eurostat-news/-/ddn-20220104-1 (accessed on 25 December 2024).
13. Zargarzadeh, N.; Mousavi, S.M.; Santos, H.O.; Aune, D.; Hasani-Ranjbar, S.; Larijani, B.; Esmaillzadeh, A. Legume Consumption and Risk of All-Cause and Cause-Specific Mortality: A Systematic Review and Dose-Response Meta-Analysis of Prospective Studies. *Adv. Nutr.* 2023, *14*, 64–76. [CrossRef] [PubMed] [PubMed Central]
14. Rimm, E.B.; Appel, L.J.; Chiuve, S.E.; Djoussé, L.; Engler, M.B.; Kris-Etherton, P.M.; Mozaffarian, D.; Siscovick, D.S.; Lichtenstein, A.H.; on behalf of the American Heart Association Nutrition Committee of the Council on Lifestyle and Cardiometabolic Health; et al. Seafood long-chain n-3 polyunsaturated fatty acids and cardiovascular disease: A science advisory from the American Heart Association. *Circulation* 2018, *138*, e35–e47. [CrossRef]
15. Nestel, P.; Clifton, P.; Colquhoun, D.; Noakes, M.; Mori, T.A.; Sullivan, D.; Thomas, B. Indications for Omega-3 Long Chain Polyunsaturated Fatty Acid in the Prevention and Treatment of Cardiovascular Disease. *Heart Lung Circ.* 2015, *24*, 769–779. [CrossRef] [PubMed]
16. González-Pérez, R.; García-Iruretagoyena, L.; Martinez-Perez, N.; Telleria-Aramburu, N.; Telletxea, S.; Padoan, S.; Torheim, L.E.; Arroyo-Izaga, M. Prevalence and Predictors of Food Insecurity among Students of a Spanish University during the COVID-19 Pandemic: FINESCOP Project at the UPV/EHU. *Nutrients* 2023, *15*, 1836. [CrossRef] [PubMed] [PubMed Central]
17. Mukaka, M.M. Statistics corner: A guide to appropriate use of correlation coefficient in medical research. *Malawi Med. J.* 2012, *24*, 69–71. [PubMed] [PubMed Central]
18. Saha, S.; Okafor, H.; Biediger-Friedman, L.; Behnke, A. Association between diet and symptoms of anxiety and depression in college students: A systematic review. *J. Am. Coll. Health* 2021, *71*, 1270–1280. [CrossRef]
19. Iqbal, R.; Dehghan, M.; Mente, A.; Rangarajan, S.; Wielgosz, A.; Avezum, A.; Seron, P.; AlHabib, K.F.; Lopez-Jaramillo, P.; Swaminathan, S.; et al. Associations of unprocessed and processed meat intake with mortality and cardiovascular disease in 21 countries [Prospective Urban Rural Epidemiology (PURE) Study]: A prospective cohort study. *Am. J. Clin. Nutr.* 2021, *114*, 1049–1058. [CrossRef] [PubMed]
20. Farvid, M.S.; Sidahmed, E.; Spence, N.D.; Mante Angua, K.; Rosner, B.A.; Barnett, J.B. Consumption of red meat and processed meat and cancer incidence: A systematic review and meta-analysis of prospective studies. *Eur. J. Epidemiol.* 2021, *36*, 937–951. [CrossRef] [PubMed]
21. Sprake, E.F.; Russell, J.M.; Cecil, J.E.; Cooper, R.J.; Grabowski, P.; Pourshahidi, L.K.; Barker, M.E. Dietary patterns of university students in the UK: A cross-sectional study. *Nutr. J.* 2018, *17*, 90. [CrossRef]
22. Fondevila-Gascón, J.F.; Berbel-Giménez, G.; Vidal-Portés, E.; Hurtado-Galarza, K. Ultra-Processed Foods in University Students: Implementing Nutri-Score to Make Healthy Choices. *Healthcare* 2022, *10*, 984. [CrossRef] [PubMed] [PubMed Central]
23. Kim, H.; Hu, E.A.; Rebholz, C.M. Ultra-processed food intake and mortality in the USA: Results from the Third National Health and Nutrition Examination Survey (NHANES III, 1988–1994). *Public Health Nutr.* 2019, *22*, 1777–1785. [CrossRef]
24. Vilaro, M.J.; Colby, S.E.; Riggsbee, K.; Zhou, W.; Byrd-Bredbenner, C.; Olfert, M.D.; Barnett, T.E.; Horacek, T.; Sowers, M.; Mathews, A.E. Food Choice Priorities Change Over Time and Predict Dietary Intake at the End of the First Year of College Among Students in the U.S. *Nutrients* 2018, *10*, 1296. [CrossRef] [PubMed] [PubMed Central]
25. Tam, R.; Yassa, B.; Parker, H.; O'Connor, H.; Allman-Farinelli, M. University students' on-campus food purchasing behaviors, preferences, and opinions on food availability. *Nutrition* 2017, *37*, 7–13. [CrossRef] [PubMed]

26. Roy, R.; Soo, D.; Conroy, D.; Wall, C.R.; Swinburn, B. Exploring University Food Environment and On-Campus Food Purchasing Behaviors, Preferences, and Opinions. *J. Nutr. Educ. Behav.* **2019**, *51*, 865–875. [CrossRef] [PubMed]
27. van den Bogerd, N.; Peppelenbos, H.; Leufkens, R.; Seidell, J.C.; Maas, J.; Dijkstra, S.C. A free-produce stand on campus: Impact on fruit and vegetable intake in Dutch university students. *Public Health Nutr.* **2020**, *23*, 924–934. [CrossRef] [PubMed] [PubMed Central]
28. Kebbe, M.; Gao, M.; Perez-Cornago, A.; Jebb, S.A.; Piernas, C. Adherence to international dietary recommendations in association with all-cause mortality and fatal and non-fatal cardiovascular disease risk: A prospective analysis of UK Biobank participants. *BMC Med.* **2021**, *19*, 134. [CrossRef] [PubMed]
29. O'Neal, C.S.; Cocco, A.R.; Della, L.J.; Ashlock, M.Z. Pilot Intervention Using Food Challenges and Video Technology for Promoting Fruit and Vegetable Consumption. *J. Nutr. Educ. Behav.* **2022**, *54*, 707–717. [CrossRef] [PubMed]
30. Háskóli Íslands. Nemendur. Available online: https://www.hi.is/kynningarefni/nemendur (accessed on 25 December 2024).
31. PxWeb. Students by Level, Type of Education, Degree, Broad Field of Study and Sex 1997–2023. Available online: https://px.hagstofa.is/pxen/pxweb/en/Samfelag/Samfelag__skolamal__4_haskolastig__0_hsNemendur/SKO04103.px/ (accessed on 25 December 2024).
32. Háskóli Íslands. Facts and Figures. Available online: https://english.hi.is/about-ui/about-university/media-and-press/facts-and-figures (accessed on 16 January 2025).

Disclaimer/Publisher's Note: The statements, opinions and data contained in all publications are solely those of the individual author(s) and contributor(s) and not of MDPI and/or the editor(s). MDPI and/or the editor(s) disclaim responsibility for any injury to people or property resulting from any ideas, methods, instructions or products referred to in the content.

MDPI AG
Grosspeteranlage 5
4052 Basel
Switzerland
Tel.: +41 61 683 77 34

Nutrients Editorial Office
E-mail: nutrients@mdpi.com
www.mdpi.com/journal/nutrients

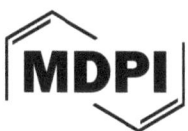

Disclaimer/Publisher's Note: The title and front matter of this reprint are at the discretion of the Guest Editors. The publisher is not responsible for their content or any associated concerns. The statements, opinions and data contained in all individual articles are solely those of the individual Editors and contributors and not of MDPI. MDPI disclaims responsibility for any injury to people or property resulting from any ideas, methods, instructions or products referred to in the content.

www.ingramcontent.com/pod-product-compliance
Lightning Source LLC
LaVergne TN
LVHW072324090526
838202LV00019B/2350